Chinese Dietary Therapy

Neither the publishers nor the author will be liable for any loss or damage of any nature occasioned to or suffered by any person acting or refraining from acting as a result of reliance on the material contained in this publication.

For Churchill Livingstone:

Commissioning editor: Inta Ozols
Project editor: Valerie Bain
Project manager: Valerie Burgess
Project controller: Nicola Haig/Pat Miller
Copy editor: Holly Gothard
Design direction: Judith Wright
Sales promotion executive: Maria O'Connor

Chinese Dietary Therapy

Main editor
Liu Jilin

Subject editor
Gordon Peck BAc CAc MRTCM

Contributing editors
Liu Yanzheng
Zhang Yueyen
Li Yaoguang

Main desk editor
Ling Yikui

Translated by
Li Shaoming Wang Huiying

CHURCHILL LIVINGSTONE
EDINBURGH HONG KONG LONDON MADRID MELBOURNE NEW YORK AND TOKYO 1995

CHURCHILL LIVINGSTONE
Medical Division of Pearson Professional Limited

Distributed in the United States of America by Churchill
Livingstone Inc., 650
Avenue of the Americas, New York, N.Y. 10011, and by
associated companies, branches and representatives
throughout the world.

First edition published in Chinese
© Shandong Science and Technology Publishing House, 16
Yuhan Road, Jinan, Shandong, People's Republic of China
1988
First edition in English based on the first Chinese edition,
revised
© Pearson Professional Limited 1995
This edition is published by arrangement with Shandong
Science and Technology Publishing House

First Chinese edition published 1988
First English edition published 1995

ISBN 0-443-04967-X

British Library Cataloguing in Publication Data
A catalogue record for this book is available from the British
Library.

Library of Congress Cataloging in Publication Data
Chung i shih liao hsüeh. English.
    Diet therapy in traditional Chinese medicine / main
editor, Liu Jilin; subject editor, Gordon Peck;
contributing editors, Liu Yanzheng, Zhang Yueyen,
Li Yaoguang; main desk editor, Ling Yikui; translated
by Li Shaoming Wang Huiying. -- 1st English ed.
        p.   cm.
    'First edition in English based on the first Chinese
edition, revised' -- T.p. verso.
    Includes bibliographical references and index.
    ISBN 0–443–04967–X
    1. Diet therapy. 2. Medicine, Chinese. I. Liu, Chi-lin.
II. Title.
    [DNLM: 1. Diet Therapy--methods. 2. Medicine,
Chinese Traditional. 3. Nutrition. WB 400 C5594
1995]
RM217.C5213 1995
615.8' 54' 0951--dc20
DNLM/DLC
for Library of Congress   94-44954
                                                  CIP

The
publisher's
policy is to use
**paper manufactured
from sustainable forests**

Produced by Longman Singapore Publishers (Pte) Ltd
Printed in Singapore

Contents

Preface

This book on Chinese Dietary Therapy is probably unique. It was compiled in China by experts in the field, using the principles of Traditional Chinese Medicine and, most importantly, quoting sources for all the information.

Practitioners in almost every field will realize the influence of diet on health and there should be something of value here for most therapists. Acupuncturists and Chinese herbal practitioners will have an understanding of the underlying principles and if this is lacking then *Foundations of Chinese Medicine* by Giovanni Maciocia (Churchill Livingstone) or *The Web That Has No Weaver* by Ted Kaptchuk (Rider) will provide useful background material. I hope my introduction will help to place the book in a Western context and give a brief overview of the contents.

My first contact with Oriental approaches to food as medicine was in 1973, when I studied macrobiotics with Michio Kushi and Bill Tara. I was grateful when Giovanni Maciocia and Julian Scott introduced Chinese Dietary Therapy as part of my training in acupuncture in 1976 and have found it invaluable in my practice ever since. I am constantly finding that even small changes in diet can profoundly enhance the effects of treatment and, as importantly, allow the patient to influence their own well-being.

In editing this volume, I have tried to make the text accessible to Western practitioners and this has meant virtually rewriting some sections which would otherwise have proved too abstruse or tedious. I apologize for any remaining peculiarities and trust the indices and footnotes will help to clarify the material. I hope you will find it useful for yourself and your patients alike.

Turbridge Wells 1994   Gordon Peck

Acknowledgements

Churchill Livingstone are grateful to the following for their kind assistance in finalizing the text of *Dietary Therapy in Traditional Chinese Medicine*:

Mr Giovanni Maciocia, who acted as advisor.

Royal Botanic Garden, Edinburgh: particularly Dr De-Zhu Li (visiting botanist and Deputy Director, Department of Plant Systematics and Phytogeography, Kunming Institute of Botany, China) who, assisted by Mr Ian Hedge and Dr Robert Mill, helped compile the Glossary of Herbs; also Mr Bill Tait who organized these translations.

The Royal Zoological Society of Scotland, Edinburgh: Anne Gallagher, Education Officer, who provided missing animal family names.

A Crombie and Son, Butcher, Edinburgh and Mrs Marguerita Bain: for advice relating to the availability of meat products.

Chinese medical terms

There is still no full agreement on the translation of Chinese medical terms into English. We have tried to use the most widely-accepted forms (capitalizing names for internal organs to distinguish them from their western counterparts, for instance), but some alternative translations have been left where they give a useful insight into a Chinese term. Both the common and pharmaceutical Latin names are given for herbs. The Pinyin name is listed in the Glossary of herbs.

Introduction: Chinese Dietary Therapy in a Western practice

Although most of the concepts used in TCM are as relevant in the modern West as when they evolved in China, some adaptation is necessary. This chapter aims to set the book in a Western context and also to clarify some of the terms used.

THE CONCEPT OF QI

Underpinning Chinese Medicine is the notion of Qi. The literal meaning, 'breath' or 'vapour', indicates an intangible immaterial quality; yet the term covers such substantial substances as Blood, and the quality of the Qi may be clearly observed in the material with which it interacts. The radiant face of a healthy person and the wholesome smell and flavor of properly grown produce reflect the unseen Qi which invigorates them. The Qi of the Seasons combines with the Qi of the earth to produce food that reflects this interaction. Traditional diets and cooking methods are based on an understanding of these processes (think of salads in summer or hot stews of root vegetables in the winter). Similarly as humans settle in different geographical locations the foods they traditionally eat reflect an awareness of the need to balance the Qi of food with the Qi of the environment. Thus Eskimos subsist on warming fatty meats whilst people in the Tropics consume large amounts of lush, cooling fruits.

In food, as in all natural phenomena as a whole, we may be constantly aware of the behavior of Qi, and Chinese Dietary Therapy depends upon the interaction of food Qi with that of the body.

FOOD OR MEDICINE?

There is a wide spectrum in the therapeutic effects of foods and medicinal herbs, ranging from relatively mild staple foods, which may be consumed regularly and frequently to nourish the body, to extremely strong and possibly poisonous substances used exclusively in herbal medicine. A rough indication of the qualities of a food or herb is the strength of taste. This could be seen to represent the relative amount of Qi contained within the food or herb. Generally, mild flavored foods are consumed as staples (grains and pulses, for example), while foods and drinks with stronger taste (tea, coffee, spices and condiments, etc.) are used less frequently because they have more of a medicinal effect (Figure 1).

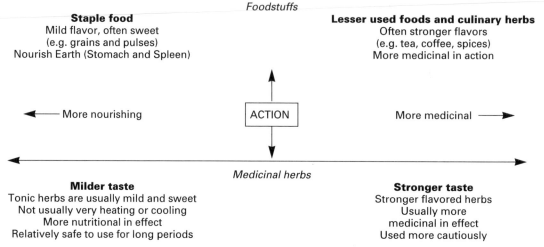

Fig. 1 Medicinal effects of foods and herbs.

The same principles apply to medicinal herbs, only a wider range of effects is involved. Qi and Blood tonics, for instance, have a sweet taste, are usually fairly mild in flavor and do not have a pronounced heating or cooling effect. With certain provisos, they may be taken over long periods of time with relative safety and are often found on sale as single herbs (Chinese angelica, milkvetch and ginseng, for example). Even within this category the slightly stronger and more pungent taste of Chinese angelica indicates its ability to move rather than purely tonify Blood.

Yin and Jing tonics are similar, with a slightly different range of tastes but still a relatively mild flavor and relatively few contraindications. It is only when we look at Yang tonics that we begin to find some strong tastes, and their dynamic action and the longer list of contraindications reflect these qualities. They are rarely used alone and inappropriate use may produce ill effects relatively quickly, so they fall into an intermediate stage, closer to medicinal herbs than to foods.

Herbs with a strong flavor and a strongly Hot or Cold nature normally have a more obvious medicinal rather than nutritional effect. They are used less frequently and for shorter periods of time and may need to be moderated by other herbs.

So we can see a gradual progression from staple foods, which nourish in a stable way, through tonic herbs which have much in common

with food, to Yang tonics and strong-tasting foods and drinks which have more of a medicinal effect. Finally come the purely medicinal herbs with a strong taste and a powerful action, which therefore need more caution in their use.

It is easy to see, then, why foods are so useful for slowly and gently supporting a person's Qi and also how they may reinforce or temper the effects of herbs used medicinally.

The following section deals with the nature of foods in terms of heating and cooling properties. The emphasis in TCM Dietary Therapy is on combining compatible foods rather than balancing foods of opposite natures. For instance, Warm foods will reinforce Warm herbs, while Cold foods would work against them. In everyday diet, however, there are many examples of the use of 'incompatible' combinations. The Warm nature of ginger helps to offset the Cold nature of melon, while yogurt is traditionally used to moderate the Hot nature of curries. In hot climates curries will induce perspiration and Cold fruits will balance the hot conditions, so the main foods are appropriate and the additions can give a finer balance. In temperate climates, it is better to avoid strongly Hot or Cold foods altogether as far as possible. A useful analogy is that of a seesaw with the most strongly heating and cooling foods at either end and those with a milder effect towards the middle.

It is far easier to keep a balance if the bulk of

the diet is drawn from foods near the fulcrum, with progressively less taken from the stronger-acting foods towards the ends. A patient with Cold symptoms could be encouraged to take predominantly more Neutral food (such as rice, soy beans or maize) with some Warm additions rather than trying to balance a Cold diet by adding Hot items. Too much Hot or Cold food will just disrupt the Qi of the body.

HOT AND COLD

The nature of foods (Hot, Cold, Cool, Warm or Neutral) is a fundamental principle in Chinese Dietary Therapy and a chart showing some examples is shown in Figure 2.

As you will see from the text, the nature of food can be affected by cooking. In general terms, frying and roasting in oil increase the heating properties of food, while baking has a similar, but less marked effect (baked foods often have a drying effect, especially on the colon).

You should note that when the term 'roasting' is applied to the ingredients used in herbal preparations it means dry-roasting in a pan over a flame. Steaming and boiling slightly counteract any cooling properties of food, but will also help to moderate the effects of some Warm or Hot foods because of the watery component. For example, raw peanuts have a Neutral nature and a propensity for the channels of the Spleen and Lung. They are also able to reinforce Spleen Qi, moisten the Lungs and dissolve Phlegm. Once they have been roasted in oil, however, they develop a distinctly Warm to Hot nature and may

actually create Phlegm. Lamb, on the other hand, has a Warm nature but if cooked in the traditional Greek way, where it is 'sweated' very slowly with the addition of a little lemon juice in a covered container, its heating nature is moderated. Herbs which are used for cooling and moistening are often administered in their fresh state (turnip juice, purslane, etc.) and even the relatively gentle process of drying them will modify their cooling and moistening nature to some extent.

How about freezing or microwaving? Well, food eaten frozen or chilled obviously has a Cold effect quite apart from its original nature. Iced drinks, cold milk, spring water from the fridge – they are all common items in the diets of many patients and should definitely be considered if you are questioning or giving dietary advice. If the patient's problem involves Cold or Yang Deficiency then simple changes in habits can make a big difference to their health and it is surprising how many people have never considered the effects of such behavior.

Microwaving is another widespread factor which is obviously not mentioned in the classics and the effects are not clearcut. On the one hand moisture is liberated during cooking and it is difficult to brown many foods which points to an effect similar to steaming. However, foods containing sugar or fat cook very rapidly and it is quite possible to caramelize sugar. Any food or drink which has been microwaved is capable of producing vicious burns or scalds if it is consumed straight from the cooker, so more of a heating effect is indicated. On balance the main effect seems more akin to steaming with all that implies, but some foods at least may have a Hot nature superimposed. From a purely Western standpoint, some modern research gives us pause for thought before we use microwaves for any sort of cookery. When human milk is microwaved even to below the temperature of blood heat some of the antibodies normally present are destroyed (Raloff 1992). Maybe those gut instincts were justified. . . .

Heating foods	Cooling foods
Dispel Cold	Clear Heat and toxins
Tonify Yang Qi	Tonify Yin fluids
Nourish Qi	Tranquilize Heart Fire
May increase Heat	Calm Liver Yang
May induce Fire	May damage Yang Qi,
Can damage Yin Body	especially the Stomach and
Fluids (e.g. in stomach,	Spleen, Heart or Kidney
Liver or Lungs)	
Examples	**Examples**
Chillies	Watermelon
Mustard	Cucumber
Horseradish	Green tea

Fig. 2   Hot and Cold foods.

MACROBIOTICS

Many people come to Chinese medicine, and

particularly Chinese dietetics, via an interest in macrobiotics and have to reconcile the Chinese concepts with those they already know. The term 'macrobiotics' was coined by George Ohsawa (1968) to describe an application of the Yin/Yang principle to health, diet and life in general. He developed the system during the 1960s from his very individual understanding of the Japanese interpretation of Chinese philosophy and science. Unfortunately many people are driven to distraction in trying to reconcile the two systems. Macrobiotics takes a much more reductionist view than TCM and classes foods purely in terms of Yin/Yang. The problem is that Ohsawa's ideas of what constituted Yin or Yang qualities do not always coincide with the general consensus (for instance, the expansive upward qualities of Yang in Chinese medicine are considered to be relatively Yin in terms of macrobiotics).

Anyone looking for tidy solutions might be tempted to class Hot and Warm foods as more Yang and Cold and Cool foods as more Yin, but there are many glaring exceptions to this rule. For instance, salt is considered to be extremely Yang in terms of macrobiotics yet in TCM it has a Neutral or Cool nature, is moistening and will lead other herbs to tonify the Kidney Yin. On the other hand, spices such as ginger and garlic which are manifestly Warm and Yang in nature in terms of Chinese medicine, are classified as Yin in macrobiotics. Each of the systems has its merits, but because of these inconsistencies the two are probably best kept separate.

If macrobiotics has a difficult time reconciling its ideas with those of TCM, theories from other cultures do not always fare better and often allocate different natures to foods. To an Iranian bananas are very Warm, yet they are Cold in Chinese medicine; while in Ayurvedic medicine rose is distinctly cooling and in TCM it has a slightly Warm nature. We can assume in both cases that the use to which the plant is put determines the nature assigned to it. Unfortunately, but perhaps inevitably, there is disagreement even among contemporary writers. Bob Flaws (1991), for instance, assigns a Cold nature to coffee based on its downward action on the colon and the fact that its diuretic action causes Qi, and therefore warmth, to be lost. Most other authors

note its effect on mobilizing Yang within the body, possibly contributing to Liver Yang or Liver Fire and aggravating such symptoms as febrile Painful Obstruction Syndrome and migraine headaches. These qualities would point more to a Hot nature. Some foods even appear to have a homoeopathic effect. For instance, baked crabs clear Damp and Heat when used medicinally, yet crab is commonly seen to aggravate skin conditions such as urticaria which involve the same factors.

What is the moral? Remember Chinese medicine takes a flexible approach.

FIVE ELEMENTS – PHILOSOPHY AND PRAGMATISM

Most practitioners will be familiar with the Five Tastes from the point of view of the Five Elements (Figure 3). In this book, as in current TCM, the Elements, their associated qualities and their interrelationships are applied when appropriate but are discarded when they are not useful descriptions of observed life. In Dietary Therapy, for example, the propensity of a food or herb to enter a particular acupuncture channel is deduced more from its precise action in the body and does not always correspond with the organ system classically associated with one of the Five Tastes according to the Five Element system. Emotions tend to run high in some acupuncture circles

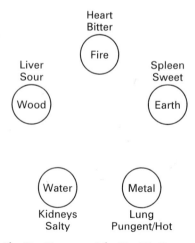

Fig. 3   The Five Flavors and the Five Yin Organs.

when the Five Elements are mentioned and as there have been some lengthy discussions on the relative merits of the system by authors such as Giovanni Maciocia (1989) and Ted Kaptchuk (1983) we will resist the temptation to join in or to elaborate on basic Five Elements theory.

However, the Five Tastes associated with the Organs *do* have a place in diagnosis and in treatment. Most early sources agree that overconsumption of any one taste will have undesirable effects and the rationale is straightforward. Moderate amounts of a given taste will strengthen the function of the associated Yin Organ and tissues (often a craving for a particular flavor will point to a problem with the related Organ). Overintake actually impairs its function and may also cause it to overact on the related Organ according to the Control Cycle (see Fig. 4). For instance, moderate intake of sour flavor nourishes the Wood element and thus the Liver and also the tendons. An excess of the same flavor will have a harmful effect on the tendons first of all and then the Liver Qi overacts to suppress the Spleen. This in turn damages the tissue associated with the second Organ (in this case, the flesh will become withered and the lips dry). For more information on this theme refer to the Nature and taste of food in chapter 2.

Food Qi is considered ultimately to form the various tissues of the body and the taste of the food will determine which Organ, sphere of activity and tissue will be affected. Further advice from the classics generally consists of using particular tastes to nourish, support or control specific Organs in terms of Five Element

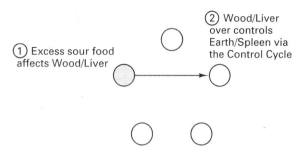

Fig. 5.   Effects of an excess of sour food.

relationships and eating a balanced range of the Five tastes to provide a healthy regime. As with Hot and Cold foods, moderation is the keynote and milder flavored foods such as grains, pulses and staple vegetables should form the central part of the diet, with progressively stronger tasting foods being eaten more sparingly.

So far, so good. It is when the therapeutic actions of the foods are discussed that contradictions begin to appear. The Liver (Wood) has a spreading quality, while the Lungs (Metal) tend to harden and contract. The sour flavor associated with the Liver, however, is astringent while the pungent flavor of the Lungs tends to disperse. Likewise bitter flavors, although they dry, also tend to cool and have a downward movement rather than the hot upward action you might expect from the Fire element.

Given these apparent contradictions it is understandable that 5 elements theory is used selectively. It is an elegant and useful system which underlies a surprising amount of TCM, but it is manmade and cannot be used as a rigid set of universally applicable rules.

FASTING, APPETITE AND ALLERGIES

Fasting is not normally recommended in modern Chinese medicine, as it is considered to deplete the Stomach and Spleen. In Chapter 32 of *The Spiritual Axis* we are treated to a graphic account of how a healthy person would die after just 7 days of fasting. This contrasts with the naturopathic approach in the West which concentrates on ridding the body of toxins and uses fasting of one sort or another as a major form of treatment. There are pros and cons for each approach and in

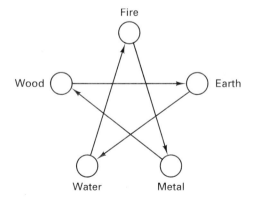

Fig. 4   The Control Cycle.

illness it is possible to be guided by a person's appetite. In acute conditions it is normal to treat the Biao, or obvious manifestation of a disease, as this is normally reliable, and if a person has no appetite at all they are usually better for fasting. If, however, they have a strong desire for a particular taste, then it may reflect a Deficiency and foods of that taste are likely to be helpful for them. In chronic disease we pay attention to the Ben, or root of the problem, and this is not necessarily obvious. It could be a distorted appetite which has contributed to the condition, either through an excess of a particular type of food affecting its related Internal Organ, or through overconsumption of exotic foods which leads to chaotic behavior of Qi and perversion of the normal appetite. In this case the patient may crave the very foods they should be avoiding, and it is interesting to see how often a person's favorite foods are those to which they are allergic or sensitive. This also reflects our national habits: milk products, refined wheat products, tea, coffee, orange juice and sugar usually head the lists when food sensitivity and allergy are discussed, and they are all consumed in large quantities.

A useful guideline for the correct amounts of food to be taken is to consider what would be available in natural circumstances and how much one would be inclined to eat if one had to prepare it from its raw state. Not everybody realizes, for instance, that a carton of orange juice contains the juice from 15 oranges and very few people would eat 50 grams of brazil nuts if they had to crack them all. Whole oranges can be very useful medicinally and brazil nuts are fine in small amounts, but problems are frequently seen in people who consume orange juice by the glass daily or eat shelled nuts by the handful.

Muesli is another concentrated food and is very popular in the West, yet many patients suffer from problems which include Spleen Qi Deficiency, and uncooked cereals and nuts are the last thing they should be consuming, particularly if (as is so often the case) sugar is included in the recipe. It is interesting to note that the original Bircher-Benner recipe for muesli was based mainly around grated apple, with a minimal amount of cereal included.

FOOD PRODUCTION IN THE WEST

Historically most countries have adulterated foods in some way or another and China is no exception. However, the amount of adulteration which was likely when the earlier texts were prepared in China pales in comparison with modern Western production methods. This should be borne in mind when using and recommending foods and also when considering the daily intake of patients. In Dietary Therapy we are dealing specifically with the Qi which is taken in the form of food and drink and everything involved in the production of food will affect this.

If a vegetable such as a carrot has been produced by intensive farming methods using chemicals to force quick growth and protect against pests it may look perfect while being virtually tasteless. Many Westerners have never enjoyed the completely different flavour of a carrot grown in good soil in its own time. When we consider that the flavour of each food is an indicator of its Qi and its therapeutic action we can understand the importance of food which tastes right as well as looking appealing.

By using the traditional Four Examinations and especially that of observation, it quickly becomes clear that a person's Qi reflects not only their lifestyle in general but their food intake. Someone with a balanced diet of healthily produced food will have a clear and radiant complexion compared with a person living on devitalized foods and stimulants. If we look at more of the modern factors involved in food production the devitalizing effects of adulterated foods on the body should become clearer.

Foods which are highly processed need to have artificial flavouring added to compensate for the loss of taste (and Qi) which occurs during processing. The end product may be so strong in taste that we gradually lose our natural ability to appreciate subtle differences in taste and our judgement of the food quality. Many studies have shown that the average Westerner prefers very strongly flavored food even when the flavoring is artificial. Is there a solution? One answer is to restrict the range of foods consumed for a while. Many people do this inadvertently by using one of the many diets currently being promoted (food combining, grape fasts and food allergy elimination diets, for example). After even a short period on one of these regimes, a person's natural ability to discriminate flavor recovers and many people find they begin to avoid or drastically reduce the amounts of some of the less useful foods they were taking in previously.

ADDED VALUE?

It is in the interests of manufacturers in the West to increase the profits gained from foods by adding fats, salt or sugar. Why these three ingredients? Fat is used in processing foods which are broken down into smaller components and can thus be sold for a higher price weight for weight. Added sugar and salt increase consumption when they are added to foods for reasons that are particularly interesting from a Chinese dietary perspective. Many people in the West have poor dietary habits (irregular meals, unbalanced diets, eating without resting afterwards, etc.) and as a result their Spleen Qi easily becomes deficient. In this situation the desire for sweet foods, which would nourish the Spleen is increased and if strongly sweet food is available the person is usually drawn to it. Unfortunately the excess of strong sweet flavor does nothing to nourish the Spleen, instead it damages it, and the continued craving creates a vicious circle. If the person works hard and continues to push themselves their Kidney Qi could become depleted and a craving for salt will develop. A small amount of salty food will stimulate the Kidneys and give a temporary increase in energy, but once again an excess will do nothing to actually nourish the Kidneys and the outcome is an exhausted and undernourished body. Nourishing the Spleen Qi by using small regular meals, including mildly sweet food such as root vegetables, and avoiding very strong flavors will usually help to bring a person back to balance.

Sugar has useful medicinal properties but it is often included as an ingredient in herbal drinks purely for extra flavor. Unless it is a necessary ingredient, it is probably better to exclude it.

FRESH OR TAINTED?

The eating of whole fruits and vegetables including the skins obviously makes a lot of sense in terms of nutrients, but once again the old rules do not apply in the modern West. Orthodox farming methods create serious problems caused by pesticides and antifungal sprays and by chemicals used to preserve foods during storage. Washing is not always sufficient to remove some of the wax-based preparations sprayed onto fruit during the growing period, for instance, and the sensible approach might be to peel food unless it is known to come from an organic source.

Pickling and drying foods to preserve them have a long history but there are many methods available in the West which are very recent. Frozen food has only been in common use for the last 40 years or so, and even canning and bottling are relatively modern. Irradiation of food has only just been introduced in Britain and certainly does not figure in any Chinese text.

Each of these techniques makes its impact on the fresh food. Bottled carrots and peas, for instance, sold very badly when customers could see the dull colour of the cooked product, and most cookery books contain sections on how badly various foods fare once frozen. From a TCM perspective all of these methods will affect the Qi of the food. Once something has been preserved in this way and is left open to the elements again, it will normally deteriorate very quickly – an indication of the lack of Qi contained within the food. This is particularly marked in irradiated food, which may look perfectly fresh when viewed through a sealed plastic container but will deteriorate very rapidly once opened because its naturally protective organisms have been destroyed by the irradiation (the equivalent of destroying its Defensive Qi). From a nutritional point of view it is the ability to support all aspects of bodily Qi which is affected by preserving. You could view it as suspending the vitalizing quality of the Qi.

One of the drawbacks of both the preservation and the easy transport of food is that it is possible to eat foodstuffs which are inappropriate for a given season or country. It is hardly surprising that the person with Spleen Yang deficient symptoms suffers during the winter if they are living on salads and tropical fruits. One of the most sensible guidelines in macrobiotics is to eat food which grows within a few hundred miles of one's home and which is either in season or can be easily stored without elaborate treatment. British macrobiotics would not be eating rice or soya products if this were the case, but in general terms the principle is very sound.

FOOD AND THE SEASONS

A good guide to the appropriate foods for any season is what types of food would normally be growing at that time. During spring and summer flowers and leaves are abundant and their nature is to float the Qi. Light, leafy vegetables are easily available and succulent fruits and vegetables are commonly consumed. The actions of these foods help to relax the skin and muscles, to cool the body and to protect and nourish the body fluids (see Figs 6 and 7). During autumn and winter,

fruits are drying, seeds are being formed and in nature the energy is tending to concentrate more in the roots of plants; it will be seen that their energy tends to sink. The fruits will help to reinforce and moisten the Lungs, which predominate in autumn, while rooty vegetables and seeds help to strengthen the Kidneys during the winter.

FOODS, FADS AND DIETS

In the West there is a problem with people becoming obsessive about food. The modern tendency is to concentrate on foods and medicines which can be taken by mouth and possibly to disregard other factors affecting health. As a practitioner, it is necessary to be cautious about giving dietary advice in case patients take it to extremes. A common question people will ask is 'Is this food good or bad?'. This reflects the linear thinking of Westerners and it is always worth explaining to patients that particular foods are appropriate or inappropriate for a given situation rather than being inherently good or bad. It is all too easy to fall back on lists of do's and don'ts in diet and this is far removed from the flexibility of TCM. Reference to the use of Chinese herbs and their specific actions, can often make the concept of dietary advice easier for patients to understand.

Nature	Part of plant
Hot and Warm foods tend to lift	Flowers and leaves (spring and summer) tend to float
Cold and Cool foods tend to lower	Roots, fruits and seeds (autumn and winter) tend to sink

Fig. 6 Actions of foods.

Summer
Nature prospering, hot weather
Skin and muscles relaxed, the Heart needs Coolness
Diet should dispel Heat from body and nourish fluids

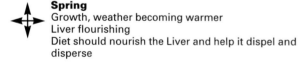

Spring
Growth, weather becoming warmer
Liver flourishing
Diet should nourish the Liver and help it dispel and disperse

Autumn
Coolness, Dryness, retreating and dying off
Inward movement of the Lungs flourishes
Diet should reinforce and moisten the Lungs

Winter
Cold, everything in hiding
Kidney Yang Qi gathered and stored
Diet should reinforce the Kidney and warm the Yang

Fig. 7 Foods and the seasons.

Faddism is common and care needs to be taken when questioning patients about food in order to get a clear idea of a person's natural appetites. All too often the reply is dictated by what the person thinks they should be eating rather than what they would actually like.

MEAT AND VEGETABLES

It is interesting to note that meat plays an important part in Chinese diet. Although large quantities are not necessarily consumed, it is considered to be one of the most useful foods for supplementing deficient Qi and particularly Blood. An informal New England study found that the addition of small quantities of meat, or poultry, to the diets of female vegetarians who were infertile through Blood deficiency led to pregnancy in a significant proportion of cases even when Chinese herbs had not helped (Valaskitgis 1978). Obviously in many cultures there are millions of healthy vegetarians, and careful choice of foods will usually compensate for the lack of meat in the diet. A problem in the West, however, is that many people assume that becoming a vegetarian automatically leads to health and spiritual development, and some people avoid meat, but eat rubbish. Mention of the fact that Hitler was a vegetarian and that food helps to form our material and energetic framework may be helpful in these cases.

COW'S MILK

Milk's sweet taste, neutral nature and propensity for the channels of the Lung and Stomach all indicate that it should be a useful tonic, so it is no surprise that it is commonly used to nourish Qi and Blood when deficiency gives rise to dizziness and fatigue.

The ability to nourish Yin fluids makes the occasional administration of milk useful in treating thirst and constipation from Dryness. Milk also reinforces the descending function of the Stomach, counteracting difficult swallowing and vomiting but this, combined with its concentrated nourishing properties and tendency to lubricate, means that it may overload a weak Spleen and give rise to Damp or Phlegm. For these reasons the use of milk is more appropriate for recuperation from illness (especially cases such as pulmonary tuberculosis involving Yin deficiency) rather than for general use. From my own experience, I would suggest that modern cow's milk has a relatively Cool nature and that it will deplete Spleen Yang if taken in large amounts.

Whatever the nature, the Phlegm-producing effects may be modified by taking garlic or ginger with the milk.

Milk as medicine or disease factor

Whole unpasteurized milk from cows reared naturally is a very concentrated food capable of forming a substantial calf very quickly. As such, it is easy to see how Chinese medicine came to view its main therapeutic uses. In the West, too, it has always played an important part in traditional medicine and has been successfully used in the treatment of such problems as pulmonary tuberculosis and gastric ulcers.

Despite this background, milk has had a very bad press over the past few decades and a look at the differences between its use in China and Europe may make the reasons clearer.

Overconsumption

Traditionally the consumption of milk was quite moderate for most of the population, however in recent times intensive farming methods and increasing economic reliance on the dairy industry have created a massive supply in the West and a subsequent overconsumption. It is well known that races such as the Japanese identify Europeans by the sour milk smell they exude. The excessive consumption of dairy products may well be a reason for the rapid increase in the average height of Western children over the last few decades, and is almost certainly implicated in the growing number of milk-related diseases. Studies of conditions as wide-ranging as chronic rhinitis, rheumatoid arthritis, ulcerative colitis and even delinquency (Kaptchuk & Croncher 1986, Samuelsson et al 1991, Riordan et al 1993, Seignnlet 1992) have all implicated milk products as triggers. If we consider Phlegm, Damp and deficient Spleen Qi or Yang as the possible results of high intake, we can usually understand the connection.

Adulteration

Overconsumption is not the only factor, however – the product consumed today is far removed from the original. Even 26 years ago a well-respected writer on naturopathy (Hewlett Parson 1968) qualified his inclusion of milk in a book with the proviso that whole unadulterated milk was very difficult to find and that it would be far better not to go near the product if it was not the real thing. The main differences are as follows:

Pasteurization

The pasteurization process, and particularly the UHT heat treatment used in long-life milk, appear to greatly increase the tendency to cause Phlegm in those who are susceptible (probably by making it more difficult for those with weak Stomach and Spleen to transform it). Many well-respected Western practitioners have documented the effects of treated versus untreated milk and whenever milk is recommended as a dietary supplement, they specify unpasteurized milk from untreated healthy cows.

Homogenization

This process distributes the fat more uniformly and has been implicated in a variety of conditions which in Western terms would relate to the gut, but in TCM would involve the Spleen. As the fat particles are smaller, they are more readily absorbed by the small intestine and may thus bypass a natural barrier in sensitive individuals. Whole milk does not present this problem.

Antibiotics

Intensive farming has meant an increase in infections and antibiotics are frequently given to cows. It is a matter of debate whether any active residues pass on in pasteurized milk but there are always financial pressures for farmers to allow milk from heavily dosed cows to be collected before the medication has fully cleared. Some authors consider these residues to be a factor in the sensitivity to dairy foods which seems so common in developed countries.

Animal feeds

Bovine spongiform encephalitis (BSE) is just one result of feeding cows animal byproducts such as sheep's brain and spinal cord. Cows are herbivores and it is hardly surprising that such obscene methods rebound on the producers.

Growth hormones are still added to the feeds of selected herds and as their identity is allowed to be kept secret, nobody knows where the pooled milk ends up or what the long-term effects on humans are likely to be.

Baby food

Babies have an inherently weak Earth. It is not until they are around 7 years old that the Stomach and Spleen are considered to be fully consolidated. Their Postnatal Qi depends on proper functioning of the Stomach and Spleen, yet they have relied until birth upon the Prenatal Qi of the mother nourishing them directly. Mother's milk is obviously the correct food for young babies and usually presents no problems to their digestive systems. However, modern pressures and preferences often result in the child having to transform something meant originally for a growing calf. As a result, the Earth is often weakened and chronic Phlegm problems may result, often with a specific intolerance of cow's milk. The use of cow's milk should be reserved for emergencies only in babies and younger children and if it has to be used, then a little ginger or garlic should be given to help balance the Phlegm-producing effects.

Added together, these modern factors go a long way to explain the discrepancy between the original uses for cow's milk and the reputation it has today. How much longer this will remain the case depends largely on consumers making clear demands for good quality products and on good quality information, rather than marketing propaganda.

Dairy products and soya milk

Milk may be processed into other products and this will affect the nature to some extent, but broadly speaking if a person is affected by milk then soft dairy foods such as buttermilk, yogurt, cottage cheese and related foods are all likely to have a similar effect. This should be borne in mind before advising yogurt after antibiotics. Skimmed milk products may be marginally less of a problem, but many slimmers have found to their cost that their Spleens do not thrive on such a diet.

Butter, hard cheeses and pungent cheeses such as Stilton seem relatively slightly Warmer. If the background problem includes deficient Spleen Yang, they may have slightly less effect than the other dairy products, but they will exacerbate Phlegm-Heat problems.

Milk from sheep and goats is increasingly used and as it is usually produced on a small scale from free-roaming animals, it is far less likely to be contaminated. Some producers are able to sell it unpasteurized and it is not surprising that many milk-sensitive people are able to consume moderate amounts of these products without problems. In larger quantities, however, similar problems occur and moderation should be the rule.

Soya milk is now widely available and, as you will see from the section on soya beans, has similar properties to cow's milk, except that instead of entering the Lung channel, it tonifies the Spleen. This means it is less Damp and Phlegm-producing in moderate amounts. When it is made into tofu, it is often considered to have a more lubricating and Cool nature and in parts of Indonesia is considered appropriate for quelling the sexual desire of celibate monks. Be warned!

I hope these notes, along with the main text, will help Western practitioners to begin using a fascinating and valuable therapy. Books have a way of crystallizing information which should really remain flexible. Please accept the ideas given in this introduction as indicators and starting points for your own studies and if any of the theory does not hold true in practice, then see how it needs to be modified to keep it alive and dynamic in the true spirit of Chinese medicine.

REFERENCES

Flaws B 1991 Arisal of the clear. Blue Poppy Press, Boulder, Colorado, p 57
Kaptchuk T 1983 The web that has no weaver. Rider, London, p 343ff
Kaptchuk T, Croncher M 1986 The healing arts. BBC Publications, London
Maciocia G 1989 The foundations of chinese medicine. Churchill Livingstone, Edinburgh
Ohsawa G 1968 The unique principle. Ohsawa Foundation, Los Angeles
Raloff J 1992 Microwaving can damage your health. Science News 141: 261
Riordan A M et al 1993 Treatment of active Crohn's disease by exclusion diet: East Anglian multicentre controlled trial. Lancet 342: 1131–4
Samuelsson S M et al 1991 Risk factors for extensive ulcerative colitis and ulcerative proctitis: a population based case-controlled study. Gut 32: 1526–30
Seignnlet J 1992 Diet, fasting and rheumatoid arthritis. Lancet 339: 68–9
Valaskitgis P 1978 New England School of Acupuncture, Boston. Personal communication

Part One

An introduction to Dietary Therapy in TCM

The concept, origin and development of Dietary Therapy in TCM 1

TCM Dietary Therapy is a newly developed use of material found in ancient Chinese dietary materia medica. This chapter gives an outline of the basic approach.

The concept of TCM Dietary Therapy

TCM Dietary Therapy deals with the properties of foods, their affects on health, and the therapeutic use of foods in the preservation of health and in the prevention and treatment of illnesses.

TCM Dietary Therapy has evolved and developed mainly through reference to books on dietetic materia medica and various medical books. In ancient China, terms most closely representing the concept of TCM Dietary Therapy are Shi liao or Shi zhi, meaning dietotherapeutics. However, what the ancients meant by the terms was not really treating diseases by using foods but using foods to maintain health or to help in the management of illnesses. The words *liao* and *zhi* (managing, treating or curing) derived perhaps from the belief that 'Food has the same action for treating diseases as herbal medicine and is based on the same principles' (BCQZ) and should not be taken too literally.

In his *Prescriptions Worth a Thousand Gold* (QJYF), Sun Simiao of the Tang dynasty categorized the properties and application of fruits, vegetables, cereals, fowl and animals, insects and fishes, while in the preface to the book he dealt with the significance and principles of Dietary Therapy and desirable and undesirable foods for specific illnesses. The contents of his works are mainly in the field of dietetic materia medica. Later works on dietetic materia medica are more or less the same in content, but they develop the idea of TCM Dietary Therapy.

It is these works we regard as the foundation for TCM Dietary Therapy, although there are some references in herbal medical works such as the *Treatises on Exogenous Febrile Diseases and Internal Diseases* (SHZBL), *Prescriptions for Emergencies* (ZHBJF), *Medical Records of an Official* (WTMY), *Peaceful Prescriptions of Holy Benevolence* (TPSHF), *Complete Collection for Holy Relief* (SJZL) and *A Complete Work of Medical Traditions* (GJYTDQ). Nowadays, the function of food in health preservation, prevention and treatment of illnesses is drawing more and more attention and medical and nutritional circles are beginning to study this subject from different points of view.

TCM Dietary Therapy is different from herbal medicinal therapy. The former mainly uses foods such as cereals, meats, fruits and vegetables, which are served as food and drink, while the latter mainly utilizes medicines in the form of herbs. The former has a wider range of application and is mainly administered to the healthy population and secondly to patients as auxiliary means to medication or other therapies, while the latter has a narrower application, mainly directed to patients and secondly to the healthy population as an important means for the treatment and prevention of diseases.

Dietary Therapy not only preserves and improves health, prevents and treats diseases, but also is a source of sensory enjoyment to the sensory organs and the mind. Dietary Therapy is very different in this aspect from herbal medicines, which usually have a disagreeable taste. Of course, as Dietary Therapy and herbal medication both have advantages and shortcomings, they are both indispensable in the prevention and treatment of diseases.

The origin and development of TCM Dietary Therapy

The ancients said that 'Food is the primary need for any people'. To maintain life and health, humans must look for foods and explore their functions in preserving health, preventing and treating diseases. Arguing from this point of view we could say that the study of Dietary Therapy has existed consciously or unconsciously as long as the human race.

Distilling was invented in the Xia dynasty in the 21st–16th centuries BC and during the Yin and Shang dynasties, the distilling and application of alcohol were widespread. Alcohol, apart from being used as a drink, was also widely used in medicine. By this time, herbal medical decoctions were developed from cooking. During the Zhou dynasty (11th century BC to 771 BC), there were official dietetic professionals working in the royal court and cooking started to become diversified.

With the accumulation of experience and knowledge, the theory of Dietary Therapy developed. In China's first works on medical theory, namely Huangdi's *Internal Classic* (HDNJ), including *The Plain Questions* and *The Miraculous Pivot* dating back to the Warring States period (2nd century BC), there were already good theories on Dietary Therapy. For instance, *The Plain Questions* (*The Relations Between the Viscera and the Seasons*) mentions that 'Medicines are used to fight the evils, cereals are used to nourish the body and fruits, meats and vegetables to aid the efforts – all the tastes working together to reinforce the vital Qi and Essence'. *The Plain Questions* (*the Five Major Principles*) also says that 'Cereals, meats, fruits and vegetables must all be taken to provide nutrition'. This is to say that foods must be consumed to assist the efforts of medicines in treating diseases and that humans should take all kinds of foods. This is consistent with the modern idea of a balanced diet.

The classics also deal with the physiological characteristics of internal organs and their relationship to the properties and tastes of foods, thus laying a foundation for Chinese Dietary Therapy.

In the Eastern Han dynasty (25–220 AD), there appeared China's first specialized book on materia medica, Shennong's *Herbal Classic* (SNBCJ). The book contains a number of foods which have the function of improving health and delaying aging. These include coix seeds, Chinese wolfberries, Chinese dates, poria, chickens, the fat of the wild goose, honey, lotus rhizome, lotus seeds, sesame and grapes. Han dynasty physician Zhang Zhongjing used foods in his medicinal recipes and formulated Cinnamon Bark Decoction, mutton soup with Chinese angelica and ginger and pig's skin soup, which are very good dietotherapeutic recipes. His methods for the treatment of exogenous Wind-Cold syndrome and Exterior deficiency syndrome by inducing spontaneous perspiration using Cinnamon Twig Decoction followed by hot gruel are very good dietetic practice. These methods, coupled with his views on food hygiene, made a valuable contribution to medicine.

In the Western and Eastern Jin dynasties and the Southern–Northern dynasties (265–589 AD), there was a marked growth in the knowledge of preventing and treating diseases with foods. In the Jin dynasty, Ge Hong, in his *Prescriptions for Emergencies* (ZHBJF), recorded a number of simple and proven recipes, many of which are dietotherapeutic.

There were also detailed recommendations on food hygiene and desirable and prohibited foods for specific diseases. In *Collective Notes to the Canon of Materia Medica* (BCJJZ) written by Tao Hongjing of the Southern dynasty, due attention was given to the specificities of foods. He classified fruits, vegetables and cereals with herbs and woody plants. In the chapter on Medicines for General Diseases, for example, for edema in the upper abdomen he enumerated such foods as kelp, kombu, red beans, soya beans, balsam pears, carp and the snakehead mullet, while for diabetes, he recommends such foods as cogongrass rhizome, wax gourd, cow's milk, mare's milk and wheat.

In the Song dynasty (960–1129 AD), it was general practice to use foods in the prevention and treatment of diseases. For example, in both the officially published formulary *Peaceful Prescriptions of Holy Benevolence* (TPSHF) and *Complete Collection for Holy Relief* (SJZL), Dietary Therapy was dealt with in special chapters which contain more than 100 diet recipes. A book called *Caring for Aged Relatives* (YLFQS) by Chen Zhi during this period deals with Dietary Therapy specially for geriatric diseases and includes diet recipes, mostly simple prescriptions.

During the Yuan dynasty (1206–1368 AD), Dietary Therapy underwent further development. Monographs on Dietary Therapy include Wu Rui's *Daily Herbal* (RYBC), Jia Ming's *A Dietetic Handbook* (YSXZ) and *Essence of Diet* (YSZY) by Hu Sihui, who was a court diet physician. The latter work put particular stress on the rational combination of daily foods and the addition of proper medicines in foods for health preservation and the prevention and treatment of diseases. There are fairly detailed and practical records on the preparation of foods.

In the Ming dynasty (1368–1644 AD), with the development of medicine and Dietary Therapy, more foods came to be recorded in works of materia medica. For example, *The Great Compendium of Materia Medica* (BCGM) records about 500 kinds of food, including cereals, vegetables, fruits, fish and reptiles, fowl and animals. More specialist works on Dietary Therapy were published, including Lu He's *Dietetic Herbal* (SWBC), Ning Yuan's *Verified Dietetic Herbs* (SJBC), Wu Lu's *A Collection of Diet*s (SPJ) and Gao Lian's *Notes on the Use of Foods and Drink*s (YZFSJ), which are all typical works on the subject.

By the Qing dynasty (1616–1911 AD), Dietary Therapy had been widely recognized by all physicians. The most valuable works include Shen Lilong's *Collection of Dietetic Herbs* (SWBCHZ), Wang Shixiong's *Recipes of Foods and Drinks from the Suixi House* (SXJYSP), Zhang Mu's *A Study on Diets for Correcting Ailments* (TJYSB) and Yuan Mei's *Diet Recipes from the Suiyuan Garden* (SYSD). These works cover a wide range of fundamental knowledge and practical applications; foods for the management of diseases and those for daily use.

TCM Dietary Therapy therefore has a history of over 3000 years and a very rich content, which is not only recorded in literature but has also been handed down from generation to generation.

In recent years, with the improvement of people's living standards and the development of Chinese medicine, Dietary Therapy is gaining strength and has attracted international attention. Significant achievements have been made in scientific research and the clinical application and teaching of TCM Dietary Therapy. In the course of modernization and the promotion of Traditional Chinese Medicine, TCM Dietary Therapy will undoubtedly develop and make a useful contribution to the health and longevity of mankind.

General properties 2
of food

According to the principles of Chinese Dietary Therapy, although herbal medicines can be included when appropriate, the basic therapeutic ingredients are commonly consumed food and drinks such as rice, soya beans, turnips, mutton and tea. It is this use of food that defines Dietary Therapy.

Many foods, apart from the ordinary items with which we are familiar, can function as both food and Chinese herbal medicine, e.g. ginger, dates, longans, Chinese wolf-berries, mulberries, pigskin and mutton. There is no clear dividing line between the two. The properties of most of the usual diet items are mild, but they do all have definite effects in preserving health and preventing or curing illnesses. However, these tendencies are not as marked as those of herbal medicines.

Dietary Therapy is based on an understanding of the tendencies or properties of foods. In this context, the principal properties of a food are its nature, taste, channel propensity and functions.

Of course, the modern scientific understanding of nutrients and the physiological effects of food are part of the basis of Dietary Therapy, but although this book lists nutritional information on foods, the emphasis is on descriptions in terms of TCM, which are derived from observations of the effects of foods we consume. For example, the beneficial effects of animal liver and carrot on the Liver and the eye can be related to the vitamin A or provitamin A which they contain; the effects of coix seeds, peanuts and soya beans on nourishing the Spleen and relieving edema can be attributable to the vitamin B1 they contain; and the effects of tomatoes, turnips and shepherd's purse in cooling the Blood and arresting bleeding can be related to the vitamin C they contain.

The nature and taste of food

Nature and taste are the most important properties of food. The nature of food is classified into Coldness, Coolness, Warmth and Heat, which are called 'the Four Natures'. In practice, these natures divide into two basic kinds, Cold or Hot. The nature of a food is defined on the same basis as in Chinese medicine, that is, by observing its effects on the human body. These are seen in both the intended therapeutic effects and in the side effects. Generally speaking, when a food acts as an antipyretic, a detoxifier or a tranquilizer, or when it can calm the Liver and impair Yang Qi (e.g. Yang Qi of the

Spleen and Stomach or of the Heart or Kidney), it is Cold in nature. Watermelons, balsam pears, turnips, pears, laver and clams are foods of this kind. On the other hand, when a food has the effects of warming the Middle Burner to dispel Cold, reinforcing Yang Qi, replenishing Fire and nourishing Qi, or when it can assist Heat and induce Fire or impair the Yin Body Fluids such as those of the Stomach, the Liver or the Lungs, it is considered as having a Warm nature. Typical foods of this kind are ginger, Chinese spring onions, Chinese chives, garlic, chillies and mutton. Only a few foods have a nature that is extremely Hot or Cold; some have only a slight tendency to Cold or Heat and are described as being Neutral in nature.

According to the classification of the dietetic materia medica, foods also have Tastes, as herbal medicines do. The categories principally employed are the Five Tastes of sourness, bitterness, sweetness, pepperiness and saltiness and pungent. These are mainly sensed by the gustatory organs but are also inferred from the food's actions. This concept is consistent with the principle of TCM that different Tastes have different actions. For example, some meats and animals' internal organs may be labeled as sweet for their function of nourishment, though in fact they do not taste sweet. Similarly, kelp, laver, clams or jellyfish do not taste salty but they are classed as salty because they have the effects of softening and dissolving hard masses. Hence the taste ascribed to a food may indicate its actions.

Generally, sourness, (which includes sourness combined with astringency) can act to arrest perspiration, stop diarrhea or cure seminal emission. Examples are plums and thorny eleagnus. Foods that are sour, or sweet and sour, such as plums, tamarind, rosehip and vinegar, have the effects of promoting the production of Body Fluids to quench thirst and assist the digestive system. Bitterness has an antipyretic effect and can relieve asthma and coughing, or act as a purgative. Foods of this description include balsam pears, Chinese olives, Chinese wolfberry shoots, mountain rorippa and dandelion. Sweetness can remedy debility, regulate the Stomach, relieve spasm and pains. Chestnuts, sweet apricot kernels, pumpkin, grapes, dates, maltose and animals' meat and viscera are all examples of foods which have these effects. Foods with a light sweetness can act as a diuretic and remove Damp; examples are coix seeds, shepherd's purse and wax gourd. The pungent Taste incorporates foods of a hot, spicy nature which are often aromatic in flavor, can induce perspiration, promote the circulation of Qi and Blood, dissolve Heat and assist digestion. Foods of this nature include Chinese spring onion, ginger, onion, rose petals, jasmine flowers and peppercorns. The chief function of saltiness is to soften and disperse hard masses. Foods of this kind include kelp and laver.

Moreover, the sourness of vinegar, the sweetness of sugar, the pungent nature of spices and the saltiness of soy sauce are indispensable seasonings in our daily cooking and are used to flavor food and make it more appetizing.

Channel propensities of food

The properties of a food are also expressed in its channel propensity, which means that a food has a clear effect on a particular channel or channels (i.e. the Internal Organs and their main and collateral channels), but has little or no effect on the other channels. Channel propensity is derived from the effects of a food on the human body considered in combination with the physiological and pathological characteristics of the Internal Organs and their channels. Four examples are given below:

1. Ginger and cassia bark are able to promote appetite; turnips and watermelons can promote the production of body fluids. As the Stomach is responsible for ingestion, likes moisture and dislikes dryness, and conditions such as loss of appetite, dehydration and thirst are categorized as Stomach symptoms, the four foods mentioned above can be classified as having a propensity for the Stomach channel.

2. Persimmon and honey can nourish Yin, moisten dryness and relieve coughing; mustard greens and water chestnut can dissolve Phlegm. As the Lung is a fragile organ in charge of respiration and at the same time is the vessel for

Phlegm, symptoms such as dry throat, coughing and coughing up of phlegm are attributed to the Lungs; hence, these four foods have a propensity for the Lung channel.

3. Chinese wolfberries and pig's liver can cure night blindness and blurred vision; shepherd's purse and crown daisy chrysanthemum can relieve redness, swelling and pain in the eyes. As the Liver opens into the eye, which has sight when it is receiving sufficient blood, such symptoms as redness, swelling and pain in the eye are attributable to Heat rising in the Liver; hence these four foods come under the propensity of the Liver channel.

4. Walnuts, almonds and bananas not only moisten dryness and arrest coughing, but also aid bowel motions. As these symptoms are attributable to the Lungs and the Large Intestine, these foods have a propensity for the Lung and Large Intestine channels.

Finally, most foods contain substances essential to the body which are the sources for the generation and transformation of Qi and Blood. Many foods have direct effects on the digestion and absorption of food and the movement of wastes about the body. Therefore, these foods have a propensity for the channels of the Spleen, Stomach and the Large Intestine. Examples of this kind are turnips, Aster Indicus, rosehips, Chinese haws, Chinese yams, lotus seeds, gorgon fruits, coix seeds, spinach, sesame seeds and almonds.

Like nature and taste, channel propensity is just one aspect of dietetic properties. All these aspects must be considered together to give a comprehensive description of a food's properties. Thus, the Chinese chive is described as sweet and pungent in taste, with a Warm nature and having a propensity for the channels of the Kidney, Stomach and Liver. When we look at these separately, it is difficult to tell what function it will perform. But when we look at the four aspects altogether, we can roughly tell that this food has the following functions:

• As it has a sweet and pungent taste, a Warm nature and a propensity for the Kidney channel, it can fortify the Kidney and benefit the Yang.

• As it is pungent, Warm and has a propensity for the Stomach channel, it can warm the Stomach and restore appetite.

• As it is pungent and has a propensity for the Liver channel, it can disperse extravasated blood.

If we know the nature and taste of a food but not its channel propensity, we cannot tell what functions it will perform. Thus, the pungent taste and Warmth of the Chinese chive do not work in the Lung channel and thus cannot disperse Cold or induce perspiration. On the other hand, we cannot tell what functions a food will perform when we know nothing but its channel propensity. In the case of the Chinese chive, though it has a propensity for the Kidney channel, it does not nourish the Kidney Yang, and though it has a propensity for the Stomach channel, it does not reinforce the Stomach and promote the production of Body Fluids. Therefore channel propensity needs to be considered together with nature and taste.

It must be stated that since a food has its properties, nature, taste, channel propensity and function, it also produces the effects of lifting, lowering, floating or sinking. Examples of these functions are; causing vomiting and resuscitation, associated with lifting and floating, or purgation and relief of spasm, associated with lowering and sinking. However, these tendencies are not as significant as in herbal medicines and we have excluded them from the body of the text (see Introduction).

A few kinds of foods, e.g. gingko, taro, garlic and chillies, are poisonous to a certain degree or have unwanted side effects. When they are used as food, these undesirable effects should be avoided by processing the food in an appropriate way, or by controlling the amount consumed. This contrasts with practice in TCM herbal medicine, where herbs can be used as 'poison to fight another poison'. Once again, we do not include this as an aspect of the properties of food.

The application 3
of foods

The importance of food in health preservation was pointed out as early as in Huangdi's *Internal Classic* (HDNJ), which also recommends that one should eat a full and balanced range of foods and that it is important to use foods properly in the treatment of disease. To illustrate these principles we may consider five aspects – the combination of foods, balanced diet, proper application of food, preparation of food and general rules of avoiding certain foods in different diseases.

The combination of foods

Foods are generally consumed with no thought for their combined actions. However, to enhance the therapeutic effect, flavor and nutritional value, different foods may be used together. Through the combination of foods either with each other or with herbal medicines, the properties of the foods may be modified. The different effects produced by these combinations are rather like the compatibility of herbs, which can be classified as mutual reinforcement, mutual assistance, incompatibility, mutual detoxification, mutual inhibition and antagonism. In Dietary Therapy, the various permutations may be summed up in the following four ways:

1. *Mutual reinforcement and assistance*. This means that foods whose nature and effect are basically the same or similar in one aspect can, to a certain degree, enhance each other in dietotherapeutic effect or edibility. For example, in mutton soup made with Chinese angelica and ginger, mutton is capable of warming and replenishing Qi and Blood, Chinese angelica root is capable of replenishing Blood and relieving pain. When the two are used together, the effects of replenishing deficiency, dispersing Cold and relieving pain are enhanced; the addition of ginger can enhance the effects of warming the Middle Burner and dispersing Cold and at the same time can moderate the flavor of mutton and make it more palatable. As another example, the fresh juice of lotus rhizome and cogongrass rhizome can both cool Blood and arrest bleeding. When they are used together, the effects of clearing away Heat, cooling Blood and arresting bleeding are enhanced, and the mixture is also more palatable than the two taken separately.

In 'pork liver soup with spinach', spinach and pig's liver can both nourish the Liver and improve the acuity of vision. When they are used together, the effects of nourishing the Liver and improving the acuity of vision are enhanced, making the remedy an effective treatment for blurred vision due to Liver Deficiency or night blindness.

2. *Incompatibility and mutual detoxification*. This means that when two foods are used together, the toxicity or side effect of one food can be partly or totally removed by the other. In this interaction, the former is regarded as incompatible with the latter while the latter is considered as detoxifying to the former. For example, garlic is thought to prevent and treat poisoning from fungi; olives to detoxify slight poisoning from puffer fish, fishes and crabs; honey and mung beans to detoxify the poison of Sichuan aconite and aconite. There are many more examples of this kind in writing and in folk lore which, however, need further research for verification.

3. *Mutual inhibition*. When two foods are used together, their original effects are lessened or even lost through interaction. Foods that have such incompatibility usually have contradictory natures. For example, if one has chillies, ginger or peppercorn after having foods such as tremella fungus, lily bulb or pears for the purpose of nourishing Yin, promoting the production of Body Fluids and moistening dryness, then these effects would be reduced; if one has mung beans, fresh turnips or watermelon after having mutton or beef for the purpose of warming and reinforcing Qi and Blood, these effects would also be reduced. In practice, such typically incompatible foods rarely appear together within one recipe in daily use but as customs vary and sometimes more than two kinds of food are served at the same time, then the above situation may still take place.

4. *Antagonism*. When two foods are used together, toxic reactions or obvious side effects can be produced. The ancient Chinese recorded such antagonisms, e.g. between honey and raw Chinese spring onion or between persimmon and crabs. Examples of antagonism between foods and herbal medicines are kelp and liquorice, carp and magnolia bark. However, these examples require further studies for verification and such antagonism between foods is rarely seen.

In short, in most cases, when foods are used together not only can their original effects be enhanced, but new effects can be produced. Therefore, by using different foods together we may obtain more dietary value and a wider range of application than by using one food at a time. Besides, proper combination of different foods can improve the coloring, smell, taste and texture, thus increasing their palatability and making them more appetizing. This is also a higher form of dietetic application.

The different relations of foods as described above could in practice determine which foods are suitable to be used together and which foods are not. Mutual reinforcement and mutual assistance could enhance the effects of foods and increase their palatability. These are the desirable effects expected of Dietary Therapy and hence this kind of combination is most often employed. Incompatibility and mutual detoxification can be useful with a few foods which are poisonous or have side effects, though they are less often employed than the first kind of combination. Mutual inhibition and antagonism could reduce the effects of foods or produce toxic side effects, which are not beneficial to Dietary Therapy and therefore should be avoided.

However, it must be stated that in some regions, people like to add ginger, Chinese spring onion, peppercorn, Sichuan peppercorn or chillies as condiments to some foods. When these condiments have a contradictory action to those of foods to which they are added, this generally is not taken as an instance of mutual inhibition. For example, when ginger, Chinese onion, Sichuan pepper or chillies is added to season foods that are Cool in nature, because these condiments are used in very small amounts, their major effects are appetizing and flavoring (see Introduction for a discussion on the balancing effects of such combinations).

Balanced diet

We may deal with this issue under two aspects, that is, the advantages of a balanced diet and the disadvantages of an unbalanced diet.

A BALANCED DIET

A balanced diet means that the kinds of foods we consume and the nutrients these foods contain should be comprehensive, adequate in amount and proportion, so that the nutrients supplied by our diet will meet the needs of the body.

Our daily diet consists of various kinds of food. A balanced diet requires that the types and amounts of foods should be present in appropriate proportions. This issue is dealt with as early as in *The Internal Classic* (NJ), which says that 'One should have cereals for nourishment, which should be assisted by fruits, meats and vegetables'. These remarks not only point out the types of food to be consumed, but also the positions of different kinds of foods in dietetic structure. According to the notes and interpretations by Wang Bing of the Tang dynasty, 'cereals' refers to unpolished rice, red beans, wheat, soya beans and millet, 'fruits' refers to peaches, plums, apricots, chestnuts and dates, 'meats' refers to beef, mutton, pork and chicken and 'vegetables' refers to cluster mallow, bean leaves, scallion, Chinese spring onion and Chinese chives. This is testimony that from a very early date, the Chinese people had a wide variety of foods and that cereals, meats, vegetables and fruits as foods should be included in suitable amounts in the diet.

AN UNBALANCED DIET

Balanced dietetic structure requires that the foods one consumes should be varied, including various tastes, suitable amounts of meat and vegetables, suitable amounts of Cold, Hot, Warm and Cool foods. If one's diet is unbalanced, irregularity of the functioning of the internal organs and an imbalance Yin and Yang can occur. The

excessive intake of certain nutrients can also affect one's health.

The Five Tastes and the Five Internal Organs of the human body have certain affinities. The intake of one food for a long time can impair certain Internal Organs and result in illness. According to *The Plain Questions* (SW):

Overintake of sourness makes the Liver Qi to be exuberant, which tends to mar the Spleen Qi; overintake of saltiness leads to exhaustion of major bones, contracture of muscles and depression of Heart Qi; overintake of sweetness causes stuffiness in the Heart and asthma, leading to darkness in the face and unbalanced Kidney Qi; overintake of bitterness leads to deficiency of Spleen Qi and exuberance of Stomach Qi; overintake of pungent taste leads to flaccidity of tendons and muscles and dispiritedness.

The Plain Questions, the Origin of the Five Zang Organs states that:

Overintake of saltiness leads to uneven pulse and change of skin color; overintake of bitterness leads to dryness of skin and hair loss; overintake of pepperiness leads to shortness of pulse and dry finger nails; overintake of sourness leads to thickened and hardened muscles and dry and scaled lips; overintake of sweetness leads to pain in the bones and hair loss.

All these remarks show that the overintake of any one taste could cause unwanted consequences to the human body.

Nor should one consume extremes of Cold or Hot foods. *The Miraculous Pivot* (LS) states that 'Food must not be extremely Hot or Cold'. *The Synopsis of the Gold Chamber* (JKYL) also points out that 'Intake of Cold or Hot food should be moderate... so that the body is not harmed'. For example, overintake of Cold or Cool foods, such as excessive consumption of raw and cold fruits and melons, could impair the Yang Qi of the Spleen and the Stomach, leading to deficiency in the Spleen and the Stomach, causing the development of Cold-Damp inside the body, and leading to abdominal pain or diarrhea.

When women take an excess of raw and Cold foods, it could cause an accumulation of Cold-Damp in the womb, leading to dysmenorrhea or irregular menstruation. Overconsumption of spicy, Warm, dry or Hot foods can lead to accumulation of Heat in the Stomach, causing thirst, fullness or pain in the abdomen or constipation.

The temperature of foods taken should not be too high. Modern medicine believes that very hot foods may trigger off carcinoma of the esophagus.

In short, imbalance in diet can interfere with the balance of Yin and Yang in the human body, impair the functioning of the Internal Organs and cause either malnutrition or an excess of unused nutritional by-products.

Appropriate use of food

In daily cooking and Dietary Therapy, the appropriate use of foods mainly consists of a rational choice of foods, rational cooking and processing of foods and the appropriate preparation of foods.

Rational choice of food is the most important of these factors. If a balanced selection of foods (in terms of flavor, nature, combination and suitability for the individual) is chosen, it will lead to health. An unbalanced selection could lead to illness. For example, for patients suffering from mental derangement, foods such as wheat, day lily, lily bulb, lotus seeds, dates, pig's heart, hen's eggs and oyster should be chosen.

Rational cooking and processing of food are also very important. They will reduce the loss of nutrients and at the same time increase the palatability of foods and make them easier to digest. For example, when cooking rice, it is not desirable to wash or rub it excessively and the water temperature should not be too high; and if there is liquid in the cooked rice, it should be consumed as well.

When cooking vegetables, it is desirable to choose fresh ones and to wash them before cutting. They should not be left to soak or stand for long after preparation. Condiments may be added to improve color, smell and taste in cooking. To reduce the loss of vitamin C, it is advisable to stir-fry vegetables quickly at a high temperature.

• Fruits or vegetables with edible skins or cores should be eaten whole if possible. As mentioned earlier, this may not be advisable unless they are from an organic source.

• Animal products are normally difficult to digest and thus should be cooked very thoroughly for easy digestion, particularly if they are for children or elderly people. Slow gentle cooking will make meat more digestible than with faster cooking methods. However, many Western sources consider that raw meat is much more easily digested than the cooked product (leaving aside matters of hygiene).

• Yeast is preferable to raising agents such as bicarbonate of soda in dough-based foods. With candidiasis becoming so widespread, the removal of any raising agents may be prefered.

Proper preparation of food is also essential. For example, when preparing foods for the prevention or treatment of the common cold, foods that have a pungent taste or aroma may be used for an infusion made with boiling water; if a decoction is made instead, the foods should not cook for too long or the aromatic substances will evaporate and the medicinal effect will be reduced. Other examples might be the use of porridge-based recipes to regulate the Spleen and Stomach or for deficiency illnesses use nourishing foods made into soups, steamed, cooked into thick pastes or made into medicinal wines by infusion.

In short, suitable preparation of foods should be used according to the patient's lifestyle and the actual condition of his or her illnesses.

The preparation of food

Most foods have to be cooked or prepared in a certain way for eating. In Dietary Therapy, common preparations of food include cooked rice, gruels, soups, steamed paste, cooked dishes, decoctions, tonics, medicinal wines, powders, electuaries (sweet medicated pastes), candied fruits and sweets. The following is a brief introduction to the concepts of preparation and their significance in Dietary Therapy.

COOKED RICE

Unpolished rice and glutinous rice are mainly used in conjunction with other foods or herbal medicines such as dates, longans, Chinese yam or pilose asiabell root, which are steamed or boiled. Generally, cooked rice has the effects of replenishing Qi and reinforcing the Spleen and nourishing Blood. An example is cooked rice with pilose asiabell root which was recorded in *The Records from the Awakening Garden* (XYL).

GRUELS

Unpolished, glutinous rice or millet are mainly used together with appropriate amounts of other foods or herbal medicines, cooked with water into a semifluid matter (gruel). If the added herbs or food are not suitable for cooking with the food (e.g. when there is residue), it is advisable to obtain juice from the added food or herb through cooking or squeezing before adding it to the main dish. Sugar, salt or lard can be added for flavor. Gruels have a wide range of applications and are suitable for patients of all ages and categories. For example, mung bean gruel and lotus leaf gruel are used in the summer to prevent sunstroke. Convalescent patients or women after childbirth are advised to take gruels for a speedy recovery.

SOUPS

Meat, eggs, milk, fish or tremella fungus are commonly used in soups with appropriate amounts of herbal medicines, boiled or stewed. Condiments such as sugar, soy sauce, ginger and peppercorn can be added for flavor according to the taste and property of the food. In Dietary Therapy, soups are mainly used as alteration or nourishment. For example, 'tremella fungus soup' can nourish the Yin and moisten the Lungs and 'mutton soup with Chinese yam', as recorded in the *Essence of Diet* (YSZY), can reinforce the Spleen and the Kidney.

COOKED DISHES

A great many kinds of food can be used in the form of cooked dishes. These may include vegetables, meats, poultry, eggs, fish and prawns. Cooking methods are also varied, including steaming, braising, stir-frying, stewing in soy sauce, stewing, roasting and quick boiling. Generally, condiments are added in cooking these dishes and may include ginger, Chinese spring onion, garlic, chillies, Sichuan pepper, pepper, mustard, salt, soy sauce, vinegar, wine or sugar. Apart from being used in prepared dishes in Dietary Therapy, specific foods and condiments are chosen and combined so as to give the dishes good coloring, taste and smell, a coherent nature and beneficial effects on health.

Generally, dishes made with meat, fish, poultry and eggs are more nourishing, while dishes made with vegetables have more varied functions.

DECOCTIONS

Foods or medicines are boiled in a suitable amount of water and the extract obtained. Except for items that cannot be cooked for long, foods or herbal medicines are usually boiled two or three times and the decoctions made each time are mixed into two or three servings.

Decoctions are made for the purpose of treating diseases but as dietotherapeutic items, their palatability should also be considered.

DRINKS

Generally, foods, tea materials and condiments that are sour and sweet, fragrant or slightly bitter are boiled in water, infused in hot water or distilled to make the desired drink. The drinks thus made can be consumed instead of tea.

Fresh, juicy and edible fruits, stems, leaves or rhizomes of some plants can also be cut up or crushed, wrapped in gauze and squeezed to obtain fresh juice for drinking immediately. Sometimes honey, sugar or wines can be added. Drinks can be taken either cold or warm.

There are also instant drinks, generally made with foods (sometimes with added herbal medicines) by boiling, removing the residue and concentration, adding dry sugar to make a dry powder which is then ready to be consumed any time by mixing with boiling water.

Drinks commonly have the effects of cooling, promoting the production of Body Fluids so as to quench thirst, and are also used as diuretics.

MEDICINAL WINES

Medicinal wines are generally transparent liquids made with foods or herbal medicines which are steeped in cold or hot liquor or in yellow rice or millet wines. There are also medicinal wines made with glutinous rice and other foods or herbs by boiling them together and then fermenting with yeast. This kind of wine is called rice wine. It is desirable to make medicinal wines with 5–10° of alcohol.

Alcohol is at the same time a food and a medicine. It has the effects of dispersing Cold, activating the Blood circulation, warming the Stomach and assisting the effects of other herbal medicines. The effects of herbal wines vary with different foods or herbs added to the wines. For example, Chinese wolfberry wine can reinforce the Liver and the Kidney; when tiger's bone and chaenomeles fruits are added, they have the effects of strengthening the tendons and the bones, relieving rheumatism and removing Damp.

POWDERS

Foods or medicines are powdered by grinding after air drying, oven baking or roasting (in this context, roasting refers to cooking dry in a wok or similar pot, without fat). Grains and dry fruits are usually used in this way. Suitable medicines can be added. Before serving, mix the powder with boiling water, add condiments such as sugar or salt to taste. For powders that are not quite palatable, take them with water or thin millet gruel. Powders are easy to take and most are rich in nutrients are appetizing and can reinforce the Spleen.

ELECTUARIES

Electuaries are generally made with nourishing foods which are boiled in water and condensed, adding refined honey, white sugar or crystal sugar and then further condensing it to a fairly semisolid state. Dissolve it in boiling water when needed.

Electuaries mainly have the effect of moistening dryness. For example, mulberry electuary nourishes the Liver and the Kidney; autumn pear electuary moistens and clears Heat from the Lungs, promotes the production of Body Fluids and relieves coughing.

CANDIED FRUITS

Generally, fruits, melons or vegetables are heated in water or herbal liquid until the water or herbal liquid is almost dry, then a large amount of honey or sugar is added. The mixture is then cooked thoroughly until the liquid is dried up.

Candied fruits are delicious and can be eaten directly or sliced and soaked in water as an infusion. The effects of candied fruits vary with different contents, but generally they are alterative, can regulate the Stomach, moisten dryness and promote the production of Body Fluids.

SWEETS

Medicinal sweets are made with white sugar, brown sugar, crystal sugar or maltose, mixed thoroughly and evenly with the juice, extracts or powder of other foods. The sugar is then boiled in water and thickened until it makes filaments when picked up and is no longer sticky when touched. Cut up into lumps when cooled.

Medicinal sweets can also be made by mixing prepared food and refined sugar syrup.

This kind of food may have different effects. For example, pear sweets can clear away Heat, moisten the Lungs and arrest coughs; peppermint sweets and puffball sweets can clear away Heat, moisten dryness and soothe the throat;

mulberry sweets and sesame sweets can reinforce the Liver and the Kidney.

Besides the preparations discussed above, there are still other forms of foods which use rice and flour as major materials, e.g. pastry, noodles, steamed stuffed buns and mung bean vermicelli. Cooked dishes are also varied in forms, but will not be discussed in this book.

Diet prohibitions

Dietetic prohibitions include the foods to be avoided by patients with certain diseases and for women during pregnancy and after childbirth.

DIET PROHIBITIONS DURING ILLNESS

Some foods can affect the healing process of diseases or the effects of medicines being taken and are therefore to be avoided. Generally, during the course of herbal treatment, all raw, cold, greasy, sticky and fishy smelling foods which are difficult to digest should be avoided.

Different diseases call for different prohibitions. For example, when patients with diarrhea and abdominal pain due to deficient Cold in the Spleen and the Stomach are taking herbal medicines for the purpose of warming the Middle Burner and dispersing Cold, such foods as raw and cold fruits or melons, foods of a Cold or Cool nature, fishy, sticky or greasy foods are to be avoided; when patients with insomnia are taking tranquilizers, they should not have such stimulating drinks as coffee or strong tea; patients with deficient Yang and excessive Cold should avoid raw, cold foods or foods with a Cold or Cool nature; patients with deficient Yin and exuberant Heat should avoid foods of a pungent and dry nature, which tend to agitate Fire; patients with edema should avoid salty foods; patients with diabetes should avoid sugar; patients with Yang syndromes, sores and ulcers, rashes or ringworm and scabies should avoid pungent, peppery, fragrant and dry foods.

In addition, when a patient has just recovered from a disease and his or her Stomach Qi is not adequately restored, he or she should avoid greasy and rich foods and take gruel instead.

Huangdi's *Internal Classic* (HDNJ) specially points out that 'When a Heat disease is being cured, taking meat can make the disease come back, and overeating can lead to diarrhea. These are to be prohibited'. These remarks should be duly noted.

In short, the foods taken during the course of an illness should aid the effects of medicines being taken; foods that have a contradictory action to the medicines being taken or which are bad for the illness are prohibited. Just as *The Synopsis of the Gold Chamber* (JKYL) says, 'Some foods benefit the cure of the disease, some are harmful to health; beneficial foods do good for health, while harmful foods cause diseases or even bring danger to life'.

DIETETIC PROHIBITIONS DURING PREGNANCY AND AFTER CHILDBIRTH

Pregnant women and women after childbirth have special physiological requirements such as nurturing the child and breast feeding and therefore dietetic prohibitions have special significance.

During the course of pregnancy, the Blood of the Internal Organs, the meridians and the collaterals all rush the Blood to the Chong and Ren vessels, leading to the deficiency of Yin to Blood and the excess of Yang Qi in the rest of the body. Therefore during pregnancy, wines, dry ginger, cinnamon bark, pepper and chillies which are pungent in taste and Warm, dry and fiery in nature should be avoided, lest they consume or impair Yin fluids and affect the fetus or pregnancy.

For women suffering from vomiting during pregnancy, foods with a fishy taste or smell, greasy foods or foods that are not easy to digest are to be avoided. Moreover, foods can be served according to the pregnant woman's taste. Attention should be paid to the nutritional value of foods. In the later phase of pregnancy, as the fetus is developing and affecting the rising and descending of the functioning Qi which is inclined to cause stagnancy of Qi, foods that could lead to Qi distension and are astringent, such as taro, sweet potatoes and pomegranates, are to be avoided.

Women after childbirth are susceptible to loss of Blood and Yin fluids, Blood stasis and deficiency syndromes and they also have to produce milk to feed the baby. Their diet should be adequate and spread evenly through the day, emphasizing nutritious foods which are easy to digest.

Foods to be avoided are those with a pungent taste (which tend to impair Yin), foods that are Cold in nature (such as melons and raw food), sour or astringent in nature. As *The Essence of Diet* (YSZY) puts it, 'The breastfeeding mother should not feed the baby when she is too full; nor when she is hungry; nor when she is too cold or hot, nor should she have Cold or Cool foods which cause disease'.

The principles of *Dietary Therapy in TCM* 4

Dietary Therapy is founded on the insight of TCM theory. In broad terms this is apparent in the holistic approach adopted in Dietary Therapy and in the application of treatment principles based on the differentiation of symptoms and signs.

Holism in Dietary Therapy

According to holism, the human body is an organic whole, and the body and its natural environment also form an organic whole. When Dietary Therapy is conducted, it is important to harmonize the interactions both between the different parts of the body and between the body and its natural environment.

THE REGULATION OF YIN AND YANG

The normal physiological activities of the human body are maintained by the coherence of its Yin and Yang. The onset and development of any illness result from a breakdown of the relative equilibrium between Yin and Yang. 'Excessive Yin produces Yang illnesses and excessive Yang produces Yin illnesses. Yin deficiency produces Heat and Yang deficiency produces Cold.'

These are the principle mechanisms of illnesses. Dietary Therapy employs methods of correcting the disequilibrium and remedying deficiencies to adjust Yin and Yang and restore their dynamic equilibrium. For example, in cases of excessive Yang Heat which tends to consume and impair Yin fluids, the established treatment in Dietary Therapy is directed to clearing the Heat and protecting the Body Fluids. Recommended diets are the 'Five-Juice Mix' (see Epidemic Febrile Diseases), celery gruel and mung bean gruel, which will purge the excessive Yang to regulate Yin. If Yang is deficient and cannot control Yin so that Cold becomes overwhelming, the method of warming the channels and dispersing Cold is used in Dietary Therapy treatments. Recommended diets are 'mutton soup with Chinese angelica and ginger', 'walnuts sauteed with Chinese chives and thick mutton soup', which will reinforce Yang to help control Yin.

In short, Dietary Therapy always emphasizes the rational arrangement of diets on the principle of regulating Yin and Yang to maintain their equilibrium.

THE COORDINATION OF THE INTERNAL ORGANS

The Internal Organs are interrelated and the Internal Organs and the body are an integrated unity. An illness in the Internal Organs may be reflected in a certain part of the body and conversely an illness in that part may reflect illness in a certain organ. In addition, if an organ is not functioning properly, it will affect the functions of the other Internal Organs.

Dietary Therapy should be aimed at coordinating the interactions between individual organs and also between the parts of the body, to restore the interrelated physiological balance of the organism. For example, blurred vision may be due to deficiency of Liver Blood, which is reflected in the eye. The Dietary Therapy treatment is to nourish and reinforce the Liver and Kidney. Recommended foods are pig's liver sauteed with Chinese wolfberry shoots and pork liver soup. When ulcers occur in the mouth and on the tongue, they are the result of excessive Heat (Fire) in the Heart and the Stomach reflected in the mouth and tongue. Treatment is to purge the Heat (Fire) in the Heart. Recommended diets are rush pith gruel and bamboo reed tea (made with bamboo leaves and reed rhizomes). Both treatments are examples where the Internal Organs are coordinated and the diverse parts of the body are harmonized.

To take another example, an illness in the Lungs may arise when the organs themselves are attacked by pathogenic Qi or as a result of illness in another organ. In the former case the Dietary Therapy treatment should be directed to the ventilation of the Lungs and the reduction of the Counter-flow Qi. Recommended food is a ginger infusion with sugar. If the illness is due to excessive Fire in the Liver which impairs the Lungs, then the treatment should be focused on purging the Liver Fire. An infusion of chrysanthemum and crown daisy chrysanthemum is recommended.

If the illness is due to the generation of Phlegm owing to deficiency in the Spleen and the Lungs being filled with Phlegm and Damp, the Dietary Therapy treatment should emphasize the reinforcement of the Spleen and the elimination of the Damp. A recommended food is Zhi-zhu rice (rice cooked with trifoliate oranges and rhizome of largeheaded atractylodes (Atractylodes macrocephala)). If the illness is due to deficiency in the Kidney Yin which fails to nourish the Lungs, then treatment should be concentrated on nourishing the Kidney and moistening the Lungs. A recommended food is a lily bulb soup with Chinese wolfberries.

For conditions such as headaches, tinnitus, flushing, red eyes and restlessness which are due to an excessive level of Liver Yang, diets such as chrysanthemum infusion and celery gruel will remove the excessive Heat from the Liver and control the excessive Liver Yang.

Diets such as Chinese yam gruel and Spleen-reinforcing cakes will protect the 'middle earth' (Zhong tu) and prevent the excessive Wood from impairing the Spleen. Mulberry electuary and pig's kidney soup can nourish the Kidney fluid which in turn nurtures the Liver Wood. Bamboo leaf gruel and rush pith infusion will purge the pathogenic Fire of the Heart in order to achieve the objective of purging a subordinate organ when the principal organ is full. Similarly, for illnesses in the other Internal Organs, suitable diets can be chosen on the basis of their interrelationships.

ADAPTING TO THE CLIMATE

Seasonal changes in climate have a significant effect on the physiological functions and pathological changes of the body. Therefore Dietary Therapy should take into account the characteristics of the climates of the different seasons.

In spring, as the weather turns warmer and everything is growing, the Liver becomes very active in its function of dispelling and dispersing. Hence the diet should aim at nourishing the Liver and reinforcing its dispelling function. Recommended foods are pig's liver sauteed with Chinese chives and an infusion made with mulberry leaves, chrysanthemum flowers and peppermint leaves. Summer is hot and everything is prospering. The skin and muscles are relaxed and the body is characterized by the Heart's craving for Coolness. The diet should therefore be concentrated on dispelling Heat and generating Body Fluids. Recommended foods are mung bean (green bean) soup and lotus leaf soup. In autumn, it is cool and dry and everything is dying or retreating and this reflects in the Lungs' inward movement. Dietary Therapy should aim at reinforcing and moistening the Lungs. Recommended foods are sundried persimmon and tremella fungus soup. Winter is Cold and everything has gone into hiding. In the body the Kidney Yang Qi is gathered and stored. The diet should reinforce the Kidney and warm the Yang and the recommended food is thick mutton soup.

When Dietary Therapy is administered for specific illnesses, seasonal climatic characteristics should also be taken into consideration. For example, the common cold in spring and summer should be treated with foods which are Cool and pungent such as an infusion of mulberry, chrysanthemum and peppermint and lotus leaf gruel, while the common cold in autumn and winter should be treated with foods which are pungent, Warm and have the effects of inducing perspiration. Such foods are hot ginger tea with brown sugar and Cong-chi gruel (made with rice, Chinese spring onion and fermented soya beans).

REGIONAL VARIATIONS

China is a large country whose altitudes, climates and lifestyles vary in different regions. People who live in different regions have thus developed different physiological activities and are characterized by different illnesses. Therefore when Dietary Therapy is administered, these factors should be taken into consideration and suitable diets should be prescribed. For example, in the south-east coastal regions of China, the climate is warm and wet and the inhabitants tend to be affected by Damp-Heat. Their diets should be plain in flavor and have the function of removing Damp from the body. In the north-west

plateau regions where the climate is cold and dry, the inhabitants tend to suffer from Coldness and Dryness. The appropriate diet is foods with a Warm nature which will dispel the Coldness or foods which generate Body Fluids and moisten the Dryness. In treating the common cold to induce perspiration, in the north-west spring onion and fermented soya bean gruel and a ginger infusion with sugar and perrila are more appropriate; while in the south-east, Gan-ge gruel (made with rice and kudzu vine roots) and an infusion of mulberry, chrysanthemum and peppermint are used.

There are also regional variations in taste. For instance, the people of Shanxi and Shannxi prefer acidic (vinegary) food, while those in Yunnan, Guizhou, Sichuan and Hunan prefer hot spicy food and those in Jaingsu and Zhejiang prefer sweet and salty food. Overall, people in the north-east and northern provinces of China prefer salty and hot spicy food, those residing in the coastal areas prefer seafood, while people in the north-west prefer dairy products such as cheese.

ADAPTING TO INDIVIDUAL NEEDS

The physiological characteristics and the conditions of a person's Qi and Blood vary with age. In Dietary Therapy treatment the food should be chosen according to the patient's age and physical characteristics.

The young are in the process of vigorous growth, but both their Yin and Yang are immature and they tend to suffer from indigestion and ascariasis. Their diets should therefore aim at reinforcing the Spleen and promoting digestion. Recommended foods are Chinese yam gruel (made with rice and Chinese yams) and preserved Chinese hawthorn apples. On the other hand, food that is Warm or Hot in nature and has the effect of reinforcing Yang should be taken with care.

The elderly are in the process of decline. Their Qi and Blood are deficient and their Yin and Yang are both gradually weakening. Their diets should be more nourishing and easier to digest. Examples are Qiong Yu Gao (an electuary) and a thick soup made with sheep's internal organs. Food that is Cold or Cool in nature and difficult to digest should be taken with care.

Individual differences in physical constitutions require different Dietary Therapies. A body which suffers from Yang excess and Yin deficiency is suited to food which is Cool in nature and Yin-reinforcing, such as tremella fungus soup, specially prepared black soya beans and mutton and honey electuary; food that is Warm in nature and Yang-reinforcing should be taken with care. A body with weak Yang and dominant Yin is suited to foods which are Warm in nature and Yang-reinforcing, such as thick mutton soup; food that is Cold or Cool in nature and harmful to Yang should be taken with care. A body whose Qi is weak is suited to food which is Qi-reinforcing such as ginseng gruel and Spleen-reinforcing cakes. A body whose Blood is weak is suited to food which is Blood-reinforcing such as Yu Ling Gao (an electuary) and mutton soup with ginger and Chinese angelica.

Men and women have different physiological characteristic and diets should reflect these differences. Women who go through menstruation, pregnancy, childbirth and breastfeeding regularly suffer from impairment of Blood. Their physical condition is usually characterized by Blood deficiency and Qi excess. Hence their day-to-day diet should be based on food which is Blood-enriching.

During menstruation and pregnancy, they should take foods which reinforce the Blood and nourish the Kidney, such as egg soup and glutinous rice gruel with donkey-hide gelatin. Foods which are greasy and Blood-activating should be taken with care. Examples are gruel with three-colored amaranth and mutton soup with ginger and Chinese angelica. For women who suffer from profuse leukorrhea as a result of Spleen deficiency, foods which reinforce the Spleen and remove Damp are recommended. Examples are Chinese yam gruel and Spleen-reinforcing cakes.

After childbirth, deficiency in Blood and Qi and deficiency in milk should be taken into consideration. Suitable diets are foods which reinforce Qi and Blood and help to generate milk. Examples

are eel soup with ginseng and Chinese angelica, stewed hen with ginseng and Chinese angelica and pig's trotters stewed with Chinese spring onion.

Administration of diets based on the differentiation of symptoms and signs

According to the theory of treatment on the basis of differentiation of symptoms and signs, illnesses are dynamic and changeable. Corresponding with the type of pathogen, physical conditions and climate, an illness may manifest different symptoms, while on the other hand different illnesses may manifest the same symptoms. This requires diet administration based on the differentiation of symptoms and signs.

DIFFERENT DIETS FOR THE SAME ILLNESS

This means that different diets are administered for the same illness because of different symptoms. Take stomach ache, for example. With differences in its causes, physical conditions, environment and case history, it may manifest different symptoms. Therefore the diet to be administered should also be different. If the problem is caused by eating bad food, Chinese hawthorn apple cakes or turnip gruel should be taken to help digestion and regulate the functions of the Stomach. If it is caused by Cold impairing the Stomach Yang, (lesser) galangal gruel or chicken cooked with round cardamon which will warm the Stomach and relieve the pain is inappropriate. If it is caused by impairment from the Liver, plum blossom gruel, fingered citron wine and rose tea should be administered to soothe the Liver and regulate the Stomach. If it is a result of deficiency and Coldness in the Spleen and Stomach, crucian carp soup and barley soup should be taken to reinforce the Spleen and warm the Stomach. If it is caused by deficiency of Stomach Yin, lady-bell gruel (made with rice and the roots of straight ladybell) and Stomach-reinforcing soup should be taken to nourish the Yin and reinforce the Stomach.

Taking another example, measles is a common infectious disease among young children after being affected by the measles toxin. Following the development of the measles pathogen, different symptoms manifest in three stages and the diet to be administered should be varied according to the different symptoms. In the initial stage, when the measles have not erupted, water chestnuts and fermented glutinous rice are desirable food for helping the eruption of the spots by means of perspiration. In the second stage, when the excess Heat is accumulated in the Lungs, food such as gypsum gruel is administered to clear the Heat and relieve the toxin. During the last stage, when the Heat lingers on, the symptoms reflect the impairment of the Yin of the Lungs and Stomach and sugarcane juice and juice of the cogongrass rhizome are recommended for nourishing the Yin and clearing the Lungs.

THE SAME DIET FOR DIFFERENT ILLNESSES

Different illnesses when manifesting the same symptoms or which are due to a common aetiology may be treated with the same diet. For instance, protracted diarrhea, prolapse of the anus, bloodstained stools, uterine bleeding and prolapsed uterus may all be caused by the decrease in Middle Qi. Food which can lift the Middle Qi is recommended and examples are ginseng and poria gruel, chicken cooked with Chinese angelica and the roots of membranous milkvetch.

The administration of different diets for the same illness or of the same diet for different illnesses is a reflection of the principle of treating a disease on the basis of differentiation of symptoms and signs. In both cases, diets are administered selectively according to the nature of the illness.

Principal methods of Dietary Therapy

5

Through appropriate selection of foods and by combining foods with Chinese herbal medicines, it is possible to create a variety of therapeutic effects. These can be described in terms of the classical herbal treatment principles such as warming, clearing Heat, purging or inducing sweating. However if we focus on the areas where Dietary Therapy can have its greatest impact we are left with four main areas of therapeutic influence.

1. Invigorating Qi and replenishing the Spleen
2. Enriching Blood and nourishing Yin
3. Tonifying the Kidney and replenishing the Vital Essence
4. Reinforcing the Stomach and promoting the production of Body Fluids.

Method of invigorating Qi and replenishing the Spleen

This method is used for syndromes involving Qi deficiency due to weakness of either the Lungs or Spleen.

INVIGORATING THE LUNG QI

This method involves selecting, preparing and cooking therapeutic foods that can invigorate the Lung Qi or combining foods with similarly targeted medicines.

For example, Qi-reinforcing gruel or sweets can be made with dates, maltose, honey, chicken, ginseng, pilose asiabell root and the root of membranous milkvetch for such symptoms as shortness of breath, a weak voice, susceptibility to the common cold and sweating due to a deficiency of Lung Qi.

INVIGORATING THE SPLEEN QI

This method involves making therapeutic foods using items that can invigorate the

Spleen Qi or preparing food with medicines with a property of reinforcing the Spleen Qi. For example, Chinese date gruel or Chinese yam noodles made with polished glutinous rice, dates, pig's tripe, chicken, quail and pilose asiabell root, the rhizome of largeheaded atractylodes and Chinese yam are used in the treatment of poor spirits, weak limbs, poor appetite and loose stools due to deficiency of the Spleen.

REINFORCING THE SPLEEN AND REMOVING DAMP

This method involves making therapeutic foods using items that have the property of reinforcing the Spleen and removing Damp or preparing food with medicines which have those properties.

For example, lotus seeds cooked with pig's tripe or red beans and crucian carp soup are made by using lotus seeds, gorgon fruit, coix seeds, red beans, flat beans, crucian carp, eel and poria and the rhizome of largeheaded atractylodes in the treatment of facial edema, heaviness in the body, swollen limbs, excessive bowel sounds and diarrhea due to weak Spleen which fails to absorb and transport bodily water.

REINFORCING AND LIFTING SINKING QI

This method uses the same principles, this time using foods or herbs which have the property of reinforcing the Qi or lifting the Yang, to treat diseases due to deficiency and collapse of Qi.

For example, chicken cooked with Chinese angelica and the root of membranous milkvetch, or a ginseng gruel, are made by using chicken, mutton, pigeon, crucian carp, dates, polished glutinous rice and ginseng, pilose asiabell root, the root of membranous milkvetch and cimicifuga rhizome in the treatment of such symptoms as shortness of breath, a weak voice, loose stool, prolapse of the anus, a prolapsed uterus, sagging of the stomach into the lower abdomen, uterine bleeding and leukorrhea, which are due to the collapse of the Central Qi.

REPLENISHING QI AND CONTAINING BLOOD

With this method, foods are used alone or with herbs to treat deficiency of Spleen Qi which is then unable to contain the Blood within the vessels.

For example, peanut and date sweets, or chicken cooked with Chinese angelica and the root of membranous milkvetch, are made by using peanuts, dates, longan aril, eel, cuttlefish and the root of membranous milkvetch and pseudoginseng in the treatment of vomiting of blood, bloodstained stool, bleeding from the gums and uterine bleeding owing to deficiency of Qi failing to control Blood.

Method of enriching the Blood and nourishing Yin

Blood enriching as a treatment principle means enhancing the Blood generating function and making up for the lack of Blood, which thereby nourishes the Heart and Liver and strengthens the physical condition as a whole. It is applied to Blood deficiency syndromes due to insufficient Blood production, after protracted illness or loss of blood.

The Yin nourishing method can nourish Yin Body Fluids, nourish the tendons and bones and astringe and hold the Yang Qi. It is applied to people with a tendency to Yin deficiency and patients with a lack of Yin Body Fluids due to Heat syndrome or protracted illnesses.

PROMOTING THE PRODUCTION OF BLOOD BY MEANS OF REPLENISHING QI

This method involves making therapeutic foods using items that can promote the production of Blood by means of replenishing Qi, or preparing food with medicines with the same nature in the treatment of deficiency in both Blood and Qi. For example, a soup made with Chinese angelica, ginseng and eel, or one made with Chinese angelica and mutton, are made by using carrots, spinach, peanuts, dates, longan aril, chicken, pig's liver, mutton and the root of membranous milkvetch and Chinese angelica in the treatment of a pale complexion, dry finger nails, faintness and palpitations owing to deficiency of both Qi and Blood.

REPLENISHING BLOOD AND NOURISHING THE HEART

This method involves making therapeutic food using items that have the property of replenishing Blood, nourishing the Heart and tranquilizing the Mind for the treatment of syndromes owing to deficiency of Blood failing to nourish the Heart. For example, Yu Ling Gao (an electuary), candied ginger, dates and longan, and pig's heart with Chinese angelica and ginseng are made with longan aril, litchi, dates, grapes, pig's heart, chicken and ginseng, Chinese angelica, the seed of wild jujube and poria for the treatment of palpitations, amnesia and insomnia owing to deficiency of Heart Blood.

REPLENISHING BLOOD AND NOURISHING THE LIVER

This method uses items which have the property of replenishing the Blood and nourishing the Liver for syndromes of deficient Liver Blood. For example, pig's liver sauteed with Chinese wolfberry shoots or Chinese wolfberry and Chinese angelica wine are made with carrots, spinach, pig's liver, chicken liver, Chinese wolfberry, mulberry, the tuber of knotweed and Chinese angelica for the treatment of blurred vision, faintness, hypochondriac pain, palpitation and muscle tremor, numbness in the hands and feet owing to deficiency of Liver Blood.

NOURISHING YIN AND CALMING THE WIND

This method involves making therapeutic foods using items that have the property of nourishing the Liver Yin and soothing the Liver Wind for

the treatment of Wind syndrome owing to deficient Yin. For example, a soup made with ingredients of the minor Wind-calming pill, Xiao Ding Feng Dan (egg yolk, E Jiao, Gui Ban and mussel), or a soup made with donkeyhide gelatin and chicken egg yolk are made by using mulberries, black beans, the meat of the soft-shelled turtle, oyster, egg yolk, and tortoise plastron, freshwater turtle shell and the root of herbaceous peony, in the treatment of tremors of the hand and foot, spasm and faintness due to agitated deficient Wind arising from deficiency of Liver Yin.

NOURISHING YIN AND CLEARING HEAT

By using foods or herbs which will nourish Yin and clear Heat, it is possible to treat deficiency of Yin and exuberance of Yang. For example, chicken cooked with the dried rhizome of rehmannia, soup made with lily bulb, or Chinese wolfberry and chicken eggs, made by using pears, lotus rhizome, cow's milk, egg yolk, dried rhizome of rehmannia, Chinese wolfberry and mulberry are used for the treatment of feverish sensations in the chest, palms and soles; hectic fever, night sweating and flushing of the cheeks due to Yin deficiency and exuberant Fire.

Methods of tonifying the Kidney and replenishing the Essence

This method has the function of tonifying the Kidney Qi, replenishing the Vital Essence, promoting Marrow and strengthening the tendons and bones. It is suitable for retarded growth, senility, seminal emission owing to deficiency of the Kidney Qi and the Essence.

TONIFYING AND NOURISHING THE KIDNEY YIN

This method involves making therapeutic foods

using items that have the property of tonifying and nourishing the Kidney Yin for the treatment of syndromes due to deficiency in Kidney Yin and Essence. For example, pig's kidney sauteed with Chinese wolfberries, soup made with tremella, and an edible fungus or prepared black soya beans, are made by using sesame, black beans, Chinese wolfberries, mulberries, cow's milk and pig's kidney for the treatment of dizziness, tinnitus, weak limbs and back, hectic fever, night sweating, frequent drinking and urination and seminal emission owing to the deficiency and impairment of the Kidney.

WARMING AND REINFORCING KIDNEY QI

This method uses items that have the property of warming and reinforcing the Kidney Qi. For example, Chinese chives sauteed with walnuts, or lamb soup are made by using walnuts, chestnuts, Chinese chives, cowpeas, lamb, pheasant, saline cistanche and longspur epimedium for the treatment of weakness of the legs and back, cold limbs and intolerance to cold, clear and profuse urination at night, impotence and seminal emission.

TONIFYING THE ESSENCE AND REPLENISHING MARROW

This method uses items that have the property of replenishing the Essence and Marrow for the treatment of deficiency in Essence and Marrow. For example, Yang Mi Gao, holy relieving soup with pig's kidney, is made by using sesame, black soya beans, turtle meat, sea cucumber, mussels, spinal cord of pig, spinal cord of sheep, saline cistanche, pilose antler and Chinese wolfberries for the treatment of pain in the spine and the back, weak feet and knees, early greying hair, general weakness, thin voice and retarded growth owing to deficiency of Kidney Essence.

Method of reinforcing the Stomach and promoting the production of Body Fluids

This method helps to protect and generate Body Fluids by nourishing the Stomach Yin, and to moisten the Lungs. It is thus useful for deficient Body Fluids and for a sore throat and a dry cough due to Dryness.

REINFORCING THE STOMACH AND PROMOTING THE PRODUCTION OF BODY FLUIDS

This method involves using items that have the property of nourishing Stomach Yin and producing Body Fluids to counteract deficiency in Stomach Yin or Dryness in the Intestines due to the lack of Body Fluids. For example, five-juice mix (see Epidemic Febrile Diseases) or Stomach-reinforcing soup are made by using pears, sugarcane, water chestnuts, lotus rhizome, cow's milk, sesame, honey, tuber of dwarf lilyturf and the stem of dendrobium for the treatment of thirst and dryness of mouth and dry stool owing to deficient Stomach Yin.

MOISTENING DRYNESS AND PROMOTING THE PRODUCTION OF BODY FLUIDS

This method involves using items that have the property of moistening Dryness and promoting the production of Body Fluids and nourishing the Lung Yin for the treatment of symptoms due to deficiency in Yin and Dryness of Lungs. For example, snow pear soup, or tremella and lily bulb soup, are made by using pears, lily bulbs, lotus rhizome, water chestnuts, persimmons, loquats, honey, crystal sugar, pig's lung, cow's milk, the root of straight ladybell and the tuber of dwarf lilyturf in the treatment of dry nose, dryness and pain in the throat, coughing without sputum or with bloodstained sputum or dry skin due to Dryness of the Lungs and impairment of Lung Yin.

Dietetic hygiene 6

Chinese medicine emphasizes dietetic hygiene, which includes two major aspects.

MODERATION OF MEALS

It is desirable to exercise temperance in taking meals. The time, frequency, quantity and quality of meals should be considered and it is important to cultivate the habit of taking three meals a day. The folk saying that 'Breakfast should be good, lunch should be adequate, while supper should be moderate in amount' and has its scientific rationale. Immoderate meals or overeating may exceed the capacity of the Stomach for digestion and absorption, hence impairing the Spleen and the Stomach, leading to retention of food, distension in the abdomen, anorexia, vomiting or diarrhea. This is in accordance with *The Plain Questions (SW), Arthralgia* which says 'Overeating impairs the Intestines and the Stomach'. Only timely meals of the right amounts will benefit the digestion and absorption of foods. Moreover, overeating may result in superfluity of nutrients, which can also cause diseases.

Longevity and Health Preservation (SSBY) says that 'Seeking pleasure and entertainment by eating rich tastes makes one look well, but a strong and severe Qi will develop inside, which tends to erode the Internal Organs and cause deficiency in spirits'. Obesity and cardiovascular diseases are examples illustrating this point. *The Essence of Diet* (YSZY) says that 'Those who know how to preserve health will eat when hungry, and never eat until full; will drink when thirsty, but never drink too much. They will eat small amounts often rather than take large meals at long intervals'. This is also not to be overlooked.

CLEAN AND HEALTHY FOOD

Food must be clean, fresh, free of poisons and harmless to meet the requirements of dietetic hygiene.

The Synopsis of Prescriptions of the Gold Chamber (JKYL) points out that 'Stale rice, rotten meat and smelly fish are harmful to eat' and 'Meat with red spots in it is to be avoided'. More broadly, all stale, deteriorated foods or foods that are contaminated by domestic flies, rats, poisonous things or bacteria or parasites should be avoided. Foods which contain toxins, such as germinated potatoes, poisonous mushrooms, puffer fish that have not undergone rational processing, and unprepared ginkgo nuts should not be eaten. When eaten by mistake, they not only cause diseases but could be life-threatening. Besides, a few foods, e.g. ginkgo nuts and kidney beans, have certain toxicity and side effects. With these foods, attention should be paid to appropriate cooking and the proper way of eating to avoid unwanted reactions.

In order to ensure dietetic hygiene and to prevent the contamination and deterioration of foods, smaller quantities of fresh foods should be purchased more often and properly stored. Long storage is to be avoided. Foods should be washed clean before eating or preparation. Most foods are eaten cooked by means of steaming, boiling, stir frying or roasting, which not only sterilize but can also aid digestion. The sterilization of cooking utensils is also an important issue in dietetic hygiene. However, this is a reasonably modern view and can be taken to extremes – in the West it may have led to lack of resistance to everyday organisms.

In addition, it is also worth noting that one should not eat if unhappy and appropriate activities should be carried out after meals. The older books, and the Daoists in particular, emphasized the importance of the correct frame of mind when eating. They advised careful chewing, with the attention on the food rather than on talking or thinking excessively.

Part Two

The properties and application of foods

Water and land *7* vegetables

Most vegetables are cultivated on the land, but we also include some wild plants and sea vegetables (seaweeds) which are commonly used for food.

Different vegetables may have different properties. Generally, apart from such vegetables as Chinese chives, Chinese spring onion and garlic which have a Warm nature and can warm the Middle Burner, disperse Cold and assist digestion, most vegetables have a Cold or Cool nature. The most common properties of these vegetables are clearing up Heat, easing defecation and urination, dissolving Phlegm and relieving cough. Vegetables that have a slippery texture can ease bowel motions (e.g. spinach and cluster mallow); many wild vegetables have the functions of clearing up Heat, detoxifying and cooling down the blood (e.g. pursane, houttuynia and shepherd's purse); juicy and sweet vegetables can promote the production of Body Fluids and ease thirst (e.g. turnips, lotus rhizomes and young shoots of Zizania aquatica); seaweeds have the function of softening hard masses inside the body and also act as diuretics (e.g. Kelps, Agar and Gracilaria verrucosa); fungi are mostly nourishing and reinforcing (e.g. mushroom, fragrant mushroom and hedgehog fungus).

In addition, as daily foods, vegetables are important sources of certain types of vitamins (carotin, vitamins B and C), inorganic salts and sugars needed by the body.

CHINESE CHIVE (MYBL)

This is the stem and leaves of *Allium tuberosum*, of the Liliaceae family, grown in most regions of China. It is gathered in the spring, the roots are removed, and it is washed clean for use.

Properties

Sweet, acrid and Warm, having a propensity for the Kidney, Stomach and Liver channels. It has the functions of reinforcing the Kidney and assisting Yang, warming the Middle Burner, aiding appetite and dissolving Blood stasis.

Application

• For male impotence due to deficiency of the Kidney, seminal emission, enuresis, pain and weakness of the back and legs, use together with walnuts sauteed in sesame seed oil (FMZZ).

• For dysphagia, vomiting and loss of appetite, use the juice of Chinese chives mixed with cow's milk and juice of raw ginger. Apart from the effects of aiding appetite, sending down Counterflow Qi and dispersing stagnation, it can also moisten Dryness (DXXF).

• For chest pain due to obstruction of Qi in the chest, squeeze to obtain juice for drinking alone or use with the juice of an onion (SLBC).

Preparation

Sauteed, decocted or juiced.

Notes

The item is more warming and reinforcing when cooked, but is better at dispersing stagnation when consumed fresh. It is not desirable to overcook it, nor should people with fever, owing to Yin deficiency, or patients with ulcers or eye disorders, use it.

Nutritional information

Chinese chives contain volatile oil, sulfides, glycosides, proteins, fat, sugar, carotin, vitamin B and C, cellulose, calcium, phosphorus and iron.

CHINESE SPRING ONION (BCJb)

Chinese spring onion is the stem and leaves of *Allium fistulosum*, of the Liliaceae family. It is cultivated in all parts of China, gathered in the winter, spring or summer. The root parts are removed and it is washed clean for use. Sometimes the stem and the leaves are separated for use.

Properties

Chinese spring onion has a pungent taste, Warm nature and a propensity for the Lung and Stomach channels. It has the effects of inducing sweating, relieving Exterior syndrome, activating Yang and dispersing Cold, expelling intestinal parasites and detoxifying.

Application

• For exogenous Wind-Cold syndrome marked by chills, fever, headache and lack of sweating, use Chinese spring onion and fermented soya beans to make a soup (BQZHF); or use the stems and roots of Chinese spring onion cooked with rice to make a gruel (JSML).

• For abdominal pain and diarrhea owing to excessive Yin Cold inside the body, use Chinese spring onion with dried ginger and prepared aconite root (restricted use – potentially poisonous) to make a decoction for activating Yang (SHL).

• For abdominal pain owing to intestinal parasites, take crushed stems of the Chinese spring onion with sesame seed oil or take sesame seed oil after eating crushed stems of the Chinese spring onion (RZTJYF). This prescription can relieve the pain and help expel parasites from the body.

• For acute mastitis, ulcers and swellings, squeeze the Chinese spring onion to obtain juice. Drink the juice and apply the residue to the affected area.

Preparation

Decocted, juiced, used as a condiment or in gruels.

Notes

It is not desirable to cook it for too long. It is not suitable for people with spontaneous perspiration due to deficiency or those with bromhidrosis (foul-smelling perspiration).

Nutritional information

The Chinese spring onion contains volatile oils which mainly consist of allicin and 2-allyl-sulfether, vitamin B1, vitamin B2, vitamin C, niacin, fat, calcium, phosphorus and iron.

The volatile oil inhibits *Bacillus diphtheriae*, stimulates sweat glands and induces perspiration, promotes the secretion of gastric juice and reinforces the Stomach.

GARLIC (MYBL)

Garlic is the bulb of *Allium sativum*, of the Liliaceae family. It is found in all parts of China, gathered in late spring and early summer. The membranous scales are removed before use.

Properties

Garlic has a pungent and sweet flavor, a Warm nature and a propensity for the Spleen, Stomach and Lung channels.

It has the effects of warming the Middle Burner, reinforcing the Stomach, aiding digestion, detoxifying and killing parasites.

Application

• For Coldness and pain in the upper abdomen and stagnation of food (mainly of meat), soak garlic in vinegar to eat on its own (BHJJF), or together with Chinese hawthorns and orange peel.

• For vomiting and diarrhea owing to contaminated meals or dysentery, eat the garlic raw or stewed. In the treatment of bacillary dysentery and amebic dysentery, use garlic to make a syrup for drinking, which is very effective.

• For TB and pertussis. For the former, use garlic to make gruel for drinking, or use with the powder of bletilla tuber; for the latter, crush the garlic and soak it in water to obtain juice for drinking. Add white sugar to taste.

• For hookworms and threadworms, eat garlic with torreya nuts and sunflower seeds.

• In addition, garlic has certain therapeutic effects in the prevention and treatment of influenza, epidemic inflammation of the brain, high blood pressure, and excess fat in the blood.

Preparation

Garlic is eaten raw, stewed, juiced or cooked in gruels.

Notes

It is best to use the single-segmented variety with purple skin.

Raw garlic is more stimulating and can cause heat and pain in the mouth and tongue, pain in the stomach and nausea. However, it is not desirable to overcook it. High intake of garlic can inhibit the secretion of gastric juice and cause blurred vision or foul breath. It is not suitable for people with excessive Fire due to Yin deficiency, accumulated Heat in the Lungs and Stomach, blurred vision and dry eyes or strong body odour.

Nutritional information

Garlic contains volatile oils, which mainly consists of allicin and garlicin, garlic glycoside, protein, fat, sugars, calcium, phophorus, iron and vitamins B1 and C.

Small amounts of garlic can promote peristalsis and the secretion of gastric acid. Garlic glycoside can lower blood pressure. Garlic fatty oil can lower blood fat and prevent atheroscleorsis. It also has antiseptic, antiamebic and anticancer effects.

ONION (BCJb)

Onion is the bulb of *Allium macrostemum* and *Allium chinense*, of the Liliaceae family. It is found in all parts of China, but the best are those found in Jiangsu and Zhejiang provinces. It is gathered in spring, summer or autumn. The leaves are removed and it is washed clean for use fresh, dried or cooked.

Properties

Onion has a pungent and bitter flavor, a Warm nature and a propensity for the Lung, Stomach and Large Intestine channels. It has the effects of activating Yang, dissolving hard masses, sending down Qi and aiding bowel motions.

Application

• For stuffiness in the chest, chest pain or chest ailments with symptoms of difficult breathing, or coughing up sputum owing to the accumulation of Cold Phlegm and Damp in the chest and Yang Qi failing to circulate, use onion on its own by drinking the juice (DXF). It can also be used with snakegourd fruit. It has significant therapeutic effects on angina pectoris, pleurisy and bronchitis.

• For Qi stagnation in the Middle Burner, distension and pain in the upper abdomen, or urgency of urination or defecation due to dysentery, use onion to make a gruel or decoction for drinking.

Preparation

Decocted, juiced or used in gruels.

Notes

It is not desirable to cook onion for too long. For patients with fever, Yin deficiency and Qi deficiency, it should be taken with care.

Nutritional information

Onion contains allicin, methyl allicin and garlic sugar.

CHILLIES (BCGMSY)

Chillies are the fruit of *Capsicum frutescens*, of the Solanaceae family, found in most parts of China. They are gathered in the summer and autumn. Immature chillies are called green chillies and mature ones are called red chillies. They are both used fresh, after washing, and red chillies are also used dried.

Properties

Chillies have a pungent flavor and a Hot nature and a propensity for the Spleen, Stomach and Heart channels. They have the effects of warming the Middle Burner, dispersing Cold, drying up Damp and inducing perspiration.

Application

• Use green chillies sauteed with fermented soya beans for deficient Cold in the Spleen and Stomach, Cold and pain in the upper abdomen, loss of appetite, loose or liquid stool. For loose and liquid stool, grind chillies into a powder for making pills to be swallowed in warm beancurd (tofu) (YZHB).

• For stagnation of Cold-Damp, fatigue and heaviness in the body and soreness in the body and limbs, use chillies as a vegetable or condiment from time to time.

• For the Wind-Cold type of common cold, with chills and lack of sweating, suitable amounts of chillies added to soups or noodles will have a significant effect.

Preparation

Chillies are sauteed as vegetables, made into soups, used as a condiment or taken in powdered form.

Notes

It is desirable to use the varieties that are not too hot but are oily and fleshy. Overintake of chillies can cause dizziness, dry eyes, pain in the digestive tract, diarrhea and rashes around the mouth. It is prohibited for patients with excessive Fire due to deficiency of Yin, coughing, loss of blood, eye ailments, skin sores and ulcerations, hemorrhoids or ulceration in the digestive tract.

Nutritional information

Chillies contain peppery principles, mainly capsicine and 2H-capsicine. They also contain volatile oil, protein, carotin, vitamin C, calcium and phosphorus.

Chillies have a strong local stimulating effect. Taking them orally can promote digestive function and aid appetite. Capsicine can stimulate gustatory receptors and cause reflexive temporary rising of blood pressure.

CORIANDER (SLBC)

Coriandrum sativum, a member of the Umbelliferae family, is found in all parts of China. The whole plant is gathered in the spring and washed clean for use.

Properties

Coriander has a pungent flavor, a Warm nature and a propensity for the Spleen, Stomach and Lung channels. It has the effects of reinforcing the Stomach, regulating Qi, inducing perspiration and promoting the eruption of measles.

Application

• For disorders of the Spleen and Stomach, loss of appetite and nausea, use coriander in salads or as a condiment.

• For a Wind-Cold type of common cold with slight fever and lack of sweating, or in the early stages of measles which fail to erupt thoroughly, use coriander on its own, or together with the stalk of Chinese spring onion, to make a decoction for drinking.

Preparation

In soups, salads or as a condiment.

Notes

It should not be overcooked. It is not suitable for patients with Qi deficiency, incomplete expression of the measles rash that is *not* caused by Wind-Cold astringing the Externals, or those with strong body odour or eye diseases.

Nutritional information

Coriander contains volatile oil, mannitol, flavonoids, proteins, vitamin C, potassium and calcium.

MUSTARD GREENS (MYBL)

Mustard greens are the young stem and leaves of *Brassica juncea*, of the Cruciferae family, found in all parts of China. Gather the young stems and leaves in the spring and wash clean for use.

Properties

Mustard greens have a pungent flavor, a Warm nature and a propensity for the Lung and Stomach channels. They have the effects of expelling Phlegm and regulating respiration, warming the Middle Burner, reinforcing the Stomach, dispersing Cold and relieving Exterior syndromes.

Application

• For cough caused by Cold Phlegm, stuffiness in the chest and diaphragm, use mustard greens on their own in sauteed dishes or together with mountain rorippa and ginger.

• For Cold in the Stomach, loss of appetite and vomiting, use mustard greens to make sauteed dishes, or use with ginger and brown sugar to make a soup for drinking.

Preparation

In soups, sauteed or juiced.

Notes

It is unsuitable for patients with eye diseases, ulcers, hemorrhoids or those with excessive Heat.

Nutritional information

Mustard greens contain carotin, vitamin B1, vitamin B2, vitamin C, niacin and calcium.

TURNIP (XXBC)

Turnip is the tuber of *Raphanus sativus*, of the mustard family, grown in all parts of China and gathered in winter. Remove the leaves and wash clean before use.

Properties

Acrid, sweet, Cool (tending to be sweet and Neutral when cooked), having a propensity for the Stomach and Lung channels.

It has the functions of clearing Heat, dissolving Phlegm, producing Body Fluids, cooling the Blood, inducing diuresis for treating spasmodic painful urination, reinforcing the Stomach and promoting digestion, sending down the Counterflow Qi and relieving the chest.

Application

• For cough with sticky sputum owing to Heat in the Lungs, use raw turnip, or its juice, taken with white sugar or ginger juice.

• For thirst or dry mouth caused by Heat syndrome or diabetes, use the juice from raw turnip. The effect will be much better when combined with the juice of lotus rhizome, sugarcane, pears or fresh reed rhizome (SYXJa).

• For nasal bleeding, coughing up blood, or bloodstained stool, take the juice of raw turnip with honey or the juice of lotus rhizome.

• For difficult urination caused by pathogenic Heat or the passage of a urinary stone, use turnip to make a Ming Xuan Gao (an electuary) by cooking the slices of turnip in honey. Eat the turnip when cooked till fragrant or take the juice from the cooked turnip (PJF).

• For fullness of the abdomen due to poor digestion of food, make a gruel with turnip. If the person is weak in the Stomach and Spleen, cook it with pig's tripe or pork.

Notes

It is not suitable for people with deficiency and Cold in the Spleen and Stomach. When taken cooked, it is good particularly for the Stomach and can send down the Counterflow Qi.

It is generally believed that when taking such tonifying medicines as ginseng, rehmannia or knotweed tuber, turnip should not be taken at the same time.

Nutritional information

Turnips contain glucose, sucrose, fructose, vitamin B, vitamin C, calcium, phosphorus, manganese, boron, various amino acids, coumaric acids, caffeic acid, raphaoside and amylase.

Alcohol extracts of turnip have a fairly inhibiting effect on Gram positive bacteria.

CARROT (BCGM)

Carrot is the root of *Daucus carota* of the Umbelliferae family. It is found in all parts of China and gathered in winter. The stems and leaves are removed and it is washed clean for use, fresh or air-dried.

Properties

Carrot has a sweet flavor, a Neutral nature and a propensity for the Spleen, Liver and Lung channels. It has the effects of reinforcing the Spleen, aiding digestion, reinforcing the Liver, promoting acuity of vision, sending down Counterflow Qi, arresting cough, clearing up Heat and detoxifying.

Application

• For indigestion, stagnancy of food, fullness in the abdomen, or difficult stool, take cooked carrots with sugar. Its effect can be enhanced when taken with turnip as well.

• For blurred vision owing to deficiency in the Liver, night blindness, infantile malnutrition, dry eyes, take carrots cooked with lard, or in a soup cooked with pig's liver.

• For cough due to Lung Heat, take carrot juice on its own or make a decoction with Chinese dates.

• For fever and measles failing to erupt thoroughly in children, take carrots with water chestnuts and coriander (LNCYZ).

Preparation

Carrot is eaten raw or cooked, in soups or as juice.

Notes

It is inadvisable for patients with deficient Cold in the Spleen and the Stomach to take carrots.

Nutritional information

Carrot is rich in carotin and also contains vitamin B1, B2, folic acid, various amino acids, sugars, boron, calcium, phosphorus, copper, iron, fluorine, manganese and mannitol.

CHINESE CABBAGE (CHINESE LEAVES) (MYBL)

Chinese cabbage is the young leaves of *Brassica pekinensis* and *Brassica chinensis*, of the Cruciferae family. It is cultivated in all parts of China and gathered in winter or spring, the roots removed and washed clean for use.

Properties

Chinese cabbage has a sweet flavor, a slightly Cold nature and a propensity for the Lung, Stomach and Bladder channels. It has the effects of clearing up Heat and aiding urination.

Application

• For Heat in the Lungs and the Stomach, restlessness and thirst, or cough owing to Heat in the Lungs, take Chinese cabbage on its own or in soups cooked with turnips; its juice can also be taken mixed thoroughly with white honey.

• For accumulated Heat in the Bladder and difficult urination, take Chinese cabbage in soups or juiced.

Preparation

It is eaten cooked, in soups or in juice form.

Notes

It is quite unsuitable for patients with deficient Cold in the Lungs and the Stomach. Though Chinese cabbage has the property of clearing and sending down, it has a Neutral nature and is delicious when cooked with pork or other meats.

Nutritional information

Chinese cabbage contains proteins, fat, vitamins B1, B2 and C, carotin, calcium, phosphorus and iron.

CABBAGE (BCSY)

Cabbage is the stem and leaves of *Brassica oleracea*, of the Cruciferae family. It is cultivated in all parts of China and gathered in spring or winter. The roots are removed and it is washed clean for use.

Properties

Cabbage has a sweet flavor, a Neutral nature and a propensity for the Spleen and Stomach channels. It has the effects of nourishing the Spleen, regulating the Stomach, and relieving spasm and pain.

Application

• For disharmony of the Stomach and Spleen or spasm and pain in the upper abdomen, obtain juice by squeezing and cook the juice with maltose or honey until they melt. The remedy is effective in abdominal pain from gastric or duodenal ulcer.

Preparation

Cabbage is used in salads and the juice is drunk.

Nutritional information

Cabbage   contains   brassine,   bioflavonoids,

chlorogenic acid, allylisothiocyanate and vitamin U-like substances which can promote the healing of ulceration.

CROWN DAISY CHRYSANTHEMUM (JYBC)

Crown daisy chrysanthemum is the stem and leaves of *Chrysanthemum coronarium var Spatiosum Bailey*, of the Compositae family. It is cultivated in all parts of China, gathered in winter, spring or early summer and washed clean for use.

Properties

Crown daisy chrysanthemum has a pungent, sweet flavor, a Neutral nature (but a slightly Cool nature when used fresh) and a propensity for the Lung, Liver and Stomach channels. It has the effects of dissolving Phlegm, arresting cough, clearing the head and eyes, harmonizing the Spleen and Stomach, and easing urination.

Application

• For cough owing to Phlegm-Heat, take crown daisy chrysanthemum on its own as a vegetable, in soups or juices with turnips and Chinese cabbage.

• For dizziness owing to Heat in the Liver, take crown daisy chrysanthemum on its own or as a decoction made with chrysanthemum or mulberry leaves.

• For disharmony of Stomach and Spleen and loss of appetite, take crown daisy chrysanthemum on its own as a vegetable.

• For difficult urination owing to accumulated Heat in the Bladder, take crown daisy chrysanthemum on its own as a juice or in salad.

Preparation

In decoctions, salads, sauteed dishes or juice.

Nutritional information

Crown daisy chrysanthemum contains volatile oil, choline, various amino acids, sugars, carotin, vitamin C, calcium, phosphorus and iron.

CELERY (BCJb)

Celery is the stem and leaves of *Apium graveolens*, of the Umbelliferae family. It is cultivated in all parts of China and gathered in spring and autumn. The roots are removed and it is washed clean for use.

Properties

Celery has a pungent, sweet flavor, a Cool nature and a propensity for the Liver, Stomach and Bladder channels. It has the effects of clearing up Heat, calming the Liver, reinforcing the Stomach, sending down the Central Qi and easing urination.

Application

• For feverish diseases or drunkenness, thirst and agitation due to Heat, take celery on its own as a juice (BCSY). For persistent fever in infants, decoct celery together with plantain seed and germinated barley (DNBC). As such, it has the effects of sending Heat down, nourishing the Stomach and assisting digestion.

• For dizziness, agitation due to Heat, and restlessness owing to Liver Heat and exuberant Yang, take celery in juice or salads. It is also used in the treatment of hypertension.

• For vomiting and loss of appetite owing to Heat in the Stomach, use celery as a vegetable or in a decoction together with orange peel and purple perilla leaves.

• For difficult urination of the Heat type or hematuria, take celery juice freshly pressed with the stems (leaves removed) (SHF).

Preparation

Celery is used in juice or salads, stir-fried or decocted. It is undesirable to overcook it.

Nutritional information

Celery contains a celery principle, volatile oil, bergamot lactone, chlorogenic acid, caffeic acid, rutin, carotin, vitamin C, niacin, various amino acids, sugars, calcium and phosphorus.

Celery principally has the function of lowering blood pressure. Alkaloid extracts of celery have a tranquilizing effect. Clinical observation shows that celery can lower serum cholesterol levels.

SPINACH (SLBC)

Spinach is the whole plant of *Spinacia oleracea*, of the Chenopodiaceae family. It is cultivated in all parts of China, gathered in winter or spring, the fibrous roots removed and washed clean for use.

Properties

Spinach has a sweet flavor, a Cool nature and a propensity for the Large Intestine, Stomach and Liver channels. It has the effects of moistening dryness, easing bowel motions, promoting the production of Body Fluids, quenching thirst, nurturing the Liver and improving acuity of vision.

Application

• For difficult motions in the fragile or the aged, or for constipation owing to Dryness in the Intestines. According to *Confucians' Duties to Their Parents* (RMSQ), 'For constipation in the aged who have suffered protracted illness... take cluster mallow, spinach and pig's blood or goat's blood, which can ease the motions of bowels'. The above mentioned items can be used selectively according to the actual condition.

• For great thirst owing to diabetes or Stomach heat, use the powdered root of spinach and chicken's gizzard membrane in equal amounts in liquid millet gruel (JYF). Spinach can also be used on its own as a decoction for drinking.

• For dizziness owing to Heat in the Liver, dizziness and bad vision owing to deficiency of Liver Yin, take spinach and pig's liver soup.

Preparation

In salads, sauteed dishes or soups.

Notes

It is not suitable for persons susceptible to loose stool owing to a weak Spleen. Spinach contains a large amount of oxalic acid and therefore it should not be cooked with foods rich in calcium (e.g. bean curd), or it will form ammonium oxalate and affect the absorption of calcium.

Nutritional information

Spinach contains carotin, vitamin C, protein, sugars, calcium, phosphorus, folic acid and oxalic acid.

CLUSTER MALLOW (MYBL)

Cluster mallow is the young stem and leaves of *Malva verticillata*, of the Malvaceae family. It is found in all parts of China. It can be gathered in any season of the year, the jackets of the stem and the petiole removed and washed clean for use.

Properties

Cluster mallow has a sweet flavor, a Cold nature and a propensity for the Lung, Heart, Small Intestine and Large Intestine channels. It has the effects of clearing Heat, moistening Dryness, inducing urination, removing Damp and assisting bowel motions.

Application

• For cough owing to Heat in the Lung, dryness and pain in the throat, macules or erysipelas, use cluster mallow to make a soup or gruel for drinking. For macules in infants, take the freshly pressed juice (SHF).

• For difficult urination owing to Damp-Heat, leukorrhea or jaundice, take a decoction made with cluster mallow alone (YXL).

• For constipation owing to Dryness in the Intestines, take a gruel or vegetable dish made with cluster mallow.

Preparation

In soups, gruels or juice.

Notes

It is not suitable for persons susceptible to loose stool owing to a weak Spleen, or for pregnant women.

Nutritional information

Cluster mallow contains monosaccharide, sucrose, maltose and starch.

Related item – *Basella rubra* (spinach)

Basella rubra is a creeping plant of the Basellaceae family. It is found in all parts of China and the young stem and leaves are gathered in summer or autumn and washed clean for use.

Basella rubra has a sweet and slightly sour flavor, a Cold nature and a propensity for the Heart, Large Intestine and Small Intestine channels. It has similar effects to cluster mallow and clears Heat, cools Blood, moistens Dryness, eases bowel motions and induces urination.

It is used for restlessness, fever, macules, bloody stools, difficult stool and urination. It is eaten cooked or in soups. For contraindications, see cluster mallow.

WATER SPINACH (BCSY)

Water spinach is the stem and leaves of *Ipomoea aquatica*, of the Convolvulaceae family. It is found in the valley of the Yangtze River and further south in Guangdong province. It is gathered in spring and summer and washed clean for use.

Properties

Water spinach has a sweet flavor, a slightly Cold nature and a propensity for the Liver, Heart, Large Intestine and Small Intestine channels. It has the effects of clearing Heat, cooling Blood, inducing urination, assisting bowel motions and detoxifying.

Application

• For nasal bleeding, coughing or vomiting of blood, blood in the urine and stools, take the juice with honey.

• For difficult urination of the Heat type or leukorrhea, take a decoction or soup.

• For difficult stool, take water spinach cooked with pork.

• For food poisoning, herpes or snake bite, take the juice or a decoction. For snake bite, the juice can also be taken with wine and the residue from juicing applied to the affected area.

Preparation

Decoction, cooked or juiced.

Notes

As is recorded in works of materia medica, water spinach is usually used for the detoxification of drugs or poisoning from foods but this claim requires further observation.

Nutritional information

Water spinach contains protein, fat, sugars, carotin, vitamin B2, vitamin C, niacin, calcium, phosphorus and iron.

THREE-COLORED AMARANTH (BCJJZ)

Three-colored amaranth is the stem and leaves of *Amaranthus mangostanus*, of the Amaranthaceae family. It is found in all parts of China and gathered in spring and summer. The roots are removed and it is washed clean for use.

Properties

Three-colored amaranth has a sweet flavor, a slightly Cold nature and a propensity for the Large Intestine and Small Intestine channels. It has the effects of clearing Heat, detoxifying, inducing urination, removing Damp and assisting bowel motions.

Application

• For pus and blood in the stool owing to dysentery, diarrhea owing to Damp-Heat, or difficult urination, take a decoction. For example, in the treatment of white and red dysentery (pus and blood in the stool), or before or after childbirth, take a gruel (the purple three-colored amaranth gruel) (SQYLXS) made with rice cooked in the juice of three-colored amaranth.

• For difficulty in passing stool in the fragile and the aged, or constipation, take sauteed three-colored amaranth.

Preparation

In decoction, gruel or as a sauteed dish.

Notes

It is not suitable for people with a weak Spleen and prone to loose stools, or for pregnant women.

Nutritional information

Three-colored amaranth contains lysine, carotin, vitamin C, calcium, phosphorus and iron.

Related item – Purslane

Purslane is the stem and leaves of *Portulaca oleracea*, of the Portulacaceae family. It grows wild in most parts of China. Purslane is common in Europe and is widely used as a salad vegetable on the continent. Gerard's *Herbal* gives very similar uses to those of the Chinese.

Purslane has strong effects of clearing Heat and detoxifying, especially in dysentery. Additionally, it can arrest bleeding. Today, it is used in profuse menstruation, abnormal uterine bleeding and postpartum bleeding. It can be used in salads, decoction or juices.

HOUTTUYNIA (MYBL)

Houttuynia is the whole plant of *Houttuynia cordata*, of the Saururaceae family. It is found in provinces south of the Yangtze River in China. It is gathered in late spring and early summer and washed clean for immediate use.

Properties

Houttuynia has a pungent flavor, a slightly Cold nature and a propensity for the Stomach, Large Intestine and Bladder channels. It has the effects of clearing Heat, detoxifying, reinforcing the Stomach and inducing urination.

Application

• For a cough with thick sputum due to a pulmonary abscess or Heat in the Lungs, take houttuynia on its own, or use its juice together with that of fresh reed rhizome.

• For Stomach Heat, accumulated Heat in the Internal Organs or loss of appetite, eat houttuynia or drink as a decoction.

• For difficult urination of the Heat type, scanty and dark urine, or abdominal pain owing to Damp-Heat, or leukorrhea, take houttuynia by itself or together with shepherd's purse, in decoctions.

Preparation

In salads, juices, hot water infusion or decoctions.

Nutritional information

Houttuynia contains volatile oils, which consist of decanoyl acetaldehyde, methyl n-nonyl ketone and myrcene. It also contains quercitol, houttuynia alkali and sylvite.

Houttuynia has inhibiting effects on Gram positive and Gram negative bacteria. It also enhances immunity, is anti-inflammatory and has the functions of inducing urination and arresting coughing and bleeding.

SHEPHERD'S PURSE (MYBL)

Sherpherd's purse is the above-ground parts of *Capsella bursa-pastoris*, of the Cruciferae family. It grows wild in all parts of China and is cultivated in provinces like Jiangsu and Anhui. It is gathered in March to May and washed clean for use.

Properties

Shepherd's purse has a light sweet flavor, a Cool nature and a propensity for the Liver, Stomach, Small Intestine and Bladder channels. It has the effects of cooling the Blood, arresting bleeding, clearing Heat, inducing urination, clearing Liver Heat and improving acuity of vision.

Application

• For bleeding owing to Heat, such as postpartum bleeding, abnormal uterine bleeding and bloody stools, take shepherd's purse on its own or with purslane.

• For Damp-Heat in the Lower Burner, such as difficult urination, marked by chyle in the urine and edema, take shepherd's purse decoction made with the pith of sunflower stalk and cogongrass rhizome.

• For blurred vision due to Liver Heat, or dizziness and headache, take shepherd's purse juice or make an omelette with it.

Preparation

In decoction, sauteed dishes, juices and stuffings for dumplings.

Nutritional information

Shepherd's purse contains alkaloids, amino acids, flavonoids, sugars, protein, carotin, vitamin B, vitamin C, calcium, phosphorus and iron.

Shepherd's purse has a stimulating effect on the womb. The effective substances are soluble in water and aqueous alcohol. It has the functions of reducing the time of blood coagulation in hemorrhage and it can also lower the blood pressure.

BRAKE (SLBC)

Brake is the young shoots of *Pteridium aquilinum*, of the Pteridaceae family. It is found in all parts of China. It is gathered in spring, washed clean and boiled lightly or air-dried for use. Before use, soak in water, bring to the boil and rinse to remove the bitterness and astringency.

Properties

Brake has a sweet and slightly bitter flavor, a Cold nature and a propensity for the Large Intestine and Bladder channels. It has the effects of clearing Heat, removing Damp and assisting bowel motions.

Application

• For difficult urination and yellow leukorrhea owing to Damp-Heat in the Lower Burner, take a decoction or soup made solely with brake.

• For constipation owing to Heat in the Large Intestine, take the brake cooked on its own or sauteed with pork and wood-ears.

Preparation

In decoctions, soups or sauteed dishes.

Notes

Brake can impair Yang Qi when eaten without adding oil or fat, or if eaten over a long period of time.

Nutritional information

Brake contains ergosterin, choline, glycosides, starch and tannin.

DAY LILY (RHZBC)

Day lily is the flower buds of *Hemerocallis fulva* or *H. flava*, of the Liliaceae family, cultivated in most parts of China. It is gathered in summer and air-dried or used fresh.

Properties

Day lily has a sweet flavor, a slightly Cold nature and a propensity for the Heart and Liver channels. It has the effects of clearing Heat, cooling Blood, removing Damp, tranquilizing the Mind and improving acuity of vision.

Application

• For bloody stools or hemorrhage from hemorrhoids, take the day lily decoction alone or mixed thoroughly with the juice of lotus rhizome and honey.

• For difficult, scanty and dark urine, take day lily as a decoction or eat it cooked as a vegetable.

• For mental depression and restlessness, it is best to use day lily with herbs that have the effect of tranquilizing the mind, such as albizia flower and poria. The recipe is called 'anxiety-relieving soup' (YCSY).

• For blurred vision or night blindness owing to deficiency and Heat in the Liver, take day lily sauteed with pork.

Preparation

Used in decoctions, sauteed dishes or plain boiled.

Notes

For cooling the Blood, it is best to use fresh day lily.

Nutritional information

Day lily contains carotin, vitamin C, niacin, protein, sugars, calcium, phosphorus and iron.

BAMBOO SHOOTS (MYBL)

The young shoots of *Phyllostachys nigra* or *P. pubescens* of the grass family Bambusoideae. They are widely distributed along the Yangtze River and in all regions in southern China. They are gathered in spring or winter, with the husks removed, for immediate use or storing.

Properties

Bamboo shoots have a sweet and slightly bitter flavor, a Cold nature and a propensity for the Lung, Stomach and Large Intestine channels. They have the effects of cooling, easing thirst and assisting bowel motions.

Application

• For coughing and discomfort in the chest owing to Phlegm Heat, take cooked bamboo shoots seasoned with ginger and vinegar.

• For great thirst owing to Heat in the Stomach, take a bamboo shoot decoction or take them plain boiled.

• For difficult stool, take bamboo shoots in gruels or cooked with other vegetables.

Preparation

In salads, gruels, sauteed dishes or decoctions.

Notes

Except for the purpose of easing bowel motions, it is best to use fresh bamboo shoots. It is not desirable for people with weak Spleen and tendency to loose stools to take bamboo shoots.

Nutritional information

Bamboo shoots contain protein, fat, sugars, calcium, phosphorus and iron.

WILD RICE SHOOTS (SLBC)

Wild rice is shoots from *Zizania aquatica*, the

fungus gall grown on the flowering stem of *Zizania caduciflora*, a hydrophyte of the grass family. They are cultivated in most regions of China and gathered in autumn. The leaves are removed and they are washed clean for immediate use.

Properties

Wild rice shoots have a light, sweet flavor, a Cool nature and a propensity for the Stomach, Bladder and Large Intestine channels. They have the effects of clearing Heat, promoting the production of Body Fluids, inducing urination, removing Damp and assisting bowel motions.

Application

• For hot sensations and thirst or drunkenness, take raw wild rice shoots liberally.

• For difficult urination owing to Damp-Heat or jaundice, take a decoction made with young wild rice shoots.

• For difficult stool, take young wild rice shoots raw or sauteed.

Preparation

In soups, sauteed dishes or salads or eaten raw.

Notes

It is not desirable for people with a weak Spleen and a tendency to loose stools or seminal emission to use young wild rice shoots.

Nutritional information

Young wild rice shoots contain protein, sugars, vitamin C, calcium, acids and iron.

TARO (MYBL)

Taro is the tuber of *Colocasia esculenta*, of the Araceae family. The plant is cultivated in all parts of China. It is gathered in autumn, the

fibrous roots removed and washed for immediate use or air-dried for storing.

Properties

Taro has a pungent, sweet flavor, a Neutral nature with a light toxicity. It has the effects of reinforcing the Spleen and the Stomach, eliminating scrofula and dissolving masses.

Application

• For loss of appetite and fatigue owing to a weak Spleen and Stomach, take taro cooked with pork, or 'with fish, which can be very effective for sending down the Central Qi, regulating the Middle Burner and nourishing deficiency' (RHZBC).

Preparation

Eaten boiled, in gruels, powder or decoctions.

Notes

Raw taro is slightly toxic. It produces a tingling sensation in the mouth, irritates the throat and should not be eaten without cooking. However, raw taro can be made into pills and powders. Overintake of taro stagnates Qi and dulls the Spleen.

Nutritional information

Taro contains protein, sugars, fat, vitamins B1, B2 and C, calcium, phosphorus and iron.

POTATO (BCSY)

Potato is the tuber of *Solanum tuberosum*, of the Solanaceae family. The plant is cultivated in most parts of China. Potato is gathered in summer and autumn and washed clean for immediate use or storage.

Properties

Potato has a sweet flavor, a Neutral nature and a

propensity for the Spleen and Stomach channels. It has the effects of reinforcing the Spleen and Stomach, relieving spasm and pain.

Application

• For weak Spleen and Stomach with indigestion, eat potatoes cooked with pork.

• For pain in the upper abdomen owing to disharmony of the Spleen and Stomach, take the freshly squeezed juice with honey. It is also used in the treatment of gastric and duodenal ulcers.

Preparation

Sauteed, boiled, steamed or consumed as fresh juice.

Notes

Germinated potatoes and potatoes whose skins have turned green or purple contain a considerable amount of solanine, which can cause poisoning, with symptoms such as headache, abdominal pain, vomiting, diarrhea or mental disorder.

Nutritional information

Potato contains protein, sugars, fat, niacin, vitamins B1, B2 and C, calcium, phosphorus and iron. It also contains a small amount of solanine, a suitable amount of which can alleviate the spasm of smooth muscles of the stomach and intestines and reduce the secretion of gastric juice.

SWEET POTATO (BCGMSY)

Sweet potato is the tuber of *Ipomoea batatas*, of the Convolvulaceae family. The plant is cultivated in all parts of China. It is gathered in winter, the fibrous roots removed and washed clean for use.

Properties

Sweet potato has a sweet flavor, a Neutral nature

and a propensity for the Spleen, Stomach and Large Intestine channels. It has the effects of reinforcing the Spleen and Stomach, assisting bowel motions, promoting the production of Body Fluids and quenching thirst (when used fresh).

Application

• For weak Spleen and fatigue, take sweet potatoes cooked with brown sugar. When 'a slice of ginger is added during cooking, it can regulate the Middle Burner as effectively as ginger and dates' (BCGMSY).

• For constipation, take sweet potatoes plain boiled.

• For great thirst, take raw sweet potatoes.

Preparation

Sweet potatoes are eaten raw, plain boiled, steamed, roasted or made into gruels.

Notes

As sweet potatoes have a Cool nature when eaten raw, uncooked ones are not suitable for people with full Cold in the Spleen and Stomach. Overintake of sweet potatoes can cause Fullness in the Stomach and excess pantothenic acid.

Nutritional information

Sweet potato contains sugars, protein, carotin, vitamins B1 and C, calcium and phosphorus.

LOTUS RHIZOME (MYBL)

Lotus rhizome is the fleshy rhizome of *Nelumbo nucifera*, of the Nymphaeaceae family. The plant is cultivated in most parts of China. It is gathered in autumn, winter or spring, washed clean and the nodules removed.

Properties

Lotus rhizome has a sweet flavor, a Cool nature

when used fresh or a slightly Warm nature when cooked and a propensity for the Spleen, Stomach and Heart channels. It has the effects of clearing Heat, promoting the production of Body Fluids, cooling Blood, arresting bleeding and dispersing Blood stasis. When cooked, it can reinforce the Spleen and the Stomach, arrest diarrhea and enrich the Blood.

Application

• For great thirst during feverish diseases, drink lotus rhizome juice with honey. It can also be used with pear juice or the juice of sugarcanes.

• For nasal bleeding, vomiting of blood or hemafecia owing to Heat in the Blood, take the raw rhizome or the juice from it. It can also be used with cogongrass rhizome.

• For difficulty in swallowing and vomiting, or dizziness due to Blood disorders after childbirth, with stuffiness and nausea, take the juice alone or with ginger juice mixed in.

• For loss of appetite and diarrhea owing to a weak Spleen and Stomach, take lotus rhizome cooked with dates and ginger.

• For Blood deficiency syndrome, take lotus rhizomes cooked with pork and Chinese angelica.

Preparation

Lotus rhizome is eaten raw, plain boiled, sauteed or juiced.

Notes

'Best lotus rhizome is fleshy, white, pure and sweet. When eaten raw, it is best to choose the young ones, but when eaten cooked, it is best to choose the more mature ones' (SXJYSP).

Nutritional information

Lotus rhizome contains sugars, protein, asparagine, vitamin C, pyrocatechol, gallic acid and neochlorogenic acid.

FENNEL SHOOTS (YXL)

Fennel shoots are the young stem and leaves of *Foeniculum vulgare*, of the Umbelliferae family. The plant is cultivated in all parts of China. It is gathered in spring and washed clean for immediate use.

Properties

Fennel shoots have a pungent, sweet flavor, a slightly Warm nature and a propensity for the Liver, Spleen and Stomach channels. They have the effects of regulating Qi, relieving pain, reinforcing the Stomach and harmonizing the Middle Burner.

Application

• For pain from hernia or distension and pain in the upper abdomen, obtain juice from fennel shoots and drink it with warm wine (SLBC).

• For stagnation of Qi in the Spleen and Stomach, distension in the upper abdomen, vomiting and nausea and loss of appetite, take ravioli stuffed with fennel shoots.

Preparation

Fennel shoots can be infused in wine or decocted and are used as stuffings for ravioli.

Nutritional information

Fennel shoots contain vitamin C and a small amount of vitamin B2, fennel glucoside, lotus glucoside, kaempferol-3-arabinose and quercitrin-3-arabinose.

ACANTHACEOUS INDIGO (BCSY)

Acanthaceous indigo is the young stem and leaves of *Kalimeris indica*, of the Compositae family. The plant is found in southern China. It is gathered in spring and washed clean for use.

Properties

Acanthaceous indigo has a pungent flavor, a slightly Cold nature and a propensity for the Liver, Lung, Stomach, Large Intestine and Bladder channels. It has the effects of clearing Heat, detoxifying, cooling Blood and arresting Bleeding, inducing urination, removing Damp and promoting digestion.

Application

• For diarrhea and dysentery owing to Damp-Heat take, take acanthaceous indigo on its own or with purslane.

• For sore throat, swellings and sores, take a decoction made with dandelion.

• For nasal bleeding, vomiting of blood or bloody stools, take acanthaceous indigo juice alone or with capsella.

• In the treatment of Damp-Heat jaundice take acanthaceous indigo with mountain rorippa. For edema with difficult urination, take acanthaceous indigo cooked with black soya bean and wheat in water and wine (JBDF).

• For retention of food, with dullness in the upper abdomen, take acanthaceous indigo in salads or in a decoction made with non-glutinous rice (roasted until brown) or with turnips.

Preparation

In decoctions, sauteed dishes, salads and juiced.

Nutritional information

Acanthaceous indigo contains volatile oils, protein, sugars, carotin, vitamin B2, vitamin C, niacin, calcium, phosphorus and iron.

CHINESE WOLFBERRY SHOOTS (YXBC)

Chinese wolfberry shoots are the young stem and leaves of *Lycium chinense* of the Solanaceae family.

Properties

Chinese wolfberry shoots have a slightly bitter and sweet flavor, a Cool nature and a propensity for the Liver and Kidney channels. They have the effects of clearing deficient Heat, nourishing the Liver and the Kidney and improving acuity of vision. The shoots are slightly more cooling than Chinese wolfberries themselves.

Application

• For hectic fever, thirst and dry mouth, make a decoction with the wolfberry shoots. It can also be combined with mulberries and pears to enhance the effect of clearing Heat and promoting the production of Body Fluids.

• It is used in the treatment of redness, astringency and pain in the eyes, with nebulae developing in the eyes owning to Heat in the Liver, or blurred vision or night blindness owing to deficiency of Liver Yin or Kidney Yin. For the former, take Chinese wolfberry shoots together with dandelion and capsella; for the latter, it is best to combine the wolfberry shoots with Chinese wolfberries and Korean raspberries.

• For loose teeth or toothache owing to deficient Fire in the Kidney channel, take Chinese wolfberry shoots in salads as much as possible.

Preparation

Used in salads, gruels or decoctions.

Nutritional information

Chinese wolfberry shoots contain betaine, rutin, vitamin C, glutamic acid, aspartic acid, proline and arginine.

EGGPLANT (SLBC)

Eggplant is the fruit of *Solanum melongena*, of the Solanaceae family. The plant is cultivated in most parts of China. Pick the fruits in summer and autumn when they are ripe and wash clean for use.

Properties

Eggplant has a sweet flavor, a slightly Cold nature and has a propensity for the Stomach and Large Intestine channels. It has the effects of clearing Heat, cooling Blood and assisting bowel motions.

Application

For bloody stools due to Heat in the Blood, hemorrhage from hemorrhoids, or difficult stool, take eggplants decocted or steamed. When treating bloody stools due to intestinal wind, eggplant wine can be taken, which is made with toasted eggplants soaked in wine.

Preparation

Eggplant is taken cooked, decocted, juiced or in a wine infusion.

Nutritional information

Eggplant contains sugars, protein, vitamin C, niacin, calcium, phosphorus and various alkaloids (gynesine, stachydrine, choline and solanine).

GOURD (BCJJZ)

Gourd is the fruit of *Lagenaria siceraria*, of the Cucurbitaceae family. The plant is cultivated in most parts of China. The fruits are gathered in the autumn when ripe, peeled and washed clean for immediate use.

Properties

Gourd has a light, sweet flavor, a slightly Cold nature and a propensity for the Lung, Spleen and Small Intestine channels. It has the effects of clearing Lung Heat and inducing urination.

Application

• For cough owing to Dry Heat, hot sensation and thirst, take gourd juice or a decoction of the flesh.

• For difficult urination owing to Damp-Heat, edema or jaundice, take a gourd decoction made with the skins of wax gourd and watermelon.

Preparation

In decoctions, juices or plain boiled.

Notes

It is not suitable for people with deficient Cold in the Spleen and Stomach.

Nutritional information

Gourd contains sugars, vitamin B and C, fat and protein. Animal tests show that gourd has a significant ability to induce urination.

WAX GOURD (MYBL)

Wax gourd is the fruit of *Benincasa hispida*, of the Cucurbitaceae family. The plant is cultivated in all parts of China. The ripened fruits are gathered in late summer and early autumn, peeled, washed clean and the pulp and seeds removed.

Properties

Wax gourd has a mild sweet flavor, a slightly Cold nature and a propensity for the Lung, Stomach and Bladder channels. It has the effects of clearing Heat, dissolving Phlegm, relieving thirst, inducing urination and relieving edema.

Application

• For asthma and cough owing to Phlegm-Heat, use one young fruit of wax gourd, fill it with crystal sugar and obtain the juice by steaming. Drink the juice on its own or with ginger.

• For thirst owing to feverish disease, or for diabetes, take fresh wax gourd juice liberally.

• For edema, difficult urination or obesity, take a wax gourd decoction.

• When used for edema of the deficiency type, take a soup with wax gourd cooked with carp or red beans.

Preparation

In decoctions, juices or plain boiled.

Notes

Generally the ripened fruit with skin that has an uneven appearance is the best. It is not suitable for people with deficient Cold or emaciation due to Yin deficiency.

Nutritional information

Wax gourd contains sugars, protein, vitamins B and C, niacin, calcium, phosphorus and iron.

CUCUMBER (BCSY)

Cucumber is the fruit of *Cucumis sativus*, of the Cucurbitaceae family. The plant is cultivated in all parts of China. It is gathered in summer and autumn and washed clean for immediate use.

Properties

Cucumber has a sweet flavor, a Cool nature and a propensity for the Stomach and Bladder channels. It has the effects of clearing Heat, quenching thirst and relieving edema.

Application

• For great thirst, eat the young fruits fresh or in salads.

• For edema and difficult urination, select one cucumber, cut it into two halves, boil in water and vinegar in equal amounts till it is well cooked and soft. Drink the juice at meal times. The juice is also excellent when applied externally for eczema and other skin problems if they are Heat related.

Preparation

Eaten fresh, boiled, in salads or decoctions.

Notes

It is not suitable for people with deficient Cold in the Spleen and Stomach.

Nutritional information

Cucumber contains glucose, mannose, rutin, isoquercitrin, caffeic acid, chlorogenic acid, amino acids, vitamins B2 and C, cucurbitacins A, B, C and D. In animal tests, cucurbitacin C had antitumour effects.

TOWEL GOURD (BCGM)

Towel gourd is the young fruit of *Luffa cylindrica* or *L. acutangula*, of the Cucurbitaceae family, cultivated in provinces such as Guangdong and Guangxi in China. It is gathered in summer and autumn, the rough peel removed and it is washed clean for immediate use.

Properties

Towel gourd has a sweet flavor, a Cool nature and a propensity for the Lung, Stomach and Liver channels. It has the effects of clearing Heat, dissolving Phlegm and cooling the Blood.

Application

• For thirst and sore throat in feverish diseases, take the boiled juice with a little white sugar added to taste.

• For cough with yellow and sticky sputum owing to Heat in the Lungs, take towel gourd plain boiled or the fresh juice.

• For bloody stools owing to Heat in the Blood or for hemorrhage from hemorrhoids, take towel gourd plain boiled or the fresh juice.

Preparation

Juiced, decocted or plain boiled.

Notes

It is not suitable for people with loose stool or diarrhea owing to deficient Cold in the Spleen and Stomach.

Nutritional information

Towel gourd contains saponin, mucus, citrubline, xylan, fat, protein, vitamins B and C. The variety *Luffa acutangula* contains hydrocyanic acid.

BALSAM PEARS (JHBC)

Balsam pears are the fruits of *Momordica charantia*, of the Cucurbitaceae family. The plant is cultivated in all parts of China. Note that balsam pears áre a vegetable, not related to the fruit.

They are gathered in autumn when the fruit is ripe. The fruit is cut into two halves, the pulp is removed and washed clean for immediate use.

Properties

Balsam pears have a bitter flavor, a Cold nature and a propensity for the Stomach, Heart and Liver channels. They have the effects of clearing Heat, relieving summer Heat and improving acuity of vision.

Application

• For thirst owing to feverish diseases or summer Heat, take balsam pears sauteed or decocted.

• For redness or pain in the eyes owing to Liver Heat, take balsam pears alone or with chrysanthemum and mulberry leaves.

Preparation

Balsam pears are taken sauteed, decocted or juiced.

Notes

The item is not suitable for people with deficient Cold in the Spleen and Stomach.

Nutritional information

Balsam pears contain balsam pear glycoside, 5-hydroxytryptamine, glutamic acid, alanine, proline, aminobutyric acid, citrubline, galacturonic acid and pectin. Balsam pear glycoside has the effect of lowering blood sugar.

PUMPKIN (DNBC)

Pumpkin is the fruit of *Cucurbita moschata*, of the Cucurbitaceae family. The plant is cultivated in all parts of China. Gather in summer and autumn when the fruits are ripe. Remove the fruiting stem, cut into two halves and discard the seeds for immediate use.

Properties

Pumpkin has a sweet flavor, a Warm nature and a propensity for the Spleen and Stomach channels. It has the effects of reinforcing the Middle Burner, replenishing Qi, dissolving Phlegm, promoting the discharge of pus and expelling roundworms.

Application

• For a weak Spleen or malnutrition, take pumpkin steamed with glutinous rice or boiled with ginger and brown sugar.

• For coughing up thick sputum due to a pulmonary abscess, take pumpkin boiled with beef (LNCYZ). The recipe does not only have the effects of dissolving Phlegm and promoting the discharge of pus, but also rectifies debility and enhances the body's resistance.

• For worm infestation, eat fresh pumpkin (500 g at a time for adults, 250 g for children). Two hours after eating, take some laxative or sesame seed oil to help expel the roundworms. This remedy should be administered for two consecutive days. Pumpkin seeds, chewed well, also assist in expelling all types of worms from the intestines.

Preparation

Pumpkin is to be steamed, plain boiled or eaten raw.

Notes

It is not suitable for people with stuffiness in the chest owing to obstruction by Damp or stagnation of Qi. Eating pumpkin continuously for over 2 months will cause yellowing of the skin due to the unabsorbed carotin discharged by sweat. Generally the xanthochromia will fade away gradually 2 or 3 months after stopping intake of pumpkin. This is consistent with the record in *The Great Compendium of Materia Medica* (BCGM) which says 'Overintake of pumpkin...causes jaundice'.

Nutritional information

Pumpkin contains citrubline, arginine, asparagine, gynesine, carotin, vitamins B and C, fat, glucose, sucrose, pentose, starch, mannitol, calcium and iron.

Fungi

Many fungi are eaten in China and they may often be found in oriental foodshops in the West. Some species grow in Britain and if they are collected from the wild, it is vital to identify them properly as some very poisonous species are similar.

WOOD-EARS (BCJb)

Wood-ears are the fruiting body of *Auricularia auricula* of the Auriculariaceae family. They are found in most parts of China, growing wild or cultivated, gathered in summer and autumn. In Britain they are known as Jew's ear, found on elder trees.

Properties

Wood-ears have a sweet taste, a Neutral nature and a propensity for the Lung, Stomach and Liver channels. They have the effects of moistening the Lungs, nourishing Yin and arresting bleeding.

Application

• For a dry cough without sputum or with a little sticky sputum owing to Yin deficiency and Dryness in the Lungs, stew wood-ears with crystal sugar until the sugar melts or with lily bulbs or honey.

• For a dry throat and mouth owing to deficiency of Stomach Yin, or constipation, take wood-ears alone or with spinach or carrots.

• For vomiting of blood, bloody stools, dysentery or hemorrhage from hemorrhoids and abnormal uterine bleeding. Wood-ears are especially good in the treatment of cases due to Yin deficiency or feverish diseases. Take wood-ears stewed with sugar or powdered. They are also used in combination with drugs that can arrest bleeding.

Preparation

Wood-ears are decocted, boiled, cooked in dishes or powdered.

Notes

They are not suitable for people with loose stool or diarrhea.

Nutritional information

Wood-ears contain sugars, protein, crude fiber, phosphorus, iron, calcium, niacin, carotin, vitamins B1, B2, ergosterin, lecithinase, cephalin and sphingomyelin and black thorn-fungus substance. The sugars include mannite, mannose, glucose, xylose and glucocerebroside acid.

Hot water extracts of wood-ears have the effect of inhibiting mouse sarcoma-180. The black thorn-fungus substance found in the wood-ear extracts has an antifungus effect.

TREMELLA (BCZX)

Tremella is the fruiting body of *Tremella fuciformis* of the Tremellaceae family. It is a jelly fungus, found in most parts of China, growing wild or cultivated. It is gathered in the early morning or late afternoon or on cloudy or wet days in the summer or autumn, washed clean, dried in the air or away from direct sunshine.

Properties

Tremella has a sweet taste, a Neutral nature and a propensity for the Lung and Stomach channels. It has the effects of moistening the Lungs, nurturing Yin, promoting the production of Body Fluids and arresting bleeding.

Application

• For a dry cough with no sputum or with a little sticky sputum that is difficult to cough up, owing to Yin deficiency and Dryness in the lungs, or for bloodstained sputum, take stewed tremella alone or decocted with glehnia roots, lilyturf roots and lily bulbs. It can also be made into a syrup for the above conditions.

• For dry throat and thirst owing to insufficiency of Stomach Yin or constipation, take tremella stewed into a thick sauce with white sugar.

• For coughing or vomiting of blood, bloody stools, or abnormal uterine bleeding, take stewed tremella alone or together with rehmannia root and E Jiao.

Preparation

Tremella is stewed into a thick sauce or powdered.

Notes

It is not suitable for patients with a cough owing to Phlegm-Damp or for people with loose stool or diarrhea.

Nutritional information

Tremella contains protein, fat, crude fiber, calcium, sulfur, phosphorus, iron, magnesium, potassium, sodium, vitamin B, xylose, fucose, mannose, glucocerebroside acid, glucose and antineoplastic polysaccharides A, B, C.

Animal tests show its spore preparation has the effects of dissolving Phlegm; tremella syrup can significantly enhance the phagocytic function of macrophages and can protect from radiation injury. The antineoplastic polysaccharides A, B, C have the function of inhibiting mouse sarcoma-180.

FRAGRANT MUSHROOM (RYBC)

Fragrant mushroom is the fruiting body of *Lentinus edodes* of the Pleurotus family. It is found in Sichuan, the middle and lower reaches of the Yangtze River and regions south of the Yangtze River in China. It is gathered in spring, summer or autumn and washed clean for immediate use or air-dried for storage.

Properties

Fragrant mushroom has a sweet flavor, a Neutral nature and a propensity for the Spleen and Stomach channels. It has the effects of reinforcing the Spleen and Stomach and replenishing Qi.

Application

• For a weak Spleen and Stomach, loss of appetite, shortness of breath and fatigue, or frequent urination, take fragrant mushroom by itself or stewed with chicken. Fragrant mushroom is also used for rickets, excess fat in the blood, gastric cancer or cervical carcinoma.

Preparation

Fragrant mushroom is decocted, sauteed or stewed.

Nutritional information

Fragrant mushroom contains protein (albumin, glutelin, prolamin), amino acids (glutamic acid, histidine, alanine, benzedrine acid, leucine, aspartic acid), fat, crude fiber, vitamins B1, B2 and C, niacin, calcium, phosphorus and iron. It also contains fragrant mushroom substance, fragrant mushroom acid, butyric acid, asparagine, choline, linoleic acid, ergosterin, fungus sterol, mannitol, lentinan and fragrant mushroom 'Tai sheng'.

The ergosterin contained in fragrant mushroom will turn into vitamin D2 when irradiated with the sun or ultraviolet rays; therefore it is one of the recommended foods for rickets. The fragrant mushroom 'Tai sheng' and butyric acid can lower blood fat. The lentinan or hot water extracts have a high inhibition rate on sarcoma-180.

OYSTER MUSHROOM (ZGYYZJ)

Oyster mushroom is the fruiting body of *Pleurotus ostreatus* of the Pleurotus family. It is found in Hebei, Jilin, Shanxi, Hunan, Sichuan and Yunnan, growing wild or cultivated. It is gathered in summer or autumn, washed clean for immediate use or air-dried for storage. It is commonly found in Britain, especially in parks, growing on both living and dead deciduous trees such as poplar and beech.

Properties

Oyster mushroom has a sweet taste, a slightly Warm nature and a propensity for the Spleen, Stomach and Liver channels. It has the effects of reinforcing the Spleen, removing Damp and relieving spasm.

Application

• For a weak Spleen and Stomach and loss of appetite, take oyster mushroom alone or cooked with chicken or lean pork.

• For Bi syndrome with such symptoms as soreness or pain in the joints and spasm in the limbs, take oyster mushroom alone or with Job's tears seeds, *Semen coix lachryma jobi*.

Preparation

Oyster mushroom is decocted, boiled or powdered.

Nutritional information

Oyster mushroom contains protein, fat, polysaccharide, D-mannitol, D-sorbite, cellulose, vitamins B1, B2, C, PP, calcium, phosphorus and iron. It contains 18 kinds of amino acids, including the eight essential ones.

The extracts of oyster mushroom have an inhibition rate of 75.3% on mouse sarcoma-180.

MUSHROOM (RYBC)

Mushroom is the fruiting body of *Agaricus campestris*. It is found in most parts of China, growing wild or cultivated and gathered in spring, summer or autumn. The mud is removed and it is washed clean for immediate use or air-dried for storage. It is commonly seen in fields all over Britain, especially after August rains.

Properties

Mushroom has a sweet flavor, a slightly Cold nature and a propensity for the Spleen, Stomach and Lung channels. It has the effects of reinforcing the Spleen and replenishing Qi, moistening Dryness and dissolving Phlegm.

Application

• For a weak Spleen and Stomach, with loss of appetite, fatigue and general weakness, or for lack of milk in the breastfeeding woman, take cooked mushroom on its own or with chicken or pork.

• For coughing and shortness of breath owing to Yin deficiency and Dryness in the Lungs, take plain-boiled mushrooms alone.

Preparation

Mushroom is decocted, plain-boiled or powdered.

Nutritional information

Mushroom contains protein, fat, polysaccharides, crude fiber, calcium, phosphorus, iron, copper, zinc, manganese, folic acid, niacin, vitamins A, B1, B2, C, E and K, amino acids such as alanine and glutelin. There is more linoleic acid than oleic acid.

The alcohol extract of mushroom can lower blood sugar. The culture fluid of mushroom has an inhibiting effect on *Staphylococcus aureus*, typhoid bacillus and *E. coli*.

HEDGEHOG FUNGUS (ZGYYZJ)

This is the fruiting body of *Hericium erinacaus* of the Hydnaceae family. It is found in north China, north-east China, middle and southern China, Sichuan, Yunnan, Gansu and Zhejiang provinces of China. It is also cultivated in Jiangsu and Shanghai in China. It is gathered in summer and autumn. The fruiting body of the cultivated varieties will be ripe and ready for collecting when the fungus is 3 or more months old. It is air-dried for storage or used immediately. A rare species in Britain, its large mass is distinguished by crowded white fleshy spines and it is found on beech trunks.

Properties

Hedgehog fungus has a sweet flavor, a Neutral nature and a propensity for the Spleen and Stomach channels. It has the effects of reinforcing the Spleen and Stomach and assisting digestion.

Application

• For a weak Spleen and Stomach, loss of appetite, indigestion or fatigue, take cooked hedgehog fungus or a decoction made with water and wine in equal amounts.

• It is also used in the treatment of carcinoma in the digestive tract, such as carcinoma of the esophagus, gastric cancer or intestinal cancer. Hedgehog fungus is taken on its own or with the root of kiwi fruit and spreading hedyotis to enhance the anticancer effect.

Preparation

Hedgehog fungus is used in decoctions, eaten boiled, in alcohol infusions or in tablets.

Nutritional information

Hedgehog fungus contains volatile oil, protein, polysaccharides and amino acids.

It has inhibiting effects on mouse sarcoma-180 and on the Ehrlich ascites tumor by inhibiting the composition of its DNA, obstructing the mix of thymine deoxyriboside and uridylic acid. The intensity of this effect is related to its concentration.

Seaweeds

As a group, seaweeds have many uses. As well as being a prime source of iodine, they contain a useful spectrum of vitamins and minerals and in at least one trial have been successfully used as the sole source of trace nutrients for patients.

The agar and alginates in seaweeds have the ability to chelate both heavy metals like lead and radioactive elements such as strontium 90 and so allow the body to eliminate them. Research carried out in 1965 and reported in *Nature* showed that kelp could not only inhibit absorption of strontium 90 by up to seven-eights of the dose received but would leach existing doses from body tissues. *Macrocystis pyrifera* has proved the most effective agent in terms of protection against radiostrontium, but many other species give 50% or more protection.

Many seaweeds act as natural antibiotics, particularly when harvested in the spring, with *Polysiphonia fastigiata* affecting the widest spectrum of bacteria.

See *Vegetables From The Sea* by Seibin and Teruko Arasaki (Japan Publications) for a comprehensive survey of the uses of seaweed.

KELP (JYBC)

Kelp is the fronds of *Laminaria japonica* of the

Laminariaceae family. It is found along the coasts of Shandong, Liaoning, Zhejiang and Fujian in China and is also cultivated. It is gathered in summer or autumn and generally air-dried until ready to be used.

Kombu, which is widely consumed in Japan, covers ten varieties of Laminaria (including *L. japonica* which is the variety usually sold as kombu in Europe). The therapeutic uses are similar in all the species.

Properties

Kelp has a salty flavor, a Cold nature and a propensity for the Liver, Stomach and Kidney channels. It has the effects of dissolving Phlegm, softening hard masses and relieving edema.

Application

• For goiters and scrofula, use kelp on its own or with kombu and *Undaria pinnatifida* (wakame in Japanese; sold in Europe by macrobiotic suppliers and some health food shops) to enhance the effect of dispersing hard masses.

• For difficulty in swallowing, kelp and amomum fruit are powdered together and taken in cow's milk, which not only dissolves Phlegm and softens masses but also replenishes the Stomach.

• For hernia or edema and pain in the testicles, use kelp with sargassum and badian.

• For edema and beriberi, use kelp together with diuretic drugs.

• It is also used for hypertension, coronary heart diseases and carcinomas. For these purposes, use kelp by itself or with other suitable drugs.

Preparation

Kelp is made into decoctions, salads and pills and is eaten boiled, powdered or candied.

Notes

It is not suitable for people with deficient Cold in the Spleen and the Stomach or emaciated people.

Nutritional information

Kelp contains phycocolloid acid, a kombu principle, mannitol, galactan, larminarin, laminine, potassium oxide, iodine, calcium, cobalt, iron and carotin, vitamins B1, B2, C, phosphorus, protein and amino acids such as proline, glutamic acid, aspartic acid.

The iodine and iodine compounds can be used to reduce the enlarged thyroid gland by correcting the hypothyroidism arising from the lack of iodine; at the same time it can alleviate the symptoms of hyperthyroidism by temporarily inhibiting the metabolic rate of the disease.

Iodine can promote the absorption of inflammatory exudates. Laminine has the effect of lowering blood tension and larminarin has the effect of lowering blood fat.

LAVER (BCJJZ)

Laver is the fronds of *Porphyra tenera*, *P. suborbiculata* or *P. dentata*. It is found on the shores of Liaoning, Shandong, Jiangsu, Zhejiang, Fujian and Guangdong in China. It is also cultivated, gathered in autumn or winter and air-dried, avoiding direct sunlight, for use.

British laver is usually *P. umbilicalis*, but other more delicately flavoured varieties are also found in coastal waters and all have similar properties. The Japanese nori covers several varieties of laver.

Properties

Laver has a sweet, salty flavor, a Cold nature and a propensity for the Liver, Lung, Stomach and Kidney channels.

It has the effects of softening hard masses, clearing Heat, dissolving Phlegm and inducing urination.

Application

• For goiters and scrofulas, use laver on its own or with yellow-root yam make an alcohol infusion to enhance the effect of softening hard masses.

• For a cough with yellow sputum owing to Heat in the Lungs, take laver in a decoction made with turnips.

• For edema and beriberi, use laver by itself or with Chinese cabbage or river snails.

Preparation

Laver is made into decoctions, medicinal wines, pills or powder or is eaten boiled.

Nutritional information

Laver contains protein, fat, carotin, vitamins B1, B2, B12, C, niacin, choline, amino acids (including alanine, glutamic acid, aspartic acid), iodine, calcium, phosphorus and iron. It is a food rich in nutrients.

AGAR (SJBC)

Agar is the algite of *Gelidium amansii* of the Gelidiaceae family or *Eucheuma gelatinae*. The plant is found along the coasts of the Yellow Sea, East Sea, Guangdong in Taiwan and China. It is gathered in summer or autumn, air-dried and exposed to the dew at night, then stored until ready for use.

G. amansii is one of several seaweeds used to produce agar. It grows commonly in the USA, while the cooler British waters yield *G. sesquipedale* and *G. latifolium*. Properties are similar, but agar yields vary.

Properties

Agar has a sweet, salty flavor, a Cold nature and propensity for the Lung and Large Intestine channels. It has the effects of moistening Dryness, dissolving Phlegm, clearing Heat and assisting bowel motions.

Application

• For cough owing to Dryness in the Lungs or Phlegm Heat, with yellow and sticky sputum, use agar on its own or with turnips to make a salad or with lilyturf root and glehnia root to enhance the effect of clearing Heat, moistening Dryness and dissolving Phlegm.

• For constipation owing to Dryness and Heat in the Intestine, or bloody stools, or hemorrhage from hemorrhoids, agar is used by boiling with white sugar to make a syrup. It is also used to make a salad with wood-ears.

Preparation

Agar makes salads, decoctions or soups.

Notes

It is not suitable for people with a weak Spleen and Stomach or with susceptibility to loose stools.

Nutritional information

Agar contains agar-agar, calcium, manganese, potassium, sodium and various inorganic salts and polysaccharides.

The sugar compounds contained in agar have an inhibiting effect on the B-type influenza virus and the mumps virus. The variety *Eucheuma gelatinae* has the function of lowering serum cholesterol levels in mice with excess fat in the blood.

GRACILARIA VERRUCOSA (BCGM)

This is the algite of *Gracilaria verrucosa*. It is found along the coasts of China, gathered in summer or autumn and air-dried until ready for use. Distinguished by its red stringy stems covered with distinctive wartlike reproductive bodies, *G. verrucosa* is a common sea vegetable in Britain.

Properties

Gracilaria verrucosa has a sweet and slightly salty flavor, a Cold nature and a propensity for the Liver, Stomach and Bladder channels. It has the effects of dissolving Phlegm, dispersing hard masses, clearing Heat and inducing urination.

Application

• For goiters, use *G. verrucosa* by itself or with kelp in a salad; it is also used with kombu and selfheal to make decoctions.

• For sensations of hot and difficult urination, use *G. verrucosa* to make a salad or a decoction with plantain. When the decoction is ready, remove the plantain and add sugar and vinegar to taste.

Preparation

G. verrucosa is made into salads, steamed or decocted.

Nutritional information

G. verrucosa contains phycoerythrobilin, cholesterin, galactose, polysaccharides and pyruvic acid.

Fruits (cultivated and wild) 8

The term 'fruits' in this context covers not only those commonly seen, such as pears, oranges, peaches, plums and loquats, but some that grow wild or which are not so commonly served for food, e.g. Chinese actinidias and gooseberry.

Most fruits have a sweet and sour flavor and a Cold or Cool nature and their most commonly seen effects are promoting the production of Body Fluids, clearing Heat, moistening Dryness, dissolving Phlegm and as diuretics.

Some fruits such as litchi, grapes and figs, however, are very sweet and have a Warmer nature. They are able to replenish Blood or reinforce the Liver and Kidney.

Most fruits and fresh fruits have similar nutrients to vegetables. They mainly supply vitamins (the most common one is vitamin C), inorganic salts, sugars and organic acids.

PEAR (XXBC)

Pears are the ripe fruits of *Pyrus bretschneideri* or *P. ussuriensis* of the Rosaceae family. The plant is cultivated in most parts of China. Gather the fruit in autumn and wash clean for use. Note that balsam pear, mentioned earlier, is a vegetable.

Properties

Pears have a sweet and slightly sour flavor, a Cool nature and a propensity for the Lung and Stomach channels.

They have the effect of clearing Heat, promoting the production of Body Fluids, moistening Dryness and dissolving Phlegm.

Application

• In the treatment of great thirst owing to impairment of Body Fluids by feverish diseases or dry mouth. For the former use the five-juice mix (see Epidemic Febrile Diseases) (WBTB), made with pears, water chestnuts, lotus rhizome and lilyturf root, for the latter, use pears to make an electuary with honey (PJF).

• For cough owing to Heat in the Lungs or Phlegm-Heat, remove the cores and steam the pears with Sichuan fritillary bulbs or use pear juice and ginger to make an electuary with honey. For Phlegm-Heat, varieties which have a distinct 'pear drop' taste will have a stronger effect than those with a bland flavor. In the absence of fresh pears, the concentrated juice sold in health food shops makes an excellent substitute.

Preparation

Pears are eaten fresh, steamed, stewed, decocted, juiced or in an electuary.

Notes

They are not suitable for people with weakness in the Spleen and Stomach, loose stool or diarrhea, or cough without Heat.

Nutritional information

Pears contain malic acid, citric acid, fructose, glucose, sucrose, calcium, phosphorus, iron, vitamins C, B and niacin.

ORANGES (BCSY)

Oranges are the ripe fruits of *Citrus chachiensis* or *C. suavissim* of the Rutiaceae family. The plant is cultivated in Guangdong, Guangxi, Fujian, Taiwan and Sichuan in China. Gather fruits in the winter, peel and use the pulp.

Properties

Oranges have a sweet and sour flavor, a Cool nature and a propensity for the Stomach and Bladder channels. They have the effects of promoting the production of Body Fluids, quenching thirst and inducing urination. In the editor's experience, large quantities of orange juice can have the opposite effect and will frequently aggravate hot conditions, particularly those involving Damp or Phlegm.

Application

• For Heat in the Stomach, thirst or excessive intake of alcohol, eat fresh oranges liberally or drink the juice with honey.

• For accumulation of Heat in the Lower Burner and difficult urination, eat fresh oranges or drink the juice with tea.

Preparation

Oranges are eaten fresh, made into decoctions by boiling in water or juiced.

Notes

They are not suitable for people with weakness in the Spleen and Stomach, or cough owing to Cold in the Lungs.

Nutritional information

Oranges contain sugars, vitamin C, niacin, citric acid, calcium, phosphorus and iron.

KUMQUAT (BCGM)

Kumquat is the ripe fruit of *Fortunella margarita* or *F. crassifolia* of the Rutiaceae family. The plant is cultivated in Zhejiang, Jiangxi, Guangdong, Guangxi and Sichuan in China. Gather the fruit in winter and wash clean for use fresh.

Properties

Kumquat has a pungent, sweet and sour flavor, a slightly Warm nature and a propensity for the Lung, Stomach and Liver channels. It has the effects of dissolving Phlegm, relieving cough, regulating Qi and relieving stagnation.

Application

• For cough with sputum, eat kumquat. For cough owing to Cold in the Lungs, cut the fruit open, steep in boiling water with ginger and drink the infusion; for cough owing to Heat in the Lungs, drink kumquat and turnip juice mixed.

• For retention of food, stagnation of Qi, stuffiness in the upper abdomen and loss of appetite, eat kumquat fresh or candied. It is also used with Chinese hawthorn and germinated barley to make a decoction.

• For stuffiness or pain in the hypochondria and chest owing to depression of Liver Qi, use kumquat candied in honey or with fingered citron and Seville orange flower to make an infusion in boiling water, with white sugar added to taste.

Preparation

Kumquat is candied with honey or sugar, eaten fresh, made into tea or decoctions.

Nutritional information

Kumquat contains kumquat glucocide, vitamins B and C (80% of which is contained in the pericarp), calcium, phosphorus, iron, protein and sugars.

TANGERINE (BCSY)

Tangerine is the ripe fruit of *Citrus tangerina* or *C. erythrosa* of the Rutiaceae family. The plant is grown in Anhui, Zhejiang, Jiangsu, Hubei, Hunan, Sichuan and Fujian in China. Gather fruits in winter, peel and use the segments.

Properties

Tangerine has a sweet and sour flavor, a Neutral nature and a propensity for the Lung and Stomach channels. It has the effects of promoting the production of Body Fluids, quenching thirst, assisting appetite, sending down Counterflow Qi, moistening the Lungs and dissolving Phlegm.

Application

• For thirst owing to deficiency of Stomach Yin or excessive intake of alcohol, eat plenty of the fruit or drink the juice diluted with water, with sugar added to taste.

• For vomiting and loss of appetite owing to disharmony of Stomach Qi, cut the fruit into small pieces, boil them in water and drink the decoction. Tangerine can also be made into dried orange cakes by adding sugar to the fruit (with peel on), which are then made into an infusion for drinking.

• For cough with profuse sputum owing to Heat in the Lungs, make a decoction in water with the whole fruit (with peel on). Drink the decoction with honey added to taste.

Preparation

Tangerines are taken fresh, juiced or decocted.

Notes

It is not suitable for people with weakness in the Spleen and Stomach.

CANTONESE ORANGE (SXBC)

Cantonese oranges are the ripe fruits of *Citrus junos* and *Citrus sinensis* of the Rutiaceae family. The plant is cultivated in eastern China, southwest China, Hunan and Hubei. Gather fruits in the autumn and winter and peel before use.

Properties

Cantonese oranges have a sweet and sour flavor, a slightly Cool nature and a propensity for the Lung and Stomach channels. They have the effects of promoting the production of Body Fluids, quenching thirst, assisting appetite and sending down Counterflow Qi.

Application

• For thirst owing to deficiency of Stomach Yin or excessive intake of alcohol, eat plenty of the fruit or drink the juice.

• For vomiting and loss of appetite owing to disharmony of Stomach Qi, according to the *Kaibao Herbal* (KBBC), cut the fruits into thin slices and add salt and honey to make a decoction for drinking. Cantonese oranges can also be made into dried orange cakes by candying the whole fruit with the peel on, which can then be taken in an infusion.

Preparation

Cantonese oranges are eaten fresh, juiced or decocted.

Nutritional information

Cantonese oranges contain citric acid, malic acid, vitamin C and sugars.

GRAPEFRUIT (RHZBC)

Grapefruits are the ripe fruits of *Citrus grandis* or its variety *C. grandis var. wentanyu* of the Rutiaceae family. The plants grow in south China, Guangdong, Guangxi, Sichuan, Shannxi and Taiwan. Gather the fruit in autumn and winter and remove the peel before use.

Properties

Grapefruits have a sweet and sour flavor, a Cold nature and a propensity for the Stomach and Lung channels. They have the effects of promoting the production of Body Fluids, easing thirst, restoring appetite, sending down Counterflow Qi, dissolving Phlegm and arresting cough.

Application

• For great thirst owing to deficiency of Stomach Yin or excessive intake of alcohol, eat plenty of fresh grapefruits.

• For vomiting and loss of appetite owing to disharmony of Stomach Qi, make a decoction with grapefruit (with peel on) for drinking after adding sugar to taste.

• For cough owing to Phlegm, cut grapefruits into pieces, remove the seeds, soak in wine for one night, boil until soft and mix with honey to be sipped from time to time.

Preparation

Grapefruits are eaten fresh, juiced, decocted or made into an electuary.

Nutritional information

Grapefruits contain sugars, vitamin C, citric acid, calcium and phosphorus.

It is reported that the fresh juice of grapefruits contains insulinlike substances which can lower blood sugar.

PERSIMMON (MYBL)

Persimmons are the ripe fruits of *Diospyros kaki* of the Ebenaceae family. The plant is found in the eastern, middle and southern parts of China and in Sichuan, Shaanxi, Gansu and Hebei. Gather the fruit in autumn and winter, store until they become red and ripe to reduce the astringent taste, or else use green.

Properties

Persimmons have a sweet and slightly astringent flavor, a Cold nature and a propensity for the Lung, Stomach and Large Intestine channels. They have the effects of moistening the Lungs, dissolving Phlegm, promoting the production of Body Fluids, easing thirst and astringing the Intestines.

Application

• For cough owing to Dryness in the Lungs, eat fresh or dried persimmon.

• For thirst owing to deficiency of Stomach Yin, take crisp and sweet green persimmons preferably. The ripe red persimmon can also be used for the purpose.

• For bloody stools from dysentery or hemorrhage from hemorrhoids, use fresh or dried persimmon alone or together with persimmon leaves to make a decoction for drinking.

Preparation

Persimmons are eaten fresh or dried.

Notes

It is not desirable for people with a weak Spleen and Stomach, loose stools or a cough owing to excessive Phlegm-Damp, to use persimmon.

Nutritional information

Persimmons contain sucrose, glucose, fructose, protein, carotin, vitamin C, citrubline, iodine, calcium, phosphorus and iron. Unripe fruits of persimmon contain tannin.

PEACHES (MYBL)

Peaches are the ripe fruits of *Prunus persica* of the Rosaceae family. The plant is extensively cultivated in all parts of China. Gather the fruit in summer and remove the kernel before use.

Properties

Peaches have a sweet and sour flavor, a Neutral nature and a propensity for the Stomach and Large Intestine channels. They have the effects of reinforcing the Stomach, promoting the production of Body Fluids and moistening Dryness. The kernel is Tao Ren, which is slightly toxic.

Application

• For deficiency of Stomach Yin, thirst and dry throat, or Dryness and Heat in the Intestines and constipation, eat peaches fresh or steamed.

Preparation

Peaches are eaten fresh, steamed or boiled in water.

Nutritional information

Peaches contain glucose, fructose, sucrose, protein, malic acid, citric acid, vitamin C, niacin, calcium, phosphorus, iron, potassium and sodium.

PLUM (MYBL)

Plums are the ripe fruits of *Prunus salicina* of the Rosaceae family. The plant is cultivated in most parts of China. Gather the fruit in summer and autumn, wash clean and remove the kernel before use.

Properties

Plums have a sweet and sour flavor, a Cold nature and a propensity for the Liver and Stomach channels. They have the effects of clearing Liver Heat and promoting the production of Body Fluids.

Application

• For deficiency and heat in the Liver or hectic fever, take fresh plums or the juice.

• For deficiency in Stomach Yin, with thirst and dry throat, eat fresh or preserved plums.

Notes

Excessive intake of plums impairs the Spleen and Stomach, causes loss of appetite and diarrhea.

Nutritional information

Plums contain sugars, protein, calcium, phosphorus and iron, carotin, vitamins B and C, and niacin; they also contain asparagine, glutamic acid, glycine, proline, threonine and alanine.

APRICOT (MYBL)

Apricots are the ripe fruits of *Prunus armeniaca P. armeniaca var. ansu* of the Rosaceae family. The plant is grown in most parts of China. Gather the fruit in summer, wash clean and remove the kernels before use. The kernel is Xing Ren, which is toxic in anything more than small doses.

Properties

Apricots have a sweet and sour flavor, a Neutral nature and a propensity for the Stomach and Lung channels. They have the effects of promoting the production of Body Fluids, easing thirst, moistening the Lungs and relieving difficult breathing.

Application

• For deficiency of Stomach Yin, with thirst and dry throat, eat fresh or preserved apricots.

• For cough and Counterflow Qi owing to Dryness and Heat in the Lung channel, eat fresh apricots or drink apricot electuary made with honey.

Preparation

Apricots are eaten fresh, as preserved fruits or made into decoctions.

Notes

Excessive intake of apricots impairs the Spleen and Stomach and harms the teeth.

Nutritional information

Apricots contain sugars, protein, calcium, phosphorus, iron, carotin, vitamins B and C, citric acid, malic acid and lycopene.

LOQUAT (SLBC)

Loquats are the ripe fruits of *Eriobotrya japonica* of the Rosaceae family. The plant is found in east, middle, south and south-west China and Shannxi, Gansu and Taiwan. Gather the fruit in spring and summer, remove the peel and kernel before use.

Properties

Loquats have a sweet and slightly sour flavor, a Cool nature and a propensity for the Lung and Stomach channels.

They have the effects of moistening the Lungs, relieving cough, promoting the production of Body Fluids and easing thirst, regulating the Stomach and sending down Counterflow Qi.

Application

• For a cough or coughing up of blood owing to Yin deficiency and Dryness in the Lungs, make a decoction with unseeded loquats and drink the juice with honey. The famous cough syrup Zhi Ke Chuan Bei Pi Pa Lu is based on loquat leaf and fritillary bulb.

• For thirst and a dry throat owing to deficiency of Stomach Yin, or dry vomiting and loss of appetite, make a decoction using loquats and loquat leaves and drink it with honey.

Preparation

Loquats are eaten fresh or made into decoctions or electuaries.

Notes

It is not desirable for people with a weak Spleen and Stomach to use loquats.

Nutritional information

Loquats contain sugars, protein, fat, cellulose, pectin, calcium, phosphorus and iron, vitamins B1 and C, malic acid, citric acid and tartaric acid.

APPLE (MYBL)

Apples are the ripe fruits of *Malus pumila* of the Rosaceae family. The plant is cultivated in north-east, northern, eastern and, north-west China and Sichuan and Yunnan. Gather the fruit in autumn when ripe and wash clean before use.

Properties

Apples have a sweet and slightly sour flavor, a Cool nature and a propensity for the Spleen and Stomach channels.

They have the effects of promoting the production of Body Fluids, easing thirst, reducing fever and relieving restlessness, reinforcing the Spleen and arresting diarrhea.

Application

• For general debility with an oppressive sensation and thirst, or excessive intake of alcohol, eat fresh apples or take apple electuary.

• For deficiency of Spleen Yin, indigestion, loss of appetite and diarrhea, take freshly squeezed apple juice or a mixture made with powdered Chinese yam, with sugar added to taste.

Preparation

Apples are eaten fresh, juiced, decocted, electuated or powdered.

Nutritional information

Apples contain sucrose, reducing sugar, malic acid, citric acid, tartaric acid, quininic acid, pectin, alcohols, phosphorus, calcium, iron, potassium, sodium and vitamin C.

In rabbits, intravenous injection of apple juice, after removing the pectin, can raise the blood sugar level, induce urination and regulate the function of the intestines; it can also help prevent the blood pressure raising effect of desoxycorticosterone in rats.

BANANA (XXBC)

Bananas are the ripe fruits of *Musa paradisiaca* of the Musa family. The plant is found in Guangxi, Guangdong, Fujian, Taiwan and Sichuan. Gather the fruit in autumn and eat peeled.

Properties

Bananas have a sweet flavor, a Cold nature and a propensity for the Stomach and Large Intestine channels. They have the effects of reinforcing the Stomach and promoting the production of Body Fluids, nourishing Yin and moistening Dryness.

Application

• For a dry throat and thirst owing to deficiency of Stomach Yin or great thirst from feverish diseases, eat raw bananas liberally.

• For constipation and dry stool owing to Dryness in the Intestines, or hemorrhage from hemorrhoids, eat bananas raw or stewed with the peel on (LNCYL).

Preparation

Bananas are eaten raw, steamed or boiled.

Notes

It is more appropriate for people with Heat in the Lungs and the Stomach to eat raw bananas. People with Phlegm from weak Stomach and Spleen should avoid bananas, especially raw.

Nutritional information

Bananas contain fructose, glucose, protein, fat, calcium, phosphorus, iron, vitamin C, pectin and 5-hydroxytryptamine (which can lower gastric acid), noradrenalin and dihydroxyphenyl ethylamine.

Bananas can also alleviate irritation to the gastric mucosa and, therefore they have a significant effect in protecting against gastric ulcer. In addition, the glucose level in the urine of diabetes patients does not go up after intake of bananas.

PINEAPPLE (TWFZ)

Pineapples are the ripe fruits of *Ananas comosus* of the Bromeliaceae family. The plant is found in Guangdong, Guangxi, Yunnan, Fujian and Taiwan. Gather the fruit in summer and remove the outer peel before use.

Properties

Pineapples have a sweet and slightly sour flavor, a slightly Cold nature and a propensity for the Stomach and Bladder channels. They have the effects of promoting the production of Body Fluids, easing thirst and inducing urination.

Application

• For thirst and a dry mouth, or vomiting owing to deficiency of Stomach Yin, eat fresh pineapples or drink the fresh juice.

• For difficult urination and edema with fever, drink a decoction made with the fruit and fresh cogongrass rhizome.

Preparation

Pineapples are eaten raw, juiced or decocted for drinking.

Nutritional information

Pineapples contain sugars, protein, calcium, phosphorus, iron, vitamin C, niacin and organic acids. They also contain a certain type of enzyme which can break down proteins. The enzyme, bromelain, acts directly on Phlegm if pineapple juice is swallowed slowly.

ARHAT FRUIT (LUOHAN FRUIT) (LNCYL)

This is the ripe fruit of *Momordica grosvenori* of the Cucurbitaceae family. It is found in Guangxi, Guangdong, Hainan and Jiangxi. Gather fruits in autumn, store them for 8–10 days until the pericarps turn from green to yellow, then dry them on a low heat. Brush off the hairs before use.

Properties

Arhat fruit has a sweet flavor, a Cold nature and a propensity for the Lung and Large Intestine channels. It has the effects of clearing Heat, arresting cough, easing the throat and moistening Dryness in the Intestines.

Application

• For a cough owing to Heat in the Lungs, whooping cough, sore throat and loss of voice,

take a decoction made with arhat fruit alone or together with dried persimmon. For a cough owing to Lung deficiency with fever, take a soup made with lean pork (LNCYL).

• For constipation owing to Dryness and Heat in the Intestines, take a decoction made with arhat fruit alone or together with boat-fruited sterculia seed.

Preparation

Arhat fruit is decocted or infused in hot water for drinking.

Nutritional information

Arhat fruit contains glucose and a triterpene-like substance that is 300 times sweeter than granulated sugar.

POMEGRANATE (MYBL)

Pomegranates are the ripe fruits of *Punica granatum* of the Punica family. The plant is found in most parts of China. Gather the fruit in autumn, take out the fleshy seeds for use, or use the whole fruit with the peel on.

Properties

Pomegranates have a sweet flavor, a slight sourness and astringency, a Neutral nature and a propensity for the Stomach and Large Intestine channels. They have the effects of promoting the production of Body Fluids, easing thirst, astringing and arresting diarrhea.

Application

• For thirst and a dry throat owing to deficiency of Stomach Yin, eat fresh pomegranates or take the freshly squeezed juice.

• For persistent diarrhea or dysentery, take the juice by crushing the whole fruit with the peel on or a decoction made with the whole fruit and water.

Preparation

Pomegranates are eaten raw, juiced or decocted.

Nutritional information

Pomegranates contain sugars, protein, fat, vitamin C, calcium, phosphorus, potassium and organic acids.

FIGS (DNBC)

Figs are the ripe fruit of *Ficus carica* of the Moraceae family. The plant is cultivated in all parts of China. Gather the fruit in autumn, wash clean for immediate use or sun-dry for storage.

Properties

Figs have a sweet flavor, a Neutral nature and a propensity for the Spleen, Lung and Large Intestine channels. They have the effects of reinforcing the Spleen and Stomach, moistening the Lungs, easing the throat, moistening the Intestines and assisting bowel motions.

Application

• For a weak Spleen, indigestion and loss of appetite, chop up the fruit, dry roast until half scorched and add brown sugar to make a decoction or make an infusion in boiling water for drinking.

• For deficiency after childbirth and lack of milk, stew figs with pig's trotters for eating.

• For constipation owing to Dryness in the Intestines, or hemorrhage from hemorrhoids, eat figs fresh or boiled with pig's large intestines.

Preparation

Figs are eaten fresh, boiled or decocted.

Nutritional information

Figs contain glucose, fructose, sucrose, citric acid, succinic acid, malonic acid, oxalic acid, malic acid, amylase, lipase, protease, vitamin C, calcium and phosphorus.

Animal tests of fig extract show that it has the effect of lowering blood pressure. The substances taken from the water extracts by activated carbon and acetone treatment have inhibiting effects on Abernethy's sarcoma.

LITCHI (LYCHEE) (SLBC)

Litchi is the ripe fruit of *Litchi chinensis* of the Sapindaceae family. The plant is found in Fujian, Guangdong, Guangxi, Sichuan, Yunnan and Taiwan. Gather the fruit in summer, remove the peel for immediate use or air-dry for future use.

Properties

Litchi has a sweet and slightly sour flavor, a slightly Warm nature and a propensity for the Spleen, Stomach and Liver channels. It has the effects of promoting the production of Body Fluids, easing thirst, reinforcing Spleen Qi and replenishing Blood.

Application

• For thirst owing to deficiency of Stomach Yin, eat fresh litchi or take litchi soup made with plenty of the fruit.

• For vomiting and loss of appetite owing to a weak Spleen and Stomach, or for diarrhea, use dried litchi flesh to make a porridge with non-glutinous rice for eating. This can be improved by using lotus seeds and Chinese yam in the porridge as well.

• For palpitations and dizziness owing to Blood deficiency, take a litchi decoction made with dates.

Preparation

Litchi is eaten raw, decocted or made into gruels.

Notes

It is unsuitable for people with excessive Fire due to deficiency of Yin.

Nutritional information

Litchi contains glucose, sucrose, protein, fat, calcium, phosphorus, iron, carotin, vitamins B and C, folic acid, citric acid, malic acid and arginine.

GRAPE (BCJB)

Grapes are the ripe fruits of *Vitis vinifera* of the Vitaceae family. The plant is cultivated in all parts of China north of the Yangtze River. Gather the fruit in late summer and early autumn for immediate use or air-dry for future use.

Properties

Grapes have a sweet and slightly sour flavor, a Neutral nature and a propensity for the Kidney, Liver and Stomach channels. They have the effects of reinforcing the Liver and Kidney, replenishing Qi and Blood, promoting the production of Body Fluids and inducing urination.

Application

• For soreness in the waist and knees owing to deficiency of the Liver and Kidney, use grapes with ginseng to make a medicinal wine (BJFY).

• For palpitation, dull spirits and night sweating owing to deficiency of Qi and Blood, use raisins to make a decoction with longan or make an electuary.

• For thirst and dry mouth, take freshly squeezed juice or an electuary made by boiling the fruit in water.

• For scanty dark urine, take fresh grape juice liberally.

• As recorded in *The Peaceful Holy Benevolent Prescriptions* (SHF), a decoction of grapes is used for the treatment of painful and dripping urine. The decoction is made with grape juice, fresh lotus rhizome juice and the juice of raw rehmannia root.

Preparation

Grapes are eaten fresh, juiced, decocted and made into medicinal wines.

Nutritional information

Grapes contain glucose, fructose, sucrose, tartaric acid, citric acid, malic acid, protein, calcium, phosphorus, iron, carotin, vitamins B and C and niacin.

CHERRY (MYBL)

Cherries are the ripe fruits of *Prunus pseudocerasus* of the Rosaceae family. The plant is found in east China, Hebei, Shanxi, Shandong, Henan and Sichuan. Gather the fruit in summer and wash clean before use.

Properties

Cherries have a sweet and slightly sour flavor, a Warm nature and a propensity for the Spleen and Liver channels. They have the effects of reinforcing the Spleen and Stomach, nourishing the Liver and Kidney and astringing seminal emission.

Application

• For weak Spleen and Stomach, loss of appetite and fatigue, take a cherry decoction or a cherry electuary with longan pulp.

• For soreness in the waist and knees owing to deficiency of the Liver and Kidney, or seminal emission, take a cherry infused medicinal wine alone or in combination with dogwood fruit and magnolia vine fruit. Cherries or cherry juice will usually ease the pain of gout if taken regularly.

Preparation

Cherries are eaten fresh or decocted, made into electuaries or alcohol infusions.

Nutritional information

Cherries contain sugars, protein, fat, calcium,

phosphorus, iron, potassium, carotin and vitamin C.

RED BAY BERRY (SLBC)

Red bay berries are the ripe fruits of *Myrica rubra* of the Myricaeae family. The plant is found in east China, Hunan, Guangdong, Guangxi and Guizhou. Gather the fruit in summer for immediate use or air-dry for future use.

Properties

Red bay berries have a sweet and sour flavor, a Neutral nature and a propensity for the Stomach and Large Intestine channels. They have the effects of promoting the production of Body Fluids and easing thirst, regulating the Stomach and arresting vomiting, astringing and arresting diarrhea.

Application

• For thirst and a dry mouth, or excessive intake of alcohol, eat plenty of fresh red bay berries or suck the salt-preserved and candied fruit.

• For vomiting and loss of appetite owing to disharmony of Stomach Qi, take red bay berry decoction made with orange peel. Salt-preserved berries can be used as substitutes.

• For diarrhea or dysentery, take dried red bay berry powder made after roasting, or take a decoction made with black plums.

Preparation

Red bay berries are eaten fresh, decocted, powdered or salt-pickled.

Nutritional information

Red bay berries contain glucose, fructose, citric acid, malic acid, oxalic acid, lactic acid, vitamin C and tannic acid.

WATERMELON (RYBC)

Watermelon is the ripe fruit of *Citrullus vulgaris* of the Cucurbitaceae family. The plant is cultivated in all parts of China. Gather the fruit in summer and use the pulp with seeds removed.

Properties

Watermelon has a sweet flavor, a Cold nature and a propensity for the Stomach, Heart and Bladder channels. It has the effects of clearing Heat, relieving Summer Heat and thirst and inducing urination.

Application

• For Summer Heat or epidemic febrile diseases, excessive Heat impairing Body Fluids and great thirst, drink watermelon juice (BCHY) or a decoction made with fresh honeysuckle flower, fresh bamboo leaves and raw rehmannia root.

• For sores in the mouth and tongue owing to Heart Fire attacking upwards, eat fresh watermelon or take a decoction made with raw rehmannia root and bamboo leaves.

• For scanty dark orange urine owing to accumulation of Damp-Heat, take watermelon alone or a decoction made with cogongrass rhizome.

Preparation

Watermelon is eaten fresh, juiced or decocted.

Notes

It is not suitable for people with deficient Cold in the Spleen and Stomach.

The compound formula 'Watermelon Frost' (Fu Fang Xi Gua Shuang) is made from watermelon juice processed with mirabilite and other ingredients to produce an extremely effective Heat-clearing agent for mouth infections and burns.

Nutritional information

Watermelon contains fructose, glucose, sucrose,

malic acid, phosphoric acid, citrubline, propionic acid, alanine, glutamic acid, arginine, carotin, vitamins B and C, niacin, calcium, phosphorus and iron.

SUGARCANE (MYBL)

Sugarcane is the stalk of *Saccharum sinensis* of the grass family. The plant is cultivated in east and south China and Sichuan, Yunnan and Taiwan. Gather the plant in autumn for immediate use.

Properties

Sugarcane has a sweet flavor, a Cold nature and a propensity for the Stomach and Lung channels. It has the effects of relieving thirst, promoting the production of Body Fluids and moistening Dryness, harmonizing the Middle Burner and sending down Counterflow Qi.

Application

• For thirst owing to heat impairing Body Fluids, or excessive intake of alcohol, suck fresh sugarcane or drink the freshly squeezed juice. *The Revised General Treatise on Febrile Diseases* (CDGWRL) contains a recipe for five-juice mix for treating exhaustion of gastric fluids and persisting fever where sugarcane, fresh rehmannia root, dendrobium, reed rhizome and pears are juiced together.

• For a cough due to Dryness in the Lungs, or a dry throat with sticky sputum, take sugarcane juice made with pears or a gruel made with sugarcane juice and millet.

• For vomiting owing to deficiency of Stomach Yin, take sugarcane juice on its own or mixed with ginger juice (MSJYF).

Preparation

Sugarcane is eaten fresh (the juice is sucked), juiced or made into gruels.

Notes

It is not desirable for people with deficient Cold in the Spleen and Stomach or cough owing to Phlegm-Damp to use sugarcane.

Nutritional information

Sugarcane contains sugars, protein, fat, calcium, phosphorus, iron, vitamins B6 and C and various amino acids including aspartic acid, alanine, and such organic acids as malic acid, citric acid, succinic acid and oxalic acid.

WATER CHESTNUT (MYBL)

Water chestnut is the bulb of *Heleocharis dulcis* of the Cyperus family. The plant is found in most parts of China. Gather the bulbs in winter, remove the parts growing above ground, wash clean for immediate use or air-dry for future use.

Properties

Water chestnut has a sweet flavor, a Cold nature and a propensity for the Stomach, Lung and Liver channels. It has the effects of clearing Heat, promoting the production of Body Fluids, dissolving Phlegm, cooling Blood, resolving food retention and improving acuity of vision.

Application

• For thirst owing to the impairment of Body Fluids by Heat, take water chestnut alone or the juice combined with fresh pears, reed rhizomes, lilyturf root and lotus rhizome.

• For cough owing to Phlegm-Heat or a sore throat, drink water chestnut juice or in a decoction made with arhat fruit.

• In the treatment of red and white dysentery and blood in the stool, take water chestnuts after soaking in wine and drink the wine in which the water chestnuts have been soaked (TYJYF); for abnormal uterine bleeding, take water chestnut powdered, after dry-roasting, with wine.

• In the treatment of dyspepsia and fullness in

the abdomen, take water chestnut alone or with the rhizome of largeheaded atractylodes and fruit of citron; for abdominal mass take water chestnuts together with turtle shell and red sage root.

• For nebula in the eyes, take Dr Chen's Jinshui pills, which are made with water chestnuts and scrophularia root, bletilla tuber, plant soot (Fuligo plantae) and cimicifuga rhizome (ZYYKLJFY).

Preparation

Water chestnuts are eaten raw, juiced, decocted, powdered or made into alcohol infusions.

Notes

It is not desirable for people with deficient Cold in the Spleen and Stomach to use water chestnuts.

Nutritional information

Water chestnuts contain sugars, protein, fat, calcium, phosphorus, iron, vitamins B and C, niacin and puchiin, which has the effect of inhibiting Staphylococcus, *E. coli* and *Pseudomonas aeruginosa*.

KIWI FRUIT (SLBC)

These are the ripe fruits of *Actinidia chinensis* of the Actinidiaceae family. The plant is found in provinces south of the Yangtze River, in northwest China and Hebei. Gather the fruit in autumn and wash them clean for immediate use.

Properties

Kiwi fruit have a sweet and sour flavor, a Cold nature and a propensity for the Stomach and Bladder channels.

They have the effects of clearing Heat, promoting the production of Body Fluids, harmonizing the Stomach, sending down Counterflow Qi and inducing urination.

Application

• For thirst in feverish diseases or dry mouth in diabetes, eat plenty of the fresh fruits or take a decoction made with the peeled fruits and honey (SLBC).

• For vomiting and loss of appetite owing to Heat accumulating in the Stomach, take kiwi fruit juice mixed with the juice of ginger (KBBC).

• For difficult urination owing to Damp-Heat, or caused by the passage of a urinary stone, eat plenty of fresh kiwi fruit or drink the juice liberally.

Preparation

Kiwi fruit are eaten fresh, decocted or juiced.

Notes

It is not suitable for people with deficient Cold in the Spleen and Stomach.

Nutritional information

Kiwi fruit contain sugars, protein, calcium, phosphorus, iron, potassium, manganese, vitamins B and C and organic acids.

Kiwi fruits can prevent the development of the carcinogen nitrosamine in the human body and lower the level of cholesterol and triglyceride.

TOMATO (LCBC)

Tomatoes are the ripe fruits of *Lycopersicon esculentum* of the Solanaceae family. The plant is cultivated in most parts of China. Gather the fruit in summer and wash clean for immediate use.

Properties

Tomatoes have a sweet and sour flavor, a Cool nature and a propensity for the Stomach and Liver channels. They have the effects of clearing Heat, promoting the production of Body Fluids, nourishing Yin and cooling Blood.

Application

• For thirst and a dry throat owing to impairment of Stomach Yin by Heat, eat peeled tomatoes fresh, or crushed with white sugar and steeped for a while before eating.

• For blurred vision and dryness of the eyes, or night blindness owing to deficiency of Liver Yin, eat fresh tomatoes or as a soup made with pig's liver.

• For bleeding gums or nasal bleeding owing to Heat in the Blood from Yin deficiency, eat fresh tomatoes, or take juice made with tomatoes, nodules of lotus rhizome and cogongrass rhizome.

Preparation

Tomatoes are eaten raw, decocted or juiced.

Nutritional information

Tomatoes contain glucose, fructose, protein, calcium, phosphorus, iron, zinc, manganese, carotin, vitamins B and C, niacin, citric acid, malic acid and gynesine. Tomatoes can lower blood pressure and reduce the permeability of the capillaries.

JAPANESE RAISIN TREE FRUIT

This is the ripe fruit of *Hovenia dulcis* of the Rhamnaceae family. The plant is found in all parts of China except the north-east. Gather the fruit in autumn, wash clean for immediate use or air-dry for storage.

Properties

Japanese raisin tree fruit has a sweet flavor, a Neutral nature and a propensity for the Stomach, Lung and Bladder channels. It has the effects of reinforcing the Stomach, promoting the production of Body Fluids, moistening Dryness of the Lungs and inducing urination.

Application

• For excessive intake of alcohol, or thirst and a dry throat owing to impairment of the Stomach by Heat or general debility with an oppressive sensation, take a decoction made with Japanese raisin tree fruit or juice made with the fruit and sugarcane.

• For coughing and a dry throat owing to Yin deficiency and Dryness in the Lungs, take an electuary made with the fruit, pears and loquat leaves.

• For difficult, dark yellow urination, take a decoction made with cogongrass rhizome.

Preparation

Japanese raisin tree fruit is eaten raw, decocted or made into an electuary.

Nutritional information

The fruit contains glucose, malic acid and calcium and it has a marked effect of inducing urination in rabbits.

TAMARIND (DNBC)

Tamarind is the almost ripe fruit of *Tamarindus indica* of the Leguminosae family. The plant is found in Guangdong, Guangxi, Fujian, Sichuan, Yunnan and Taiwan. Gather the fruit in spring, remove the seeds and dry in the air until ready to use.

Properties

Tamarind has a sour, sweet flavor, a Cool nature and a propensity for the Stomach and Large Intestine channels. It has the effects of clearing Heat, relieving Summer Heat, assisting digestion, regulating the Stomach and restoring bowel motions.

Application

• For thirst and scanty, dark yellow urine owing

to summer Heat impairing Body Fluids, take tamarind decoction with sugar added to taste.

• For indigestion, fullness in the upper abdomen, loss of appetite and diarrhea, take tamarind decoction alone or with hawthorn apples and malt.

• For constipation and Heat, take a tamarind infusion made with boiling water.

Preparation

Tamarind is decocted, infused or made into electuaries.

Nutritional information

Tamarind contains malic acid, citric acid, carotin, vitamins B and C.

LEMON (BCGMSY)

Lemon is the fruit of *Citrus limonum* of the Rutiaceae family. The plant is cultivated in Jiangsu, Zhejiang, Jiangxi, Fujian, Hunan, Guangdong and Sichuan. Gather the fruit in autumn and winter for immediate use.

Properties

Lemon has a sour flavor, a slightly Cold nature and a propensity for the Stomach, Liver and Lung channels. It has the effects of cooling and relieving summer Heat, promoting the production of Body Fluids and easing thirst, regulating the Stomach and preventing abortion.

Application

• For thirst owing to Summer Heat or Heat in the Stomach, drink the juice alone or with the juice of sugarcane.

• For disharmony of the Stomach with vomiting and loss of appetite, or threatened abortion, drink a lemon infusion, or take the fruit candied or pickled in salt.

• For a cough owing to Phlegm-Heat, take a decoction made with the fruit and boat-fruited sterculia seed, platycodon root and liquorice.

Preparation

Lemon is eaten raw, decocted, pickled or juiced.

Nutritional information

Lemon contains sugars, calcium, phosphorus, iron, vitamins B1, B2 and C, niacin, citric acid, malic acid, quininic acid, hesperitin, naringin, coumarins and volatile oil.

Feeding dogs with powdered lemon can balance the course of sexual excitation and inhibition. For the average healthy person, intake of powdered lemon orally can improve the working functions of muscles and alleviate physical strain and fatigue. For the sick, intake of powdered lemon can improve acuity of vision and adaptability to darkness.

ROSEHIP (BCGMSY)

Rosehip is the fruit of *Rosa roxburghii* of the Rosaceae family. The plant is found in southwest China, Hunan, Hubei, Jiangsu and Guangdong. Gather the fruit in autumn, remove the thorns and seeds for immediate use, or air-dry for future use.

Properties

Rosehip has a sweet and sour flavor, a Cool nature and a propensity for the Stomach channel. It has the effects of cooling, relieving Summer Heat, aiding digestion and regulating the Stomach.

Application

• For thirst and scanty dark urine due to Summer Heat impairing Yin, take a lemon decoction or infusion.

• For fullness in the upper abdomen, loss of appetite and diarrhea owing to food retention, use the fruit alone or with houttuynia.

Preparation

Rosehip is eaten raw, decocted or infused.

Nutritional information

Rosehip contains malic acid, citric acid, carotin, vitamins B and C.

CHINESE OLIVE (SLBC)

Chinese olive is the ripe fruit of *Canarium album* of the Burseraceae family. The plant is found in Guangdong, Guangxi, Fujian, Sichuan, Yunnan and Taiwan. Gather the fruit in autumn, wash clean for immediate use or dry, after pickling in salt water, to store until ready to use.

Properties

Chinese olive has a sweet and sour flavor, a Cool nature and a propensity for the Lung and Stomach channels. It has the effects of easing the lungs and throat, promoting the production of Body Fluids, easing thirst and detoxifying.

Application

• For swelling and pain in the throat owing to excessive Heat in the Lungs and the Stomach, take the Blue Dragon White Tiger decoction (WSYA) and include Chinese olives and fresh turnips or chew and suck a Chinese olive in the mouth.

• For thirst owing to Heat in the Stomach or excessive intake of alcohol, take Chinese olive juice or electuary.

• For disharmony of the Stomach and Intestines with such symptoms as vomiting and diarrhea, caused by poisoning from a puffer fish, take freshly squeezed Chinese olive juice or a thick decoction made with the fruit (SXJYSP).

Preparation

Chinese olive is chewed and sucked in the mouth, decocted, juiced or made into an electuary.

Nutritional information

Chinese olive contains sugars, protein, fat, calcium, phosphorus, iron and vitamin C.

MUME PLUM (BCJb)

Mume plums are the almost ripe fruits of *Prunus mume* of the Rosaceae family. The plant is cultivated in Sichuan, Zhejiang, Fujian, Hunan, Guizhou and Yunnan. Gather the fruit in summer, wash clean for immediate use, or air-dry after soaking in salt water. The fruit can also be oven-dried at a low temperature and then blackened by covering with a lid. Remove the stones before use.

Properties

Mume plums have a sour flavor, a Neutral nature and a propensity for the Lung, Liver, Stomach and Large Intestine channels.

They have the effects of astringing the Lungs, relieving cough, promoting the production of Body Fluids, easing thirst, astringing the Intestines, arresting diarrhea and stabilizing roundworms.

Application

• For persistent cough owing to Lung deficiency, obtain juice from the fruits, add honey or maltose and sweet apricot kernels to the mixture.

• For thirst due to lack of Body Fluids, take a mume plum decoction alone, with white sugar added to taste, or with lilyturf root and reed rhizomes. White plums can also be chewed and eaten in this instance.

• For obstinate diarrhea and dysentery, take a mume plum decoction with sugar added to taste or the fruits can be boiled with lotus seeds with sugar added to taste.

• For abdominal pain from roundworms, take a decoction or powder made with mume plums, Sichuan pepper and liquorice.

Preparation

Mume plums are decocted, powdered or eaten candied or pickled.

Notes

Excessive intake of mume plums damages the teeth and harms the Spleen and Stomach. They are not suitable for people with Damp-Heat.

Nutritional information

Mume plums contain citric acid, malic acid, succinic acid, tartaric acid, sugars and oleanolic acid.

Cereals, pulses and nuts

Cereals, pulses and nuts all supply seeds or kernels for food and contain little water compared with fruits and vegetables. This makes it possible to store them for long periods.

Most cereals, pulses and nuts have a sweet flavor and a Neutral nature and most of them have the effects of reinforcing the Spleen and Stomach, removing Dampness and arresting diarrhea. Hence the advice in the *Nei Jing* to base one's diet around cereals. Generally, nuts and beans are more nourishing. Some of them, such as pine nuts, sweet almond kernels and torreya nuts, contain a lot of oil and fat and therefore have the effect of moistening the Intestines and restoring bowel motions.

Cereals such as rice, wheat, sorghum and maize are generally rich in sugars and they also contain protein and vitamin B. Nuts and beans are generally rich in proteins and fat. They also contain sugars, vitamins and inorganic salts. All are important sources of vegetable fat for the human body and supply proteins and sugars.

WHEAT (MYBL)

Wheat is the mature seeds of *Triticum aestivum* of the grass family. The plant is cultivated in all parts of China. Gather the seeds in summer and dry in the air for future use.

Properties

Wheat has a sweet flavor, a cool Nature and a propensity for the Heart, Spleen and Kidney channels. It has the effects of nourishing the Heart, reinforcing the Spleen, relieving thirst and inducing urination.

Application

• For hysteria in women with mental health problems, take a decoction made with wheat, liquorice and dates (JGYL).

• For thirst and a dry mouth, take wheat gruel (SYXJa).

• For difficult urination with fever, take a wheat decoction made with ricepaper pith (YLSQXS).

Preparation

Wheat is used in gruels or decoctions.

Nutritional information

Wheat contains starch, protein, fat, crude fiber, sitosterol, lecithinase, arginine, amylase, maltase, protease and vitamin B.

BARLEY (MYBL)

Barley is the mature seeds of Hordeum, of the grass family. The plant is cultivated in all parts of China. Gather the seeds in summer and dry in the air for storage.

Properties

Barley has a sweet flavor, a Cool nature and a propensity for the Spleen, Stomach and Bladder channels. It has the effects of reinforcing the Spleen, regulating the Stomach, relieving thirst and inducing urination.

Application

• For weakness of the Spleen and Stomach with loss of appetite and diarrhea, oven-dried and powdered barley is taken in a decoction with plantain seed.

• For thirst, take a barley decoction or barley gruel made with millet.

• For difficult, painful and dripping urination, take a barley decoction with solids removed, mixed with ginger juice and honey (SHF).

Preparation

Barley is used in decoctions, gruels and as a powder.

Nutritional information

Barley contains starch, protein, fat, sugars, calcium, phosphorus, iron, vitamins B1, B2, niacin and allantoin.

BUCKWHEAT (MYBL)

Buckwheat is the mature seeds of *Fagopyrum esculentum* of the grass family. The plant is cultivated in all parts of China. Gather the seeds in autumn and dry in the air for storage until ready to use.

Properties

Buckwheat has a sweet flavor, a Cool nature and a propensity for the Spleen, Stomach and Large Intestine channels. It has the effects of resolving undigested foods, sending down Counterflow Qi, reinforcing the Spleen and removing Damp.

Application

• For stagnation of food in the Stomach and Intestines, fullness or pain in the abdomen, take roasted and powdered buckwheat, or in a decoction made with turnips.

• For diarrhea, dysentery, gonorrhea or profuse leukorrhea, owing to a weak Spleen and Damp-Heat, *Tanxian's Effective Prescriptions* (TXJXF) records a recipe for dysentery, in which buckwheat is powdered and taken with white sugar; the *Great Compendium of Materia Medica* (BCGM) records a treatment for gonorrhea and profuse leukorrhea, in which buckwheat is powdered and made into pills with the white of hen's eggs.

Preparation

Buckwheat is used powdered, decocted or made into pills.

Nutritional information

Buckwheat contains protein, fat, sugars, calcium, phosphorus, iron, vitamins B1, B2, niacin and salicylamide.

GLUTINOUS RICE (MYBL)

Glutinous rice is the mature seeds of *Oryza sativa*,

of the grass family, cultivated in all parts of China. The seeds are gathered in autumn, dried in air and dehusked for storage until ready to use. Short grain rice is similar but not identical. Most oriental food suppliers carry proper glutinous rice.

Properties

Glutinous rice has a sweet flavor, a Warm nature and a propensity for the Spleen, Stomach and Lung channels. It has the effects of reinforcing the Spleen, Stomach and Lung Qi.

Application

• For diarrhea and loose stool owing to a weak Spleen and Stomach, take stewed pig's tripe stuffed with glutinous rice or powdered rice and Chinese yam with white sugar and pepper added to taste (LCCJYF).

• For spontaneous perspiration and fatigue due to Qi deficiency, take roasted and powdered glutinous rice and wheat bran in liquid millet gruel or rice and bran boiled with pork.

Preparation

Glutinous rice is eaten boiled, powdered or decocted.

Notes

It is not desirable for people with Phlegm-Heat to use glutinous rice. Nor should too much be eaten in the form of cooked rice, cakes or electuaries.

Nutritional information

Glutinous rice contains protein, fat, sugars, calcium, phosphorus, iron, vitamins B1, B2 and niacin.

NON-GLUTINOUS RICE (MYBL)

Non-glutinous rice is the mature seeds of *Oryza sativa*, of the grass family, cultivated in all parts of China. The seeds are gathered in autumn, dried in the air and dehusked for storage until ready to use.

Properties

Non-glutinous rice has a sweet flavor, a Neutral nature and a propensity for the Spleen and Stomach channels. It has the effects of nourishing the Spleen, harmonizing the Stomach and relieving thirst.

Application

• For vomiting and loss of appetite owing to a weak Spleen and Stomach and disharmony of Stomach Qi, non-glutinous rice is often used in combination with such Qi-nourishing and Spleen-reinforcing foods as ginseng, Chinese yam and lotus seeds, e.g. in the Eight Immortals cake (WKZZ).

• For thirst and a dry mouth owing to the impairment of Stomach Yin by Heat, non-glutinous rice is often used in combination with some antipyretic preparations such as the White Tiger decoction (Bai Hu Tang) and the bamboo leaves and gypsum decoction (Zhu Ye Shi Gao Tang).

Preparation

Non-glutinous rice is used in gruels, decoctions, cakes or cookies.

Nutritional information

Non-glutinous rice has similar nutrients to glutinous rice, but contains more phosphorus.

MILLET (MYBL)

Millet is the mature seeds of *Setaria italica*, of the grass family, cultivated in all parts of China. The seeds are gathered in autumn, dried in air and dehusked for storage until ready to use.

Properties

Millet has a sweet, salty flavor, a slightly Cold

nature and a propensity for the Spleen, Stomach and Kidney channels. It has the effects of nourishing the Spleen and the Kidney, relieving thirst and inducing urination.

Application

• For vomiting and loss of appetite owing to a weak Spleen and Stomach, take millet gruel by itself or cooked with powdered Chinese yam, lotus seeds and poria, as in the Six Miraculous Food gruel (WYDF).

• For thirst, take millet gruel alone or millet gruel cooked with the juice of reed rhizome.

• For difficult urination with fever, employ the remedy described above.

Preparation

Millet is used in gruels or decoctions or powdered.

Nutritional information

Millet contains protein, fat, starch, calcium, phosphorus, iron, vitamins B1 and B2 and niacin. In the protein contained in millet, there are such amino acids as glutamic acid, proline and alanine.

SORGHUM (SWBC)

Sorghum is the mature seeds of *Sorghum vulgare*, of the grass family, cultivated in all parts of China. The seeds are gathered in autumn, dried in air and dehusked for storage until ready to use.

Properties

Sorghum has a sweet, astringent flavor, a Warm nature and a propensity for the Spleen and Stomach channels. It has the effects of reinforcing the Spleen and the Stomach, astringing the Intestines and arresting diarrhea.

Application

For indigestion, loss of appetite and diarrhea

owing to weak Spleen and Stomach, take roasted and powdered sorghum alone or together with *Cynanchum wilfordii*, radish seed and poria.

Preparation

Sorghum is taken powdered or decocted.

Nutritional information

Sorghum contains protein, fat, sugars, calcium, phosphorus, iron, vitamins B1, B2 and niacin.

MAIZE (BCGM)

Maize is the mature or almost mature seeds of *Zea mays*, of the grass family, cultivated in all parts of China. The seeds are gathered in summer and autumn, threshed and dried in air for storage until ready to use. Fresh maize can also be used.

Properties

Maize has a sweet flavor, a Neutral nature and a propensity for the Stomach and Bladder channels. It has the effects of reinforcing the Stomach, regulating the Middle Burner and inducing urination.

Application

• For a weak Spleen and loss of appetite, take powdered maize cooked as a gruel with nonglutinous rice, or a decoction made with rosehips.

• For difficult urination or edema, take boiled fresh maize (corn on the cob) or in a decoction made with maize tassel.

Preparation

Maize is used decocted, powdered or boiled.

Nutritional information

Maize contains starch, protein, fat, calcium,

phosphorus, iron, vitamins B1, B2, B6, niacin, pantothenic acid, biotin and quercetin.

BLACK SOYA BEAN (BCJB)

Black soya bean is the mature black seeds of *Glycine max*, of the Leguminosae family, cultivated in all parts of China. The seeds are gathered in autumn, dried in the sun and shelled for storage until ready to use.

Properties

Black soya bean has a sweet flavor, a Neutral nature and a propensity for the Spleen and Kidney channels. It has the effects of nourishing the Kidney Yin, reinforcing the Spleen, removing Damp and detoxification.

Application

• In the treatment of thirst due to diabetes involving deficiency of the Kidney, take Jiuhuowan (Reviving Pills) as mentioned in PJF, where black soya beans and snakegourd roots are powdered and made into pills, which are taken in a decoction of black soya bean.

• In the treatment of edema due to a weak Spleen and beriberi or contracture of the limbs and pain from Damp Bi. For the former, take black soya bean decoction or powdered black soya beans with coix seed and poria; and for the latter, take a decoction made with coix seed and chaenomeles fruit.

• For poisoning or untoward reactions after taking drugs that have a Hot nature such as Sichuan aconite or croton seed, a black soya bean decoction made together with liquorice (BCGM) is often used.

Preparation

Black soya beans are decocted, infused in alcohol, powdered or boiled.

Nutritional information

The black soya bean is rich in protein, fat, sugars,

calcium, phosphorus, iron, carotin, vitamins B1, B2, niacin, saponin, daiozein and genistein.

The daiozein and genistein contained in black soya beans have estrogenlike effects. Daiozein relaxes spasm in isolated small intestines of mice.

SOYA BEAN (BCJB)

Soya bean is the mature or almost mature yellow seeds of *Glycine max* of the Leguminosae family, cultivated in all parts of China.

The seeds are gathered in the autumn. For the almost mature beans, gather the seeds fresh and remove the pods for immediate use; for the mature beans, dry them in the sun and remove the pods.

Properties

Soya bean has a sweet flavor, a Neutral nature and a propensity for the Spleen and Stomach channels. It has the effects of reinforcing the Spleen, removing Damp and detoxification.

Application

• For a weak Spleen and Stomach, or deficiency of Qi and Blood with emaciation and sallow complexion, take boiled soya bean milk; it is also taken powdered with dates.

• For edema and beriberi owing to a weak Spleen, take a gruel made with peanuts and coix seed or soya bean milk.

• For poisoning or untoward reactions caused by taking poisonous food by mistake or hot-natured drugs, take soya bean milk, or in a decoction made with liquorice.

Preparation

Soya bean is ground into milk, decocted, boiled or powdered.

Nutritional information

Soya bean contains similar nutrients to black soya bean, but it is more widely used than the black bean. In addition to its rich content of nutrients, it also contains iron that is easily absorbed by the human body; therefore it is especially beneficial for growing children and people with iron deficiency anemia.

RED BEAN (KIDNEY BEAN) (BCJB)

Red bean is the mature seed of *Phaseolus calcaratus* or *P. angularis*, of the Leguminosae family, cultivated in all parts of China. Gather the beans in autumn, dry them in the sun and remove the pods before use.

Properties

Red bean has a sweet flavor, a Neutral nature and a propensity for the Spleen, Large Intestine and Small Intestine channels. It has the effects of reinforcing the Spleen and removing Damp, dispersing Blood stasis and detoxification.

Application

• In the treatment of edema, beriberi or difficult urination owing to a weak Spleen, take red beans boiled with carp (SLBC) or red beans cooked in a liquid which contains the ash of burnt mulberry twigs. For diarrhea, take powdered red bean, hyacinth bean and coix seed or their decoction.

• Use in the treatment of acute appendicitis; or for dysentery or hemorrhoids with blood in the stool. For the former, take red bean decoction made with dandelion, coix seed and liquorice; for the latter, take a decoction made with purslane and vinegar.

Preparation

Red bean is decocted, boiled or powdered.

Nutritional information

Red bean contains protein, fat, sugars, calcium, phosphorus, iron, vitamins B1, B2, niacin and saponin.

MUNG BEAN (SLBC)

Mung bean is the mature seeds of *Phaseolus radiatus*, of the Leguminosae family, cultivated in all parts of China. It is gathered in autumn, dried in the sun and the pods removed before use.

Properties

Mung bean has a sweet flavor, a Cool nature and a propensity for the Heart and Stomach channels. It has the effects of clearing Heat, relieving Summer Heat, inducing urination and detoxification.

Application

• For thirst from feverish diseases or Summer Heat, drink plenty of mung bean decoction. Honeysuckle flower (Flos Lonicerae) and unopened young bamboo leaves can also be added to this decoction.

• In the treatment of difficult urination due to Heat, take boiled mung beans and orange peel cooked in the liquid of boiled hempseeds; for edema, eat boiled mung beans alone or with coix seed and mulberry bark.

• For poisoning or untoward reactions caused by taking hot-natured drugs such as Sichuan aconite or croton seed, take powdered mung bean steeped in boiling water or together with liquorice.

Preparation

Mung bean is used decocted, boiled or powdered.

Nutritional information

Mung bean contains protein, fat, sugars, calcium, phosphorus, iron, carotin, vitamins B1, B2 and niacin.

Mung bean can prevent the rise of serum cholesterol in rabbits with experimental atherosclerosis and can rapidly lower it if already raised. In addition, mung bean also has the significant effects of detoxifying and protecting the Liver.

COW PEA (JHBC)

Cow pea is the mature seed of *Vigna sinensis* of the Leguminosae family, cultivated in most parts of China. It is gathered in autumn, dried in the sun and shelled for use. Fresh young cow pea pods are also used in summer and autumn.

Properties

Cow pea has a sweet flavor, a Neutral nature and a propensity for the Spleen and Bladder channels. It has the effects of reinforcing the Spleen and Stomach, inducing urination and removing Damp.

Application

• For indigestion, loss of appetite, fullness in the abdomen and diarrhea owing to a weak Spleen and Stomach, take cow peas decocted with glutinous rice root and the root of Japanese bindweed or boiled with pork.

• In the treatment of profuse leukorrhea owing to a weak Spleen, take cow peas stewed with chicken, water spinach and ginkgo nuts. For difficult urination due to Damp-Heat, take cow peas decocted with water spinach and capsella.

Preparation

Cow pea is eaten boiled or decocted.

Nutritional information

Cow peas contain protein, fat, sugars, calcium, phosphorus, iron, vitamins B1, B2 and niacin. Young cow peas also contain vitamin C.

PEA (YSZY)

Peas are the mature or young seeds of *Pisum sativum*, of the Leguminosae family, cultivated in all parts of China. In spring, gather the young legumes, remove the pods and use the fresh seeds; in summer, gather mature legumes, dry in the sun and remove the pods for use.

Properties

Peas have a sweet flavor, a Neutral nature and a propensity for the Spleen and Stomach channels. They have the effects of reinforcing the Spleen, relieving edema, promoting the production of Body Fluids and easing thirst (immature seeds).

Application

• In the treatment of weak Spleen and Stomach, use peas with tsaoko.

• For deficiency of Stomach Yin with a dry throat and thirst, take a young pea decoction or add white sugar to taste.

Preparation

Peas are eaten boiled, powdered, roasted or decocted.

Notes

Boiled or roasted peas can cause fullness in the abdomen.

Nutritional information

Peas contain protein, fat, sugars, calcium, phosphorus, iron, vitamins B1, B2 and niacin.

BROAD BEAN (FAVA BEAN) (JHBC)

Broad bean is the mature or young seed of *Vicia faba*, of the Leguminosae family, cultivated in most parts of China. In spring, gather the young legumes, remove the pod and use the fresh seeds; in summer, gather the mature legumes, dry in the sun and remove the pods for use.

Properties

Broad bean has a sweet flavor, a Neutral nature and a propensity for the Spleen and Stomach channels. It has the effects of reinforcing the Spleen and relieving edema.

Application

• For loss of appetite and loose stool owing to a weak Spleen and Stomach, take powdered broad bean mixed with boiling water and brown sugar.

• For edema and difficult urination owing to a weak Spleen, take a broad bean decoction, or broad beans cooked with pork and wax gourd. Broad beans can also be taken after being decocted with brown sugar.

Preparation

Broad beans are eaten boiled, powdered or decocted.

Notes

Overintake of broad beans can cause fullness in the abdomen. A very small number of people, mostly young boys, can develop acute hemolytic anemia after eating broad beans. Symptoms are hematochrome urine, shock, weakness, dizziness, disturbance of gastric and intestinal functions and the increase of urobilin excretion; in more grave cases, there can be pale complexion, jaundice, back pain and exhaustion. The symptoms generally develop 5–24 hours after eating broad beans. Sometimes the problem can occur after eating roasted broad beans. The major cause of the disease is the dissolution of blood cells which are supersensitive to the vetch alkali contained in broad beans. As food, they should always be boiled for at least 10 minutes.

Nutritional information

Broad bean contains protein, fat, sugars, calcium, phosphorus, iron, vitamins B1, B2, niacin, choline, vetch alkali and glucoside.

SWORD BEAN (TAO TUO) (JHBC)

Sword bean is the mature seed of *Canavalia gladiata*, of the Leguminosae family, cultivated in the basin of the Yangtze River and southern provinces in China. In early autumn, gather the young and soft legumes for immediate use, and in autumn, gather the legumes, dry in the sun and remove the pods before use.

Properties

Sword bean has a sweet flavor, a Warm nature and a propensity for the Stomach and Kidney channels. It has the effects of warming the Middle Burner, sending down Counterflow Qi and tonifying the Kidney Yang.

Application

• For hiccups and vomiting owing to deficient Cold in the Spleen and Stomach, *Medical Steps* (YJ) records a sword bean powder; it is also used in combination with ginger and orange peel.

• For back pain due to Kidney deficiency or distension and pain from hernia, take sword beans powdered or boiled in water. Sword bean stuffed pig's kidney can also be taken after being stewed.

Preparation

Sword bean is eaten boiled, powdered or decocted.

Nutritional information

Sword bean contains protein, fat, sugars, urease, hemocyte agglutinin and canavanine.

SESAME (BCJB)

Sesame is the mature seed of *Sesamum indicum*, of the Pedaliaceae family, cultivated in all parts of China. Gather the seeds in autumn, dry in the sun and shell before use.

Properties

Sesame has a sweet flavor, a Neutral nature and a propensity for the Liver, Kidney and Large Intestine channels. It has the effects of reinforcing the Liver and Kidney, replenishing Essence and moistening Dryness in the Intestines.

Application

• For deficiency in the Liver and Kidney and lack of Essence with premature white hair, dizziness, tinnitus, soreness and weakness in the back and knees, chew sesame seeds. Rice porridge cooked with boiled sesame can also be used to make mulberry and sesame pills (YJ) with honey and mulberry leaves. *A New Book on Caring for the Aged Relatives* (SQYLXS) contains a wine made with sesame, rehmannia root and coix seed. The recipe is especially beneficial to patients with rheumatism with the symptoms of Liver and Kidney deficiency.

Preparation

Sesame is eaten raw, in the form of gruels, pills or oil.

Nutritional information

Sesame contains a large amount of fat. Its major components are oleic acid, linoleic acid, palmitic acid, arachidic acid, sterol, sesamin, sesamol and vitamin E. It also contains protein, sugars, calcium, phosphorus, iron, folic acid and niacin.

Oral feeding of sesame extracts to rats can lower blood sugar and increase glycogen in the liver and muscles, but an overdose reduces the amount of glycogen. Feeding rats with black sesame for 10 days can increase the amount of vitamin C and cholesterin in their adrenalin.

PINE NUT (HYBC)

Pine nut is the mature kernel of *Pinus koraiensis*, of the Pinaceae family, found in the north-east of China. Gather the nuts in autumn and winter, dry in the sun and remove the shells before use.

Properties

Pine nuts have a sweet flavor, a slightly Warm nature and a propensity for the Lung and Large Intestine channels. They have the effects of nourishing deficiency, moistening the Lungs and Dryness of the Intestines.

Application

• For Yin deficiency and Dryness in the Lungs, marked by a dry cough with little or no sticky sputum, the *Medical Records of an Official* (WTMY) contains a decoction in which pine nuts and walnuts are ground together into a paste and then taken with honey.

• For constipation owing to Dryness in the Intestines, *Shicai's Three Books* (SCSS) contains a gruel made with pine nuts and non-glutinous rice. Pine nuts are also eaten raw.

Preparation

Pine nuts are eaten raw, made into gruels, soft paste or pills.

Nutritional information

Pine nuts are rich in fat, the major components of which are olein and linolein; they also contain sugars, calcium, phosphorus and iron.

CHESTNUT (MYBL)

Chestnut is the mature kernel of *Castanea mollissima*, of the Cupuliferae family, found in eastern, middle, southern and south-western parts of China and Hebei, Shannxi and Gansu provinces. Gather the nuts in autumn, dry in the sun and remove the shells to store until ready to use, or shell them before use.

Properties

Chestnut has a sweet flavor, a Warm nature and a propensity for the Spleen and Kidney channels. It has the effects of reinforcing the Spleen and Stomach and astringing and arresting diarrhea.

Application

• For weakness in the waist and feet owing to deficiency of Kidney Qi, eat raw chestnut by itself or chestnut gruel cooked together with pig's kidney (JYF).

• For loose stool or diarrhea owing to weak Spleen, or for bloody stools, take chestnut roasted or stewed or together with Chinese yam, lotus seeds, euryale seed and germinated barley.

Preparation

Chestnuts are eaten raw, boiled or powdered.

Nutritional information

Chestnut contains protein, fat, sugars, calcium, phosphorus, iron, carotin, vitamins B1, B2, C, niacin and lipase.

LOTUS SEED (BCJB)

Lotus seed is the mature kernel of *Nelumbo nucifera*, of the Nymphaeaceae family, produced in Hunan, Fujian, Jiangsu and Zhejiang. Gather the lotus pods in autumn, dry in the sun and remove seeds for use. Fresh seeds are also used.

Properties

Lotus seeds have a sweet, astringent flavor, a Neutral nature and a propensity for the Spleen, Kidney and Heart channels. They have the effects of reinforcing the Spleen and Stomach, astringing the Intestines and consolidating sperm, nourishing the Heart and tranquilizing the Mind.

Application

• For loss of appetite and diarrhea owing to a weak Spleen and Stomach, or obstinate, lasting dysentery, take powdered lotus seeds alone or, as described in *Shicai's Three Books* (SCSS), take lotus seed cakes steamed together with poria, non-glutinous rice and granulated sugar.

• For profuse leukorrhea owing to a weak Spleen, turbid urine or seminal emission owing to Kidney deficiency, take lotus seeds powdered with euryale seeds and cherokee rosehips.

• For malnourishment of the Heart with restlessness and insomnia, take fresh lotus seeds in a decoction of lilyturf root or take lotus seed decoction made with lily bulbs and lilyturf root.

Preparation

Lotus seeds are eaten raw, boiled, powdered or decocted.

Notes

They are not suitable for people with constipation.

Nutritional information

Lotus seeds contain protein, fat, sugars, calcium, phosphorus, iron, vitamins B1, B2, C and niacin.

GINKGO NUT (BCGM)

Ginkgo nut is the mature kernel of *Ginkgo biloba*, of the Ginkgoaceae family, found in all parts of China. Gather the nuts in autumn and remove the outer skin for use dried or fresh after shelling.

Properties

Ginkgo nut has a sweet, slightly bitter flavor, a Neutral nature and a propensity for the Lung, Spleen and Kidney channels. It has the effects of consolidating the Lungs, relieving difficult breathing, nourishing the Spleen, arresting diarrhea, leukorrhea and frequent urination.

Application

• For difficult breathing and cough owing to Lung deficiency, take boiled ginkgo nuts or ginkgo nut decoction made with ginger, perilla fruit and magnolia vine fruit.

• For profuse leukorrhea, turbid urine and diarrhea owing to deficiency of Spleen alone, or Spleen and Kidney, *Binhu's Collection of Simple Prescriptions* (BHJJF) contains a recipe in which ginkgo nuts are powdered with lotus seeds and glutinous rice and stuffed into a blackboned chicken, which is then cooked.

• For the treatment of turbid urine and diarrhea, use ginkgo nut with lotus seeds and euryale seed.

• For frequent urination or incontinence owing to disharmony of Kidney Qi, take ginkgo nuts cooked with bitter cardamon (removed before eating) and mutton.

Preparation

Ginkgo nuts are eaten boiled, powdered or decocted.

Notes

Ginkgo nuts cannot be eaten raw. Eating raw ginkgo nuts or overintake of cooked ones can cause poisoning, with such symptoms as headache, fever, convulsion, restlessness, vomiting and difficulty in respiration.

Nutritional information

Ginkgo nut contains sugars, protein, fat, calcium, phosphorus, iron, carotin, vitamins B1, B2, niacin and trace amounts of hydrocyanic acid.

PEANUTS (DNBC)

Peanuts are the seeds of *Arachis hypogaea*, of the Leguminosae family, cultivated in all parts of China. Gather the nuts in autumn, remove shells for immediate use or dry in the sun to store until ready to use.

Properties

Peanuts have a sweet flavor, a Neutral nature and a propensity for the Spleen and Lung channels. They have the effects of reinforcing the Spleen Qi, moistening the Lungs and dissolving Phlegm.

Application

• For Spleen deficiency and loss of appetite, emaciation and general weakness or beriberi

with edema of the shins, take boiled peanuts alone or with red beans and dates.

• For lack of milk owing to deficiency of Qi and Blood after childbirth, take peanuts stewed with pig's trotters.

• For persistent cough and deficiency of the Lungs, or cough owing to Dryness in the Lungs, take peanuts powdered with sweet almonds.

Preparation

Peanuts are eaten raw, boiled, powdered or roasted.

Notes

For moistening the Lungs and dissolving Phlegm, fresh peanuts are better. It is not desirable for people with loose stool or diarrhea to eat peanuts.

Nutritional information

Peanuts contain fats, protein, sugars, calcium, phosphorus, iron, vitamins B1, B2, niacin, pantothenic acid and triterpenoid saponin.

SWEET ALMOND (SWEET APRICOT KERNEL) (BCCX)

Sweet almond is the mature kernel of some cultivated varieties of *Prunus armeniaca* or *P. armeniaca var. ansu* of the Rosaceae family, cultivated in north and north-east China, Shandong, Henan, Sichuan and Shannxi. Gather the fruit in autumn, remove the flesh of the fruit and the shell and air-dry the kernels for use.

Properties

Sweet almond has a sweet flavor, a Neutral nature and a propensity for the Lung, Spleen and Large Intestine channels.

It has the effects of moistening the Lungs, relieving difficult breathing, reinforcing the Spleen and Stomach, moistening the Intestines and restoring the appetite.

Application

• For cough and difficult breathing owing to Dryness in the Lungs and deficiency diseases, take ground sweet almonds and walnuts with honey and boiling water.

• For loss of appetite owing to a weak Spleen, emaciation and fatigue, *Scattered Medical Golds* (YXSJL) contains a recipe for an artificial milk, in which sweet almonds are ground together with peanuts and soya beans and then decocted for drinking.

• For constipation owing to Dryness in the Intestines, eat raw sweet almonds alone or with walnuts and pine nuts.

Preparation

Sweet almond is eaten raw, powdered, made into milk or cooked in gruels.

Nutritional information

Sweet almond contains fat, protein, amino acids and a trace amount of amygdalin.

TORREYA NUT (MYBL)

Torreya nut is the mature kernel of *Torreya grandis*, of the Taxus family, found in Zhejiang, Fujian, Anhui, Hubei and Jiangsu. Gather the nuts in autumn and winter, remove the fleshy outer skin, dry in the air and remove shells before use.

Properties

Torreya nut has a sweet flavor, a Neutral nature and a propensity for the Spleen, Lung and Large Intestine channels. It has the effects of killing parasites, dissolving accumulated food, moistening the Lungs, arresting cough and moistening Dryness of the Intestines.

Application

• Used in the treatment of hookworm, roundworm and tapeworm parasites or emaciation and loss of appetite owing to infantile malnutrition. For the former, take torreya nut alone or with pumpkin seeds and quisqualis fruit. For the latter, take torreya nut with largeheaded atractylodes rhizomes, Chinese yam and aucklandia roots.

• For cough owing to Dryness in the Lungs, take ground torreya nut alone or with sweet almonds and walnuts in boiling water.

• For constipation owing to Dryness in the Intestines or for hemorrhoids, eat torreya nut.

Preparation

Torreya nut is eaten raw, powdered or roasted.

Nutritional information

Torreya nut contains fat, protein, sugars, calcium, phosphorus and iron. The fats mainly contain linoleic acid, oleic acid, histidine and stearic acid.

Fowls and animals 10

Fowls are domestic fowls and wild birds such as chickens, ducks, sparrows and quails; animals are domestic and wild animals, such as pigs, ox, sheep or goats and rabbits.

The main edible parts of larger animals are their muscles (meat). The meat of these animals is mostly mild in nature and nutritious and can enrich Qi and Blood, or reinforce the Liver and Kidney. Some internal organs such as the liver, heart, stomach, lung, kidney, brain and spinal cord are also used for food and these organs have different effects. Broadly speaking, they can nourish corresponding organs in the human body. This is the general principle of TCM in the treatment of human organ illnesses. In addition, birds' eggs are also effective in nourishing the Blood, Qi and the Kidney.

Animal meat is rich in quality proteins, fat, inorganic salts (calcium, phosphorus and iron) and vitamins (chiefly vitamin B). These nutrients are easily absorbed by the human body and therefore animal meat has a high nutritional value. However, the fat of these animals contains a large amount of saturated fatty acids and cholesterols, which are not good for the aged and for patients with circulatory disorders.

Also, animal liver is rich in vitamins A and B, while birds' eggs are rich in proteins, fat, vitamins A, D, B2 and inorganic salts. The other edible parts of animals also have certain nutrients, which merit separate coverage.

CHICKEN (BCJb)

Chicken is the meat of *Gallus gallus domesticus* of the Phasianidae family. Chickens are raised in all parts of China. They are plucked and gutted, with the outer rough skin of the feet and other inedible bits removed, and washed clean for use.

Properties

Chicken has a sweet flavor, a Warm nature and a propensity for the Spleen and Stomach channels. It has the effects of warming the Middle Burner, nourishing the Spleen, enriching and nourishing Qi and Blood and tonifying the Kidney and the Jing.

Application

• For deficiency, emaciation and persistent illnesses, or edema owing to a weak Spleen, take stewed chicken by itself. For the former, milkvetch root and Chinese angelica root can be used in combination with the chicken to enhance the effect of reinforcing Qi and Blood; for the latter, red beans can be added to reinforce the Spleen and relieve edema.

• For palpitations and dizziness owing to deficiency of Qi and Blood, or for lack of milk after childbirth, take chicken boiled with Chinese angelica root and dates.

• For frequent urination, seminal emission and tinnitus owing to Kidney deficiency, take boiled chicken cooked in equal amounts of water and rice wine (BCGM), or take chicken boiled with the seeds of Chinese chives and dodder seed.

Preparation

Chicken is eaten boiled or stewed.

Notes

It is not desirable for people with excessive syndrome caused by pathogenic factors, or with lingering pathogens, to eat chicken.

Nutritional information

Chicken contains protein, fat, vitamins A, B1, B2, C, E, niacin, phosphorus, potassium, sodium, calcium, iron and magnesium.

Related items – Chicken liver

Chicken liver is the liver of domestic chickens. Wash fresh liver clean for use.

Chicken liver has a sweet flavor, a slightly Warm nature and has the effects of nourishing the Liver and improving acuity of vision. It is used for blurred vision owing to Liver deficiency or infantile malnutrition or night blindness. It is eaten steamed or made into gruels. It also has the effect of tonifying Kidney Yang in the treatment of male impotence. *Prescriptions Worth a Thousand Gold* (QJYF) contains such a recipe, in which rooster liver is used with dodder seed and sparrows' eggs to make pills.

Use one or two livers at a time.

Chicken eggs

Chicken eggs are the eggs of domestic chickens, washed clean for use. The yolk has a higher therapeutic value than the white.

Chicken eggs have a sweet flavor, a Neutral nature and have the effects of nourishing Yin and Blood and preventing abortion. Yolks have a Warm nature while whites are Cool or Neutral. If an egg is hard-boiled, halved and the yolks removed, the cooled whites may be placed directly over closed eyes to treat acute conjunctivitis. They are used for deficiency after a long illness, dizziness, poor vision, lack of milk after childbirth and threatened abortion owing to deficiency of Blood during pregnancy. Use chicken eggs by themselves with drugs such as donkey hide gelatin (Gelatinum Corii Asini). When they are used alone, there are many ways of cooking them, e.g. boiling, steaming, stir-frying and poaching in boiling water.

BLACKBONED CHICKEN (BCGM)

Blackboned chicken is the meat of *Gallus gallus domesticus Brisson* of the Phasianidae family, found in all southern provinces of China and also raised in some regions in north China. They are plucked, gutted and washed clean for use. Bantams are probably the nearest Western equivalent.

Properties

Blackboned chicken has a sweet flavor, a Neutral nature and a propensity for the Liver, Spleen and Kidney channels. It has the effects of nourishing the Liver and Kidney, clearing Heat and reinforcing the Spleen and Stomach.

Application

• In the treatment of high fever owing to

deficiency of Yin and Blood, stuff the chicken with Chinese angelica root, common peony root, *Anemarrhena asphodeloides* and cooked wolfberry bark, sew it together with a piece of string, then cook it in water and eat the meat after removing the stuffing. For anemia due to Blood deficiency, take blackboned chicken soup cooked with Chinese angelica root and dates.

• For profuse leukorrhea, spermatorrhea and turbid urine owing to deficiency of the Kidney or deficiency of both the Spleen and the Kidney, use blackboned chicken together with lotus seeds, glutinous rice and ginkgo nuts.

Preparation

Blackboned chicken is eaten boiled, steamed or made into medicinal pills or powders.

Nutritional information

Blackboned chicken contains protein, fat, calcium, phosphorus, iron, vitamins B1, B2 and niacin.

QUAIL (SLBC)

Quail is the meat of *Coturnix coturnix* of the Phasianidae family, found in east and north-east China. It is plucked, gutted and washed clean for use.

Properties

Quail has a sweet flavor, a Neutral nature and a propensity for the Spleen and Liver channels. It has the effects of reinforcing the Spleen Qi, relieving edema, removing Damp and strengthening the bones and tendons.

Application

• For loss of appetite and fatigue owing to a weak Spleen and Stomach, take boiled quail cooked with pilose asiabell root and Chinese yam.

• For edema owing to a weak Spleen, take boiled quail cooked together with red beans and ginger.

• For soreness and weakness of the waist and the knees owing to deficiency of the Liver and Kidney, make a quail decoction with eucommia bark and Chinese wolfberry. Take the meat and the decoction after removing the drugs.

Preparation

Quail is eaten boiled, stir-fried or decocted.

Nutritional information

Quail contains a large amount of protein and little fat.

Related item – Quail eggs

Quail eggs have a sweet flavor, a Neutral nature and the effect of nourishing Qi and Blood. They are used for deficiency of Qi and Blood from TB together with bletilla tuber. For deficiency of Qi and Blood in infants with a yellow complexion and emaciation, take millet porridge with beaten quail eggs stirred in while still cooking. Quail eggs contain 30% more protein than chicken eggs, 20% more vitamin B1, 83% more vitamin B2, 46.1% more iron and 5–6 times more lecithinase.

DUCK (MYBL)

Duck is the meat of *Anas domestica* of the Anaticae family, raised in all parts of China. It is plucked and gutted, with inedible parts including the outer rough skin of the feet removed, and washed clean for use.

Properties

Duck has a sweet and salty flavor, a Neutral nature and a propensity for the Lung, Spleen and Kidney channels. It has the effects of nourishing Yin and reinforcing the Stomach, relieving edema and removing Damp. A classic (and expensive) dish served in the Dietary Therapy Restaurant in Chengdu uses Dong Chong Xia (Cordyceps) with duck as a strong tonic for

Kidney Yin and Yang (see also 'Pulmonary Tuberculosis').

Application

• For fever owing to Yin deficiency, cough and dry throat, use duck with asparagus root to enhance the effects of nurturing Yin and moistening the Lungs.

• For edema and difficult urination owing to weak Spleen and Stomach, take boiled duck cooked with lotus seeds, wax gourd and coix seed.

Preparation

Duck is eaten boiled or steamed.

Notes

It is not desirable for people with exogenous Cold syndrome and loose stool or diarrhea to eat duck.

Nutritional information

Duck contains protein, fat, vitamins B1, B2 and niacin.

Related item–Duck eggs

Duck eggs have a sweet flavor, a Cool nature and have the effects of nourishing Yin and clearing the Lungs. They are used with Dryness in the Lungs, Yin deficiency, cough with little sputum, dry mouth and thirst. Duck eggs are used with tremella and crystal sugar. In the treatment of nasal bleeding owing to Heat in the Lungs, use duck eggs with acanthaceous indigo.

GOOSE (MYBL)

Goose is the meat of *Anser anser domestica* of the family, raised in all parts of China. It is plucked and gutted and with inedible parts including the outer rough skin of the feet removed and washed clean for use.

Properties

Goose has a sweet flavor, a Neutral nature and a propensity for the Spleen and Lung channels. It has the effects of enriching Qi, reinforcing deficiency, nourishing the Stomach and easing thirst.

Application

• For emaciation, fatigue and loss of appetite owing to a weak Spleen and Stomach, take boiled goose cooked with milkvetch root, pilose asiabell root and Chinese yam.

• For thirst, fatigue, shortness of breath owing to deficiency of Qi and Yin, or for diabetes, take boiled goose cooked with lean pork, Chinese yam, glehnia root and fragrant solomonseal rhizome.

Preparation

Goose is eaten boiled or decocted.

Notes

For nourishment or for the treatment of diabetes, white geese are better.

Nutritional information

Goose contains protein, fat, calcium, phosphorus, iron, manganese, vitamins A, B1, B2, and C.

PIGEON (SLBC)

Pigeon is the meat of *Columba livia domestica*, *C. livia Gmelin* or *C. rupestris pallas* of the Columbidae family. *C. livia domestica* are raised in all parts of China and *C. livia Gmelin* and *C. rupestris pallas* are found in northern parts of China. It is plucked, gutted and washed clean for use.

Properties

Pigeon has a salty flavor, a Neutral nature and a propensity for the Liver and Kidney channels. It has the effects of reinforcing the Liver and Kidney and enriching Qi and Blood.

Application

• For thirst, shortness of breath and fatigue owing to Yin deficiency, take stewed pigeon cooked with Chinese yam and fragrant solomon-seal rhizome.

• For anemia or scanty menstruation owing to deficiency of Liver and Kidney Yin, take stewed pigeon cooked with Chinese angelica root, achyranthes root and dates.

• For deficiency of Central Qi, with shortness of breath, fatigue and loss of appetite, take decocted pigeon cooked with milkvetch root and pilose asiabell root.

Preparation

Pigeon is eaten boiled or stewed.

Nutritional information

Pigeon contains crude proteins and fat.

Related item – Pigeon eggs

Pigeon eggs have a sweet and salty flavor, a Neutral nature and the effects of reinforcing the Kidney, nourishing the Heart and detoxification. They are used for soreness and weakness in the back and knees, seminal emission, dizziness or palpitation and insomnia owing to deficiency of Kidney Yin and Heart and Kidney imbalance. They are often eaten steamed with longan, Chinese wolfberries, magnolia vine fruit or cordyceps. For the prevention of measles, take two steamed pigeon eggs a day for two consecutive weeks or more.

PORK (MYBL)

Pork is the meat of *Sus scrofa domestica* of the Swidae family. Pigs are raised in all parts of China. The meat of male pig is better in quality and fresh pork is better than preserved.

Properties

Pork has a sweet, salty flavor, a Neutral nature and a propensity for the Lung, Spleen and Liver channels. It has the effects of nourishing Yin, moistening Dryness, and enriching Blood.

Application

• For a dry cough, a dry mouth and throat owing to Yin deficiency and Dryness in the Lungs, take pork boiled with glehnia root, lily bulbs and almonds.

• For emaciation, fatigue and dizziness owing to deficiency of Qi and Blood, take boiled pork with milkvetch root, Chinese angelica root and Chinese wolfberries.

• For constipation owing to deficiency of Blood and other Body Fluids, take pork (fat and lean) soup by itself.

Preparation

Pork is eaten cooked or made into soups for drinking.

Notes

It is not desirable for people with Exterior syndromes, with accumulated Damp-Heat or obesity to eat pork.

Nutritional information

Pork contains protein, fat, sugars, calcium, phosphorus, iron, vitamins B1, B2 and niacin.

Related items – Pig's spinal cord

Choose a fresh spinal cord. Remove the skin and membranes and wash it clean for use.

Pig's spinal cord has a sweet flavor and a Neutral nature. It has the effects of nourishing Yin and the Kidney. According to *Recipes of Suixiju* (SXJYSP), it is used 'for hectic fever, profuse leukorrhea and spermatorrhea, and is a good recipe for the aged'. For thirst from diabetes, take pig's spinal cord decocted alone, or cooked with dates, lotus seeds and dogwood fruit.

Pig's lung

Choose a fresh lung, clean it by pouring water through the trachea, or by cutting it into small pieces and washing it clean for use.

Pig's lung has a sweet flavor, a Neutral nature and a propensity for the Lung channel. It has the effects of moistening the Lungs and reinforcing deficiency. For protracted cough with little sputum, shortness of breath or coughing up of blood owing to Lung deficiency, boil pig's lung together with glehnia root, lily bulbs and magnolia vine fruit. Eat the lung and the soup.

Pig's lungs can also be made into a gruel with turnips.

Pig's heart

Pig's heart has a sweet and salty flavor, a Neutral nature and a propensity for the Heart channel. It is often used in medicinal diets to nourish the Heart, tranquilize the Mind and to control perspiration. For palpitation, insomnia and spontaneous perspiration owing to deficiency of Heart Qi, boil pig's heart stuffed with pilose asiabell root, Chinese angelica root and magnolia vine fruit. Eat the heart and drink the soup.

Pig's liver

Choose a fresh liver. Remove the fascia and bile duct and wash clean for use.

Pig's liver has a sweet and bitter flavor, a Warm nature and a propensity for the Liver channel. It has the effects of nourishing the Liver and improving acuity of vision. For blurred vision owing to deficiency of Liver Blood, take pig's liver with Chinese wolfberry and eat boiled or stir-fried.

Pig's spleen

Choose a fresh spleen and wash it clean for use.

Pig's spleen has a sweet flavor, a Neutral nature and has the effects of reinforcing the Spleen and Stomach. For deficiency of the Spleen and Stomach Qi, take boiled pig's spleen together with pig's tripe and non-glutinous rice.

Pig's tripe

Choose a fresh tripe. Wash away the dirt, slime and grease.

Pig's tripe has a sweet flavor, a Warm nature and a propensity for the Spleen and Stomach channels. It has the effects of reinforcing the Spleen and Stomach. For loss of appetite, loose stool, fatigue or infantile malnutrition owing to deficiency of Spleen and Stomach, take boiled tripe stuffed with amomum fruit, lotus seeds and coix seeds.

Pig's intestines

The large intestines of pig are normally used. Wash away the dirt, slime and grease for use.

Pig's intestines have a sweet flavor and a Neutral nature. It has the effect of 'consolidating the intestines'. For protracted diarrhea, prolapse of the anus and hemorrhage from hemorrhoids, take stewed pig's intestines alone. For the latter, also take boiled intestines stuffed with powdered pagoda tree flower in rice vinegar. In ancient recipes, the cooked material was made into pills.

Pig's kidney

Choose a fresh kidney. Remove the fascia and after cutting it up, wash clean for use.

Pig's kidney has a salty flavor, a neutral nature and a propensity for the Kidney channel. It has the effect of reinforcing the Kidney.

For soreness in the back owing to Kidney deficiency, take pig's kidney cooked with walnuts or eucommia bark stuffed in it. It is also used in protracted diarrhea owing to Kidney deficiency, where pig's kidney is taken after being stewed with drynaria rhizome.

Pig's bladder

Choose a fresh bladder and wash clean for use.

Pig's bladder has a sweet salty flavor and a Neutral nature. For incontinence owing to deficiency of Kidney Qi or dripping urination, take boiled pig's bladder together with euryale seed and glutinous rice.

Pig's trotters

Remove the nails and hairs, and wash clean for use.

Pig's trotters have a sweet and salty flavor, a Neutral nature and have the effects of activating blood circulation and promoting the production of milk. For lack of milk after childbirth owing to deficiency of Qi and Blood, take stewed pig's trotters by themselves or with Chinese angelica root or milkvetch root.

MUTTON AND GOAT (MYBL)

Mutton is the meat of *Capra hircus* or *Ovis aries* of the Bovidae family, raised in most parts of China. After the animal is killed, choose a good cut and wash clean for use. Mutton, when used in the text, refers to both sheep and goat meat. Goat meat is far more common in many regions of China and is considered by some sources to have a slightly Warmer nature than sheep. See also Sheep's milk.

Properties

Mutton has a sweet flavor, a Warm nature and a propensity for the Spleen and Kidney channels. It has the effects of warming the Middle Burner and enriching Qi and Blood.

Application

• For male impotence, soreness and weakness in the back and knees, intolerance to cold, profuse urination at night and profuse and clear urine owing to deficiency of Kidney Yang, take mutton stewed with garlic and ginger added for flavor.

• For abdominal pain, cold limbs, fatigue and dull spirits owing to deficiency of Blood with Cold syndrome after childbirth, take boiled or decocted mutton alone or in combination with ginger and Chinese angelica root (JGYL).

• For loss of appetite or diarrhea owing to deficient Cold in the Spleen and Stomach, with cold limbs and fatigue, take mutton gruel cooked with non-glutinous rice.

Preparation

Mutton is eaten stewed, boiled, in gruels or decoctions.

Notes

It is not desirable for people with exogenous epidemic pathogens or with susceptibility to fevers to eat mutton.

Nutritional information

Mutton contains protein, fat, calcium, phosphorus, iron, vitamins B1, B2 and niacin.

Related items – Lamb's liver

Choose a fresh liver, remove the fascia and wash clean for use.

Lamb's liver has a sweet, bitter flavor, a Cool nature and has the effects of reinforcing the Liver and improving acuity of vision. It is interesting to note that while pork has a Neutral nature and mutton is Warm, pig's liver is Warm and lamb's liver is Cool. For night blindness or blurred vision owing to deficiency of Liver Blood, take boiled Lamb's liver by itself or with largeheaded atractylodes with the herb removed after cooking.

Lamb's kidney

Choose a fresh kidney, cut it open and wash clean for use.

Lamb's kidney has a sweet flavor, a Warm nature and a propensity for the Kidney channel. It has the effects of reinforcing Kidney Qi and enriching the Essence. It is used in male impotence, frequent urination, incontinence and weakness in the waist owing to Kidney deficiency. Take the boiled kidney cooked with eucommia bark and saline cistanche. Black beans and common fennel fruit are also used in the preparation.

Sheep's milk

Choose fresh milk for use.

Sheep's milk has a sweet flavor, a Warm nature and has a propensity for the Lung and Stomach channels. It has the effects of nourishing deficiency, reinforcing the Stomach and moistening Dryness. It is used in debility, emaciation and weakness or thirst and in vomiting owing to deficiency of Stomach Yin. Goat's milk, by contrast, is used to tonify Heart Yang.

Sheep's milk can be used on its own or boiled with Chinese yam powder.

BEEF (MYBL)

Beef is the meat of *Bos taurus domestica* or *Bubalus bubalis* of the Bovidae family, raised in all parts of China. After the animal is killed, select the meat and wash clean for use.

Properties

The meat of *Bos taurus domestica* has a sweet flavor and a Warm nature; the meat of *Bubalus bubalis* has a sweet flavor and a Neutral nature. Both have a propensity for the Spleen and Stomach channels and the effects of reinforcing the Spleen and Stomach and enriching Qi and Blood.

Application

• For loss of appetite, diarrhea, edema and fatigue owing to deficiency of Spleen and Stomach, take beef soup; for pain in the abdomen, loss of appetite and loose stool, take stewed beef cooked together with amomum fruit, old mandarin peel, ginger and cinnamon bark.

• For general weakness and emaciation, shortness of breath, spontaneous perspiration and fatigue, take decocted beef cooked with milkvetch root, pilose asiabell root and Chinese angelica root.

Preparation

Beef is eaten boiled and decocted.

Nutritional information

Beef contains protein (consisting of essential amino acids), fat, calcium, phosphorus, iron and vitamins B1 and B2.

Related items – Ox tripe

Select a tripe and wash for use.

Ox tripe has a sweet flavor, a Neutral nature and a propensity for the Spleen and the Stomach. It has the effect of reinforcing the Spleen and the Stomach. It is used in loss of appetite, fullness of abdomen and diarrhea after eating owing to weak Spleen and Stomach Qi. Take boiled ox tripe cooked together with amomum fruit, old mandarin peel and ginger. For deficiency after illness, with shortness of breath and fatigue, take boiled ox tripe cooked together with milkvetch root.

Ox liver

Choose a fresh liver and wash clean for use.

Ox liver has a sweet flavor, a Neutral nature and a propensity for the Liver channel. It has the effects of nourishing Blood, reinforcing the Liver and improving acuity of vision. For palpitation, fatigue, dizziness and bad vision owing to deficiency of Liver Blood, take ox liver decocted with dates. For blurred vision owing to deficiency of Liver Blood, take ox liver decoction cooked with Chinese wolfberries.

Calf's brain

Choose a fresh calf brain, remove the meninges and fine blood vessels with a bamboo pick and wash clean for use.

Calf's brain has a sweet flavor, a Cold nature and a propensity for the Kidney channel. It has the effects of nourishing the Kidney and the brain. For dizziness, tinnitus and amnesia owing to Yin deficiency in the Liver and Kidney and deficiency of the Sea of Marrow (the brain), take calf's brain boiled as a soup or food by itself or steamed with gastrodia tuber and Chinese wolfberry. It is not desirable for the aged and middle aged to take calf's brain for a long period of time or in a large amount because it contains a lot of cholesterol.

Cow's milk

Use fresh cow's milk. The nature and effects given here refer to unpasteurized raw milk. The same characteristics will not necessarily apply to the commercial product used in the West (see section on milk in the introductory chapter).

Cow's milk has a sweet flavor, a Neutral nature and a propensity for the Lung and Stomach channels. It has the effects of nourishing and reinforcing the Stomach and moistening Dryness. For dizziness and fatigue owing to deficiency of Qi and Blood, or difficult swallowing, vomiting, thirst and constipation, drink cow's milk from time to time or in a gruel made with non-glutinous rice and dates.

RABBIT (MYBL)

Rabbit is the meat of *Oryctolagus cuniculus domesticus*, *Lepus tolai pallas*, *L. mandschuricus*, *L. sinensis* or *L. oiostolus* of the Leporidae family. Rabbits are found or raised extensively in China. After the animal is killed, remove the skin, feet, and viscera and wash clean for use.

Properties

Rabbit meat has a sweet flavor, a Cool nature and a propensity for the Spleen and Stomach channels. It has the effects of reinforcing the Spleen and enriching Qi.

Application

• In the treatment of weak Spleen and Stomach, with loss of appetite, fatigue or thirst, for the former, take rabbit decoction made together with pilose asiabell root, milkvetch root and dates; for the latter, use rabbit with Chinese yam and snakegourd root.

Preparation

Rabbit is eaten boiled or decocted.

Notes

It is not desirable for people with weak Spleen and Stomach to eat rabbit frequently.

Nutritional information

Rabbit contains protein, fat, maltose, glucose, sulfur, potassium, phosphorus and sodium. It contains more protein and much less fat than beef, mutton or pork.

FROG'S MEAT (MYBL)

Frog's meat is the meat of *Rana plancyi lataste* or *R. nigro maculata* of the Ranidae family, found in all parts of China. After the frog is killed, remove the skin and viscera and wash clean for use.

Properties

Frog's meat has a sweet flavor, a Cool nature and a propensity for the Spleen, Stomach and Bladder channels. It has the effects of reinforcing deficiency, reinforcing the Stomach, relieving swelling and removing Damp, clearing Heat and detoxification.

Application:

• For weakness and emaciation, infantile malnutrition and loss of appetite, take a gruel made with frog's meat and non-glutinous rice.

• In the treatment of edema, stuff the frog with amomum fruit and radish seed, wrap it in yellow clay or vegetable leaves and bake it dry. Remove the clay and powder the meat. For abdominal distension, gently roast dried frog's meat with mole crickets and old gourd and powder them for taking in warm wine.

• Frog's meat is also used in the treatment of mumps or sores and swelling caused by epidemic diseases.

Preparation

Frog's meat is eaten stir-fried, boiled, decocted or used in medicinal powders or pills.

Nutritional information

Frog's meat contains protein, fat, calcium, phosphorus, iron, vitamins A, B1, B2, C and niacin.

11

Fish, turtle, clam and crab

This chapter deals with edible water creatures including fish, turtles, tortoises, clams and crabs. In Chinese herbalism, they are all included under the general category of 'Fish'.

Most of the fish referred to in Chinese herbalism are Neutral or Mild in nature and are characterized by their functions of reinforcing the Spleen and Stomach, relieving edema and expelling Damp. Many fish are good appetizers. Sea cucumber and shrimps can tonify the Kidney and reinforce Yang; turtles and tortoises can reinforce the Liver and Kidney; clams are Cold in nature and most varieties have the functions of nourishing Yin, improving acuity of vision and promoting the production of Body Fluids. Jellyfish and crabs, however, are not known as tonics.

Fish nutrients are similar to those of animal meats, containing rich quality proteins, amino acids, fats (composed mostly of unsaturated fatty acids) and inorganic salts which are higher in calcium than in animal meats. Oyster, prawns and sea cucumber contain proteins, fats, calcium, phosphorus and iron. Eels and crabs contain more vitamin B2, while prawns, crabs and clams contain more vitamin A. Their nutritional values also vary in degrees.

CARP (BCJb)

Carp is the meat of *Cyprinus carpio* of the Cyprinidae family, found in the waters of all regions in China except Tibet. They are scaled and gutted, the gills are removed and they are washed clean for use.

Properties

Carp has a sweet flavor, a Neutral nature and a propensity for the Spleen and Stomach channels. It has the effects of relieving edema and activating the production of milk.

Application

• For edema, beriberi and difficult urination owing to Spleen deficiency, carp is often combined with red beans, boiled until the beans and fish are well cooked. Eat all the fish and beans with the juice. Do not add salt.

• For jaundice, remove the internal organs but leave the scales on, stew the fish and take the cooked fish at meal times.

• For lack of milk after childbirth, take boiled carp on its own or together with chaenomeles fruit. Carp soup is famous in Japan as a Spleen tonic after childbirth and during convalescence after prolonged illness. The gallbladder is removed and the whole fish cooked with used green tea leaves and burdock root for several hours and eaten complete with bones and scales. See also 'Hiccups'.

Preparation

Carp is eaten boiled, decocted or stewed.

Nutritional information

Carp contains protein, fat, sugars, calcium, phosphorus, iron, 19 kinds of free amino acids, vitamins including vitamins B1, B2, niacin, A and C. It also contains cathepsin.

SILVER CARP (BCGM)

Silver carp is the meat of *Hypophthalmichtys molitrix* of the Hypophthalmicthyinae subfamily, found in the waters of the Yangtze, Heilongjiang, Zhujiang and Xijiang Rivers of China. It is scaled and gutted, the gills are removed, and it is washed clean for use.

Properties

Silver carp has a sweet flavor, a Neutral nature and a propensity for the Spleen channel. It has the effects of reinforcing the Spleen, enriching Qi and warming the Stomach.

Application

• For loss of appetite and fatigue owing to deficient Cold in the Spleen and Stomach, take silver carp decocted or steamed with ginger and pepper.

Preparation

Silver carp is eaten boiled or decocted.

Nutritional information

Silver carp contains protein, fat, sugars and vitamins.

Related items – Variegated carp (bighead)

This is the meat of *Aristichthys nobilis* of the Cyprinidae family. Preliminary preparation is the same as above.

Variegated carp has a sweet flavor, a Warm nature and the effects of reinforcing the Spleen, warming the Stomach and enriching Qi. It acts in a similar way to silver carp. For dizziness owing to deficiency, pan-fry the head of variegated carp, add rice wine, Chinese spring onion and water and bring to the boil.

Gran carp

This is the meat of *Ctenopharyngodon idellus* of the Cyprinidae family. Gut and trim, and wash for use.

Gran carp has a sweet flavor, a Warm nature and the effects of reinforcing the Spleen and warming the Stomach. For shortness of breath, fatigue and loss of appetite owing to pulmonary tuberculosis, take gran carp or its head only steamed.

Black carp

This is the meat of *Mylopharyngodon diceus* of the Cyprinidae family. Gut, trim and wash for use.

Black carp has a sweet flavor, a Neutral nature and the effects of reinforcing the Spleen and Stomach and removing Damp. For loss of appetite owing to a weak Spleen or for beriberi, take the fish cooked on its own or decocted with coix seed.

CRUCIAN CARP (MYBL)

Crucian carp is the meat of *Carassius auratus* of

the Cyprinidae family, found in the waters of all regions of China except the western plateau. It is scaled and gutted, the gills are removed and it is washed clean for use.

Properties

Crucian carp has a sweet flavor, a Neutral nature and a propensity for the Spleen and Stomach channels. It has the effects of reinforcing the Spleen, restoring appetite, relieving edema and removing Damp.

Application

• For loss of appetite, fatigue or vomiting owing to weak Spleen and Stomach, take crucian carp decocted with pepper, dried ginger and orange peel.

• For edema and difficult urination owing to a weak Spleen, take stuffed crucian carp, amomum fruit and liquorice steamed in a bowl over water.

Preparation

Crucian carp is eaten decocted, stewed or boiled.

Nutritional information

Crucian carp contains protein, some fat, calcium, phosphorus, iron, vitamins A and B.

YELLOW CROAKER (BCGM)

Yellow croaker is the meat of *Pseudosciaena crocea* of the Sciaenidae family, found in the waters of the south and east China Sea and the Yellow Sea. It is scaled and gutted, the gills are removed and it is washed clean for use.

Properties

Yellow croaker has a sweet flavor, a Neutral nature and a propensity for the Spleen and Stomach channels. It has the effects of reinforcing the Spleen, enriching Qi and restoring appetite.

Application

• For loss of appetite or diarrhea owing to a weak Spleen and Stomach, take yellow croaker decocted by itself or with Chinese yam. For edema due to a weak Spleen, take boiled yellow croaker by itself, or with coix seed and red beans.

Preparation

Yellow croaker is eaten boiled or decocted.

Nutritional information

Yellow croaker contains protein, 17 kinds of amino acids, fat, sugars, calcium, phosphorus, iron, vitamins B1, B2 and niacin.

BUTTERFISH (BCSY)

Butterfish is the meat of *Stromateoides argenteus* of the Stromateidea family, found along the Chinese coast, mostly in the waters of the south and east China Sea. It is gutted, the fins are removed and it is washed clean for use.

Properties

Butterfish has a sweet flavor, a Neutral nature and a propensity for the Spleen and Stomach channels. It has the effects of reinforcing the Spleen and Stomach and enriching Qi.

Application

• For a weak Spleen and Stomach and deficiency of Qi and Blood, take butterfish decocted together with a suitable amount of ginger and Chinese spring onion or cooked into a gruel with rice.

Preparation

Butterfish is eaten boiled or decocted.

Nutritional information

Butterfish contains protein, fat, sugars, calcium, phosphorus and iron.

PERCH (SLBC)

Perch is the meat of *Lateolabrax japonicus* of the Serranidae family, found in the waters of China's shores and rivers. It is scaled, gutted and washed clean for use.

Properties

Perch has a sweet flavor, a Neutral nature and a propensity for the Spleen, Stomach, Liver and Kidney channels. It has the effects of reinforcing the Spleen and Stomach and nourishing the Liver and Kidney.

Application

• For loss of appetite or diarrhea owing to a weak Spleen and Stomach or edema owing to a weak Spleen, take perch decocted with rhizome of largeheaded atractylodes and old mandarin peel.

• For fragile tendons and bones owing to deficiency of the Liver and Kidney, take perch decocted with eucommia bark and loranthus mulberry mistletoe.

Preparation

Perch is eaten boiled or decocted.

Nutritional information

Perch contains protein, fat, sugars, calcium, phosphorus, iron, copper, vitamins A, B1, B2 and niacin.

MANDARIN FISH (KBBC)

Mandarin fish is the meat of *Siniperca chuatsi* of the Serranidae family, found in the waters of China's rivers. It is gutted, the gills and fins are removed and it is washed clean for use.

Properties

Mandarin fish has a sweet flavor, a Neutral nature and a propensity for the Spleen and Stomach channels. It has the effects of enriching Qi and Blood and reinforcing the Spleen and Stomach.

Application

• For general weakness and emaciation, deficiency of Qi and Blood or TB, take boiled mandarin fish by itself.

• For loss of appetite owing to a weak Spleen and Stomach, take decocted mandarin fish.

Preparation

Mandarin fish is eaten boiled or decocted.

Nutritional information

Mandarin fish contains protein, fat, calcium, phosphorus, iron, vitamins B1, B2 and niacin.

WHITEBAIT (RYBC)

Whitebait is the meat of *Hemisalanx prognathus* of the Salangidae family, found in the waters of Shandong and Zhejiang. Wash the fish clean for immediate use, or dry until ready to use.

Properties

Whitebait has a sweet flavor, a Neutral nature and a propensity for the Spleen and Stomach channels. It has the effects of reinforcing the Spleen and Stomach and moistening the Lungs.

Application

• For loss of appetite and diarrhea owing to a weak Spleen and Stomach, or for infantile malnutrition with emaciation and fatigue, take whitebait decoction made with Chinese spring onion and ginger. For infantile malnutrition, take decocted whitebait with Chinese hawthorn and germinated millet.

• For a cough with no sputum owing to deficiency and pulmonary tuberculosis, take whitebait decoction on its own.

Preparation

Whitebait is taken boiled or decocted.

Nutritional information

Whitebait contains protein, fat, sugars, calcium, phosphorus, iron, vitamins B1, B2 and niacin.

LONG-TAILED ANCHOVY (SLBC)

Long-tailed anchovy is the meat of *Coilia ectenes* of the Engraulidae family, found in the middle and lower reaches of the Yangtze River and its tributary lakes in China. It is gutted, the fins are removed and it is washed clean for use.

Properties

Long-tailed anchovy has a sweet flavor, a Neutral nature and a propensity for the Spleen and Stomach channels. It has the effects of enriching Qi and reinforcing the Spleen.

Application

• For shortness of breath and fatigue owing to a weak Spleen and Stomach, take boiled long-tailed anchovy alone or with old mandarin peel, rhizome of largeheaded atractylodes and pilose asiabell root.

Preparation

Long-tailed anchovy is eaten boiled or decocted.

Notes

It is not desirable for people with sores and scrofulas due to Damp-Heat to eat long-tailed anchovy.

Nutritional information

Long-tailed anchovy contains protein, fat and vitamins B1, B2.

SNAKEHEADED MULLET (BCJb)

Snakeheaded mullet is the meat of *Ophiocephalus argus* of the Ophiocephalydae family, found in most rivers and lakes in China. It is scaled and gutted, the fins are removed and it is washed clean for use.

Properties

Snakeheaded mullet has a sweet flavor, a Cold nature and a propensity for the Spleen and Stomach channels. It has the effects of reinforcing the Spleen, enriching Qi and relieving edema.

Application

• For edema, beriberi and difficult urination owing to a weak Spleen, take decocted snakeheaded mullet together with wax gourd and scallion stalk (the white of spring onion).

• For protracted Wind sores and chronic eczema, stuff snakeheaded mullet with the leaves of canger and stew over a low heat. Take the cooked fish with the skin and bones removed and do not add salt.

Preparation

Snakeheaded mullet is eaten boiled or stewed.

Nutritional information

Snakeheaded mullet contains protein, fat, calcium, phosphorus, iron, vitamins B1, B2 and niacin.

EEL (MYBL)

Eel is the meat of *Anguilla japonica* of the Anguilla family, found in the waters of the Yangtze, Minjiang and Zhujiang Rivers and the Hainan Islands. It is gutted, the gills are removed and it is washed clean for use.

Properties

Eel has a sweet flavor, a Neutral nature and a propensity for the Liver and Kidney channels. It has the effects of reinforcing deficiency, enriching Blood, expelling painful obstruction syndrome and parasites.

Application

• For deficiency diseases or TB, with high fever, take eel boiled in water and wine, with salt, vinegar and ginger added for flavor.

• For bloody stools from hemorrhoids complicated by anal fistula, take sliced eel stir-fried with salt and pepper.

• For Wind-Damp Bi or swelling and pain from beriberi, take eel gruel (SLBC).

Preparation

Eel is eaten boiled, decocted or powdered.

Notes

It is not desirable for people with a weak Spleen and Kidney, after illness or with profuse sputum and diarrhea to eat eel.

Nutritional information

Eel contains protein, fat, calcium, phosphorus, iron, vitamins A, B1, B2 and niacin.

FINLESS EEL (MYBL)

Finless eel is the meat of *Monopterus albus* of the Fruta Alba family, found in the waters of all regions of China except the north-west. It is gutted, the head and/or bones are removed and it is washed clean for use.

Properties

Finless eel has a sweet flavor, a Warm nature and a propensity for the Spleen and Kidney channels. It has the effects of reinforcing Qi and Blood, strengthening tendons and bones and expelling Wind-Damp syndrome.

Application

• For fatigue, palpitation, shortness of breath and dizziness owing to deficiency of Qi and Blood, take finless eel boiled with lean pork and milkvetch root.

• For protracted dysentery, bloody stools or hemorrhage from hemorrhoids, use finless eel oven-baked then powdered, to be taken orally with brown sugar for flavor. Finless eel is also taken boiled with seasonings added for flavor.

• For protracted rheumatism with soreness and pain in the body and limbs, weakness in the back and feet, take finless eel decocted with eucommia bark, loranthus mulberry mistletoe and acanthopanax bark.

Preparation

Finless eel is eaten boiled, decocted, made into medicinal powder or pills.

Nutritional information

Finless eel contains protein, fat, calcium, phosphorus, iron, vitamins B1, B2 and niacin.

LOACH (DNBC)

Loach is the meat or whole fish of *Misgurnus anguillicaudatus* of the Cobitidae family, found in the lakes in southern China. It is gutted and washed clean for use.

Properties

Loach has a sweet flavor, a Neutral nature and a propensity for the Spleen and Kidney channels. It has the effects of warming the Middle Burner, enriching Qi, removing Damp and tonifying Kidney Yang.

Application

• For emaciation and fatigue owing to a weak Spleen and deficient Qi, take loach decocted together with pilose asiabell root, Chinese yam and dates.

• For jaundice of the Damp-Heat type with difficult urination, take stewed loach with bean-curd.

• For male impotence due to deficiency of Kidney Qi, take decocted loach with pepper and the seeds of Chinese chives.

Preparation

Loach is eaten boiled, decocted or powdered.

Nutritional information

Loach contains protein, fat, phosphorus, iron, vitamins A, B1, B2 and niacin.

HUSO STURGEON (SLBC)

Huso sturgeon is the meat of *Huso dauricus* of the Acipenseridae family, found in the waters of north-east China, especially in the Heilongjiang River. It is gutted, the gills and fins are removed and it is washed clean for use.

Properties

Huso sturgeon has a sweet flavor, a Neutral nature and a propensity for the Spleen channel. It has the effects of reinforcing Qi and deficiency.

Application

• For loss of appetite, diarrhea and emaciation owing to a weak Spleen, take huso sturgeon boiled together with rhizome of largeheaded atractylodes, Chinese yam and old mandarin peel.

Preparation

Huso sturgeon is eaten boiled or decocted.

Notes

Overintake of huso sturgeon can cause Phlegm-Heat syndrome.

Nutritional information

Huso sturgeon contains protein and fat.

CATFISH (MYBL)

Catfish is the meat of *Parasilurus asotus* of the Scluridae family, found in the waters of the Heilongjiang, Yangtze and Zhujiang Rivers of China. It is gutted, the fins are removed and it is washed clean for use.

Properties

Catfish has a sweet flavor, a Neutral nature and a propensity for the Spleen and Stomach channels. It has the effects of reinforcing the Spleen and enriching Qi, promoting the production of milk and inducing urination.

Application

• For lack of milk after childbirth owing to deficiency of Qi and Blood, take catfish decocted with chicken eggs.

• For edema owing to a weak Spleen, take catfish decocted by itself or with red beans.

Preparation

Catfish is eaten boiled or decocted.

Nutritional information

Catfish contains more fat than any other fish. It also contains protein and vitamins.

HAIRTAIL (BCCX)

Hairtail is the meat of *Trichiurus haumela* of the Trichiuridae family, found in all the seas of

China. It is gutted, the head and fins are removed and it is washed clean for use.

Properties

Hairtail has a sweet flavor, a Warm nature and a propensity for the Spleen and Stomach channels. It has the effects of reinforcing the Spleen and acts as an alterative.

Application

• For lack of milk after childbirth, take hairtail decocted together with chaenomeles fruit.

• For hepatitis with loss of appetite and fatigue, take the top layer of fat of fresh hairtail after steaming.

Preparation

Hairtail is eaten boiled, decocted or powdered.

Nutritional information

Hairtail contains protein, fat, calcium, phosphorus, iron, iodine, vitamins B1, B2 and niacin.

SHARK (BCJJZ)

Shark is *Mustelus manazo* or other sharks of the Triakidae family, found in the waters of the Yellow and East China Seas. It is skinned, gutted, and washed clean for use.

Properties

Shark has a sweet flavor, a Neutral nature and a propensity for the Spleen channel. It has the effects of enriching Qi and Blood.

Application

• For shortness of breath, fatigue or persistent sores owing to deficiency of Qi and Blood, take shark's meat stir-fried or boiled or together with Qi and Blood enriching herbs.

Preparation

Shark is eaten boiled or decocted.

Nutritional information

Shark contains protein, fat, a number of inorganic salts and vitamins.

Related items – Shark's fin

Shark's fin is the dried fin of the shark. It has a sweet flavor, a Neutral nature and the effects of enriching Qi, nourishing deficiency and restoring appetite. For indigestion, abdominal pain or diarrhea owing to a weak Spleen and Stomach, take shark's fin powdered or decocted.

Shark's liver

Shark's liver has a sweet flavor, a Neutral nature and the effects of nourishing the Liver and promoting acuity of vision. For night blindness, take shark's liver decocted with largeheaded atractylodes.

CUTTLEFISH (MYBL)

Cuttlefish is the meat of *Sepia esculenta* of the Sepiidae family, found in the northern seas of China. Remove the bone and wash clean for use.

Properties

Cuttlefish has a sweet flavor, a Neutral nature and a propensity for the Liver and Kidney channels. It has the effects of nourishing the Liver and Kidney and nurturing Yin and Blood.

Application

• For anemia caused by deficiency in the Liver, Kidney or Blood, take cuttlefish decocted together with Chinese angelica root and peach kernels.

• For lack of milk after childbirth, take cuttlefish boiled with pork.

Preparation

Cuttlefish is eaten boiled, decocted or powdered.

Nutritional information

Cuttlefish contains protein, some fat and vitamin B.

SEA CUCUMBER (BCCX)

Sea cucumber is the whole body of *Stichopus japonicus selenda* or other varieties of the Stichopodidae family, found in the waters of the Yellow Sea and the Bohai Sea. Remove the internal organs, wash away the dirt and sand inside the cavity, boil in slightly salty water and dry in air for use. Soften in warm and then in boiling water before use.

Properties

Sea cucumber has a sweet, salty flavor, a Warm nature and a propensity for the Liver and Kidney channels. It has the effects of enriching Jing and Blood, reinforcing Kidney Qi and moistening Dryness in the Intestines.

Application

• For deficiency of Jing and Blood with emaciation, fatigue or anemia, take sea cucumber decocted with lean pork, with salt and ginger added for flavor.

• For male impotence and frequent urination owing to Kidney deficiency, take sea cucumber decocted with mutton, salt and ginger added for flavor.

• For deficiency of Yin and Blood, with Dryness in the Intestines and constipation, take sea cucumber decocted with tremella.

Preparation

Sea cucumber is used in decoctions and medicinal boluses or eaten boiled.

Nutritional information

Sea cucumber contains protein, calcium, iron, vitamins B1, B2 and niacin.

FRESHWATER SHRIMP (MYBL)

Freshwater shrimp is the whole shrimp or meat of *Macrobrachium nipponensis* and many other species of the Palaemonidae family, found in the waters of all regions in China. Wash clean for immediate use or air-dry until ready to use.

Properties

Freshwater shrimp has a sweet flavor, a slightly Warm nature and a propensity for the Liver and Kidney channels. It has the effects of nourishing the Kidney, tonifying Yang, and promoting the production of milk and the discharge of pus.

Application

• For male impotence owing to Kidney deficiency, take freshwater shrimp stir-fried with Chinese chives, with salt added for flavor.

• For lack of milk after childbirth, take freshwater shrimps, slightly fried, in pig's trotter soup, yellow rice or millet wine.

• For measles or smallpox that fail to erupt thoroughly owing to deficiency, take powdered freshwater shrimps.

Preparation

Freshwater shrimp is used boiled, decocted or powdered.

Nutritional information

Freshwater shrimp contains protein, fat, calcium, phosphorus, iron, vitamins A, B1, B2 and niacin.

Related item – Prawn

Prawn is the whole body or meat of *Penaeus orientalis* of the Peneidae family or *Panulirus stimp-*

soni holthuis of the Palinuridae family, found in the Yellow Sea, the Bohai Sea and the coastal areas north of the mouth of the Yangtze River or around the shores of Zhejiang, Fujian and Guangdong. Remove dirt and internal organs and wash clean for use.

Prawn has a sweet and salty flavor, a Warm nature and a propensity for the Kidney and Liver channels. It has similar functions to freshwater shrimps, but is more nourishing.

For male impotence owing to Kidney deficiency or lack of milk after childbirth due to deficiency of Qi and Blood, take prawns stir-fried after being killed by steeping in wine.

SOFT-SHELLED TURTLE (MYBL)

Soft-shelled turtle is the meat of *Trionyx sinensis* of the Trionychidae family, found in regions from north-east China to the Hainan Islands, including Hubei, Anhui, Sichuan, Yunnan, Shannxi and Gansu provinces.

Properties

Soft-shelled turtle has a sweet flavor, a Neutral nature and a propensity for the Liver and Kidney channels. It has the effects of nourishing Yin and cooling Blood.

Application

• For dizziness, pain in the back and seminal emission owing to deficiency of Liver and Kidney, take turtle meat boiled by itself or in combination with Chinese wolfberry, glossy privet fruit and prepared rehmannia root.

• For loss of blood from abnormal uterine bleeding due to deficiency and impairment of the Chong and Ren vessels, take soft-shelled turtle decocted with rehmannia root and E Jiao.

Preparation

Turtle meat is eaten boiled or used in medicinal pills.

Notes

It is not desirable for people with deficiency of Spleen and Stomach Yang to eat turtle meat.

Nutritional information

Turtle meat contains protein, fat, calcium, phosphorus, iron, vitamins A, B1, B2 and niacin.

CRAB (BCJb)

Crab is the meat or whole body of *Eriocheir sinensis* of the Grapsidae family, found in the waters of all China's coastal regions and in the basin of the Yangtze River. It is gutted, the claws are removed and it is washed clean for use.

Properties

Crab has a salty flavor, a Cold nature and a propensity for the Liver channel. It has the effects of activating Blood circulation, dispersing Blood stasis and relieving Damp. Other sources regard fresh crabmeat as having a Warm and Damp nature, which is borne out by its effect on many people with skin diseases involving Damp-Heat. It is possible that baking and powdering modify its action.

Application

• For traumatic injuries or bone fracture, take an infusion made with crab soaked in yellow rice or millet wine (TYJYF).

• For jaundice owing to Damp-Heat, take crab baked and powdered in yellow rice or millet wine. It is also baked, powdered and made into a pastelike wine preparation.

Preparation

Crab is taken in wine infusions, powdered or made into pills.

Nutritional information

Crab contains protein, fat, calcium, phosphorus,

iron, vitamins A, B1, B2, niacin and trace amounts of cholesterol.

OYSTER (SNBCJ)

Oyster is the meat of *Ostrea rivularis* or other species of the Ostreidae family, found extensively from the mouth of the Yalu River to the Hainan Islands.

Properties

Oyster has a sweet and salty flavor, a Neutral nature and a propensity for the Liver channel. It has the effects of nourishing Yin, enriching Blood, clearing Heat and removing Damp.

Application

• For pulmonary tuberculosis or abnormal uterine bleeding, take oyster boiled by itself.

• For erysipelas or thirst after drinking alcohol, take cooked oyster seasoned with ginger and vinegar.

Preparation

Oyster is taken boiled, decocted or in salads.

Nutritional information

Oyster meat contains protein, fat, glycogen, taurine, eight kinds of essential amino acids, vitamins A, B, C, D, E, copper, zinc, manganese, barium, phosphorus and calcium.

CLAM (SLBC)

Clam is the meat of *Anodonta woodiana*, *Crisaria plicata* or *Hyriopsis cumingii* found in the rivers and lakes in all regions of China. Shell for use.

Properties

Clam has a sweet, salty flavor, a Cold nature and a propensity for the Liver and Kidney channels. It has the effects of clearing Heat, nourishing Yin, nurturing the Liver and promoting acuity of vision.

Application

• For thirst owing to deficiency of Liver and Spleen Yin, take cooked clam on its own in salads.

• For dizziness and blurred vision owing to Heat in the Liver or deficiency of Liver Yin, take clams cooked in dishes, or decocted with selfheal and cassia seeds.

Preparation

Clam is eaten boiled or decocted.

Notes

It is not desirable for people with deficient Cold with loose stool or diarrhea to eat clam.

Nutritional information

Clam contains protein, fat, sugars, calcium, phosphorus, iron, vitamins A, B1 and B2.

MUSSEL (SLBC)

Mussel is the meat of *Mytilus crassitesta* and other species of the Mytilidae family, found in the Yellow Sea, the Bohai Sea and the East China Sea.

Properties

Mussel has a salty flavor, a Warm nature and a propensity for the Liver and Kidney channels. It has the effects of nourishing the Liver and Kidney and enriching Jing and Blood.

Application

• For dizziness, headache or night perspiration owing to deficiency of both the Liver and the Kidney, take mussels decocted with capsella or celery or boiled with preserved eggs.

• For abnormal uterine bleeding, take mussels decocted with rehmannia root and E Jiao Asinii Gelatinum.

• For pain in the back, impotence and dripping urine owing to deficiency of the Liver and Kidney, take rice wine soaked mussels boiled with Chinese chives.

Preparation

Mussel is eaten boiled or decocted.

Nutritional information

Mussel contains protein, fat, calcium, phosphorus, iron, iodine, vitamin B2 and niacin.

RIVER SNAIL (MYBL)

River snail is the meat of *Bellamya quadrata* or other species of the Viviparidae family, found in all regions of China. Wash away the dirt and use the snails raw, slightly steamed or boiled and shelled.

Properties

River snail has a sweet flavor, a Cold nature and a propensity for the Liver and Bladder channels.

It has the effects of clearing Heat, removing Damp and promoting acuity of vision.

Application

• For thirst in fevers, take river snails mixed with yellow rice or millet wine and boiled in water.

• For difficult urination of the Heat type and incontinence, take river snails boiled in millet wine (FSJF).

• For red eyes owing to Heat in the Liver, take decocted river snails alone or with chrysanthemum flowers.

Preparation

River snail is eaten boiled, decocted or juiced.

Notes

It is not desirable for people with deficient Cold in the Spleen and Stomach to eat river snail.

Nutritional information

River snail contains protein, fat, calcium, phosphorus and iron.

Condiments and miscellaneous

12

Condiments refer to such special food items as sugar, vinegar, soy sauce, ginger and cinnamon. Unlike vegetables, grains, fruits and meats which are generally used in large amounts as food, condiments are auxiliary items. Other items, such as fragrant flowers and tea, are used in daily drinks and have special properties, therefore they are also illustrated here.

Condiments flavour food and can make it more appetizing and more easily absorbed. They also have specific functions. For example, sugar can reinforce the Spleen and Stomach, ease spasm and relieve pain. Wine can activate the circulation of Blood and disperse Cold. Spices such as ginger and cinnamon can warm the Middle Burner, reinforce the Stomach, disperse Cold and relieve pain. As for fragrant flowers and tea, they function differently. For example, fragrant flowers are Mild and can dissolve Damp and regulate the Middle Burner. Green tea is Cold in nature and can clear Heat, relieve the sensation of heat and induce urination.

Sugar products contain sugars; vinegar contains amino acids; soy sauce contains amino acids, vitamins and inorganic salts; table salt contains inorganic salts. Therefore, these condiments also have significant nutritional values. As for such condiments as fragrant flowers and tea, they generally do not add specific nutrients to food. Their true value lies with their therapeutic effects.

BROWN SUGAR (XXBC)

Brown sugar is the brown crystals refined from sugarcane juice (see p. 84).

Properties

Brown sugar has a sweet flavor, a Warm nature and a propensity for the Spleen, Stomach and Liver channels. It has the effects of nourishing the Middle Burner, easing spasm, harmonizing the Blood and activating stagnation of Blood. A tea made from mugwort mixed with brown sugar may be used to warm, move and ease the pain of dysmenorrhea from Cold. Most acupuncturists have a ready supply of mugwort in the form of moxa.

Application

• For abdominal pain and vomiting owing to a weak Spleen and Stomach, take brown sugar decoction made with orange peel and fresh ginger.

• *Selected Medical Prescriptions* (ZYF) records the use of brown sugar in the treatment of fasting dysentery or vomiting where the patient is given a brown sugar decoction made with black plums.

• For excessive bleeding after childbirth, take brown sugar cooked with Chinese hawthorn and fermented glutinous rice.

Preparation

Brown sugar is taken decocted, dissolved or powdered.

Notes

It is not desirable for people with Phlegm-Damp or Damp-Heat to use brown sugar. It should be avoided by patients with diabetes. Patients with obesity or high blood fat should control their use of brown sugar.

Nutritional information

Brown sugar contains sucrose, protein, calcium, iron, vitamin B2 and niacin.

WHITE SUGAR (XXBC)

White sugar is the white crystals refined from the juice of sugarcane.

Properties

White sugar has a sweet flavor, a Neutral nature and a propensity for the Lung, Spleen and Stomach channels. It has the effects of moistening the Lungs, promoting the production of Body Fluids, reinforcing the Middle Burner and easing spasm.

Application

• For cough owing to Dryness in the Lungs, take white sugar boluses made with dates and sesame seeds (SLBC) or take a white sugar decoction made with straight ladybell roots, pears and tendrilled fritillary bulbs.

• For thirst and dry throat owing to deficiency of Stomach Yin, take white sugar decocted with straight ladybell roots, lilyturf roots, fragrant solomonseal or fresh lotus rhizome, pears, persimmon, oranges and watermelon.

• For dull pain in the upper abdomen owing to weak Spleen and Stomach, take white sugar syrup made with boiling water (SXJYSP).

Preparation

White sugar is taken dissolved, made into medicinal powders or pills.

Notes

Same as brown sugar.

Nutritional information

White sugar mainly contains sucrose. Today, white sugar is also refined and processed from *Sorghum vulgare var. saccharatum* of the grass family or sugar beets of the Chenopodiaceae family.

MALTOSE (INCLUDING MALT EXTRACT) (MYBL)

Maltose is a sugar product made from grains such as glutinous or non-glutinous rice, wheat, millet or maize through fermentation. Soft maltose is a yellowish brown, thick liquid and hard maltose is a yellowish white, porous solid formed by mixing air with the soft product through stirring.

Properties

Maltose has a sweet flavor, a Warm nature and a

propensity for the Spleen, Stomach and Lung channels. It has the effects of reinforcing the Middle Burner, easing spasm, moistening the Lungs to arrest cough, and detoxifying.

Application

• For loss of appetite, fatigue and abdominal pain owing to a weak Spleen and Stomach, the *Synopsis* of *Prescriptions of the Gold– Chamber* (JKYL) has the following recipe: maltose is decocted with cinnamon twigs, root of common peony, ginger, dates and liquorice.

• For deficiency of the Lung with dry cough, sore throat and shortness of breath take maltose on its own or steamed with turnip juice until the maltose melts.

• For poisoning or unwanted reaction caused by overintake of Sichuan aconite root or prepared aconite root, according to *Prescriptions Worth a Thousand Gold* (QJF), maltose should be taken immediately.

Preparation

Maltose is taken chewed, sucked or decocted.

Notes

It is not desirable for people with fullness in the abdomen and vomiting due to accumulation and stagnation of Damp-Heat in the Spleen and Stomach to eat maltose.

Nutritional information

Maltose mainly contains malt sugar.

VINEGAR (MYBL)

Vinegar is an acidic liquid seasoning made from millet, rice, wheat, sorghum or distiller's grains through fermentation.

Properties

Vinegar has a sour, sweet flavor, a Neutral nature and a propensity for the Stomach and Liver channels. It has the effects of assisting digestion, dispersing Blood stasis, arresting bleeding and detoxification.

Application

• For retention of greasy food, loss of appetite or inclination to eat sour things, take diluted liquid vinegar orally or use vinegar in salads with houttuynia or, as recorded in *Rihuazi's Herbal* (RHZBC), use fresh ginger crushed and mixed with vinegar to be taken orally.

• For hard masses in the abdomen, vinegar is often used in the preparation of drugs that have the effects of dissolving hard masses, e.g. burreed tuber, zedoary or turtle shells. Sometimes these drugs are made into boluses with vinegar.

• For vomiting of blood, bloody stools or nasal bleeding, take vinegar by itself or with purslane and acanthaceous indigo in salads.

• For discomfort caused by eating fish, meat or vegetables, take vinegar by itself, or crushed garlic with vinegar mixed in thoroughly. This will counteract mild food poisoning.

Preparation

Vinegar is taken alone or in soups, as a condiment or in the preparation of drugs.

Notes

It is not desirable for people with Damp obstructing the Middle Burner, Damp Bi or with the onset of exogenous syndrome to use vinegar.

Nutritional information

Vinegar contains acetic acid, succinic acid, oxalic acid, sugars, high grade alcohols, aromatic esters and amino acids.

Vinegar can assist digestion, restore appetite and can be used as an antiseptic and for sterilization. It has certain effects on the prevention and treatment of viral hepatitis and biliary ascariasis.

SOY PASTE (MISO) (MYBL)

Miso is a thick paste made from flour or beans through steaming and fermentation, mixed with salt and water. There are mainly two types of misos, the thick paste and the sweet paste made from fermented flour (plum sauce). The thick paste is described below.

Properties

Miso has a sweet, salty flavor, a Neutral nature and a propensity for the Spleen, Stomach and Kidney channels. It has the effects of reinforcing the Stomach, harmonizing the Middle Burner and detoxification.

Application

• For disharmony of Stomach Qi with loss of appetite, miso is often used as a condiment in dishes. It is also used by itself as a relish.

• For poisoning or discomfort in the Stomach and Intestines caused by eating fish, meat, vegetable or mushrooms, take miso diluted with boiling water.

Preparation

Miso is taken alone, diluted in water or used as a condiment.

Nutritional information

Miso contains protein, fat, sugars, calcium, phosphorus, iron, vitamins B1, B2 and niacin. It also contains amino acids such as cystine, alanine, formic acid, acetic acid, propionic acid, lactic acid, succinic acid and alcohol.

Related item – Soy sauce

This is a liquid condiment prepared on the basis of miso. It has similar effects to miso, but has a higher nutritional value. It is widely used as a condiment. Both miso and soy sauce are available in various grades. The best quality is made from soya beans, salt and water fermented together for weeks or months (some varieties of miso may also incorporate rice or barley). Unpasteurized, they contain many useful enzymes and bacteria which strengthen the function of the digestive system. Cheap products may include sugar, caramel or flavourings and may have been pasteurized for export. As these products are virtually useless therapeutically, labels should be checked carefully and cheap products viewed with suspicion.

TABLE SALT (BCJb)

Table salt is a crystal formed from sea or other salt water. Some table salts are obtained through further refining processes.

Properties

Table salt has a salty flavor, a Neutral nature and a propensity for the Spleen and Kidney channels. It has the effects of adding flavor to food, harmonizing the Middle Burner, reinforcing the Kidney and moistening Dryness.

Application

• For salt deficiency in the body after excess sweating, vomiting or diarrhea, with loss of appetite, fatigue and faintness, take table salt solution mixed with white sugar and boiling water. Commercially produced electrolyte replacement mixtures are available, but a useful substitute is $\frac{1}{2}$ teaspoon salt (low sodium salt containing sodium and potassium chloride is preferable – use slightly more) mixed with 2–3 teaspoons of sugar or honey in a little boiled water. Make up to 1 litre with lukewarm or cool boiled water.

• For deficiency of Kidney Yang or Yin, take Kidney tonifying drugs such as Shenqi pills or Liuwei Dihuang pills in salt water.

• For constipation due to hyperactivity of Fire arising from deficiency of Yin, take slightly salty boiled water before meals.

Preparation

Table salt is used as a condiment or taken in water solution.

Notes

It is strictly prohibited for patients with difficult breathing, cough, edema or diabetes (BCGM). Patients with hypertension should also control their intake of table salt.

Nutritional information

Table salt mainly consists of sodium chloride. It also contains magnesium chloride, magnesium sulfate, sodium sulfate.

Sodium chloride is the major substance for maintaining the osmotic pressure of the human body. When the body lacks this salt, symptoms such as fatigue, dizziness, anorexia, vomiting and abdominal pain will appear, which are signs of low salt syndrome.

LIQUOR (MYBL)

Liquor is a drink made from millet, rice, maize, sorghum and distiller's yeast through fermentation. These are different kinds of liquors made from different materials, by different processes and storing conditions. Classified by the process of fermentation, there are distilled liquor and non-distilled liquor. The former includes colorless liquor (Bai-jiu) and yeast liquor (Qu-jiu) and the latter includes rice wine, yellow rice or millet wine and fruit wine. Here we describe the common Bai-jiu as the standard (non-distilled liquors with a certain concentration of alcohol have the same function as Bai-jiu).

Properties

Bai-jiu has a pungent, sweet flavor, a Warm nature and a propensity for the Heart, Liver, Lung and Stomach channels.

It has the effects of activating Blood circulation, warming the Middle Burner, expelling Cold and aiding the affects of herbs.

Application

• For spasm and pain in the limbs from Bi syndrome, Bai-jiu is often used in medicinal infusions that have the effects of expelling Wind-Damp syndrome and activating the channels and collaterals, e.g. clematis root, chaenomeles fruit and snake. The infusion is to be taken orally. Sometimes Bai-jiu itself is taken with these drugs.

• For deficiency of Qi and Blood, stagnation of Blood with knotted or intermittent pulse, take a liquorice decoction made with ginseng, rehmannia root, cinnamon twig and liquorice boiled in water and Bai-jiu.

• For numbness or dull pain in the chest or a chest pain radiating to the back, take a decoction made with snakegourd fruit and onion in Bai-jiu.

• For excessive Yin Cold with cold and pain in the abdomen, take a small dose of warmed Bai-jiu.

Preparation

To be taken alone, decocted or mixed with herbs or accompanied by certain medicines, pills and powders.

Notes

It is not desirable for people with Damp-Heat or the accumulation of Phlegm-Damp, loss of blood, Yin deficiency and hemorrhoids to use hard liquors. Liquor should also be avoided by patients with nervous or mental disorders, hypertension, arteriosclerosis, hepatitis, cirrhosis of the liver or TB. Pregnant women are advised not to drink alcohol. Moreover, it is not desirable to drink alcohol before a meal or take a large amount in a short time. Long term overintake of alcohol can lead to alcoholic poisoning.

Nutritional information

Bai-jiu contains ethanol, high grade alcohol, fatty acids, aldehyde, esters, volatile and non-volatile acids.

Moderate drinking can promote digestion and

absorption of food, activate blood circulation and dilate blood vessels in the skin. It can reduce the inhibiting functions of the brain.

GINGER (BCJb)

Ginger is the fresh root of *Zingiber officinale*, of the Zingiberaceae family, cultivated in most parts of China. Gather in autumn, remove the fibrous roots and wash clean for use.

Properties

Ginger has a pungent flavor, a slightly Warm nature and a propensity for the Lung, Spleen and Stomach channels. It has the effects of warming the Middle Burner, arresting vomiting, warming the Lungs, arresting cough and relieving invasion at the Wei/Tai Yang level by inducing sweating.

Application

• For loss of appetite owing to weakness in the Spleen and Stomach or disharmony of Stomach Qi, take ginger decoction made with orange peel and brown sugar or ginger juice.

• For cough owing to Cold in the Lung or Cold-Phlegm, take ginger decoction made with maltose (BCHY).

• For the Wind-Cold type of common cold with chills, fever and headache, take ginger decoction made together with purple perilla leaves. Brown sugar can be added to the decoction (BCHY).

Preparation

Ginger is decocted, juiced or used as a condiment.

Notes

It is not desirable for people with Yin deficiency, Internal Heat, eye disease or hemorrhoids to use ginger.

Nutritional information

Ginger contains volatile oil, gingerol, amino acids and starch.

Ginger can promote the secretion of digestive fluids and improve appetite, increase intestinal tension and peristalsis of bowel motions and act as an antiemetic. It can also activate the circulation of blood.

CINNAMON (HYBC)

Cinnamon is the tree bark of *Cinnamomum japonicum* or *C. burmannii* of the Lauraceae family, found in Guangdong, Fujian, Hunan, Hubei, Zhejiang and Sichuan. Gather the tree bark in winter and dry in the shade for use.

Cinnamon bark from *Cinnamomum cassia* is widely used in Chinese herbalism and comes in two grades – the coarse outer bark, called Gui Pi, and the higher grade inner bark called Rou Gui. They are sometimes found in Eastern food shops as cassia (which is technically the correct name for Rou Gui/Gui Pi). When cinnamon is mentioned in recipes elsewhere in this book, it normally refers to this product. The cinnamon used in the West for cooking has milder action and comes from *C. zeylanicum*, a native of Sri Lanka and other countries.

Properties

Cinnamon has a pungent flavor, a Warm nature and a propensity for the Spleen, Stomach and Liver channels. It has the effects of warming the Middle Burner, dispersing Cold, warming and unblocking the channels and collaterals.

Application

• For a weak Spleen and Stomach and loss of appetite, take cinnamon powder. It is also very effective when used together with common fennel fruit, resurrection lily and Sichuan pepper as condiments.

• For deficient Cold in the Spleen and Stomach, with cold and pain in the upper abdomen or vomiting and diarrhea, take cinnamon by itself powdered or in combination respectively with common fennel fruit, Sichuan pepper, ginger, orange peel, amomum fruit or rhizome of large-headed atractylodes.

• For Bi syndrome, traumatic injuries or abdominal pain caused by Blood stasis after childbirth, take cinnamon together with herbs that have the effect of expelling Wind-Damp, activating blood circulation and relieving pain.

Preparation

Cinnamon is used decocted, powdered or as a condiment.

Notes

It is not desirable for people with Fire due to Yin deficiency or for pregnant women to use cinnamon.

Cinnamon can increase the secretion of digestive fluids and help remove intestinal gas.

Nutritional information

Cinnamon contains volatile oil.

PEPPER (XXBC)

Pepper is the fruit of *Piper nigrum*, of the Piperaceae family, cultivated in southern and south-west China. It is gathered from autumn to spring. Due to different times of gathering and methods of processing, there is a difference between white and black pepper.

Properties

Pepper has a pungent flavor, a Hot nature and a propensity for the Spleen, Stomach and Large Intestine channels. It has the effects of reinforcing the Stomach, restoring appetite, warming the Middle Burner, dispersing Heat and relieving pain.

Application

• For loss of appetite owing to a weak Spleen and Stomach, take carp soup with pepper and salt added for flavor.

• For deficient Cold in the Spleen and Stomach, with cold and pain in the upper abdomen or vomiting and diarrhea, according to *Herbal Mirror* (BCJa), pepper stuffed into dates, steamed then powdered and made into boluses can be taken orally. In *The Peaceful Holy Benevolent Prescriptions* (SHF), pepper is used in vomiting, where it is taken in decoctions made with ginger. In *Simple Recipes for Health Preservation* (WSJYF), pepper is used in diarrhea, where pepper boluses made with cooked rice are taken orally.

Preparation

Pepper is used decocted, powdered or in pills.

Notes

It is not desirable for people with Fire due to Yin deficiency, eye diseases or hemorrhoids to use pepper.

Nutritional information

Pepper contains volatile oil, piperine and chavicine. Pepper intake in small amounts can increase the secretion of digestive fluids, improve appetite and help in removing intestinal gas.

JASMINE (BCGM)

Jasmine is the flower of *Jasminum sambac*, of the Oleaceae family, found in Jiangsu, Zhejiang, Fujian, Guangdong, Sichuan and Yunnan. Gather the flowers in summer for use dried or fresh.

Properties

Jasmine has a pungent flavor, a slightly Warm nature and a propensity for the Spleen and Stomach channels. It has the effects of dissolving Damp, harmonizing the Middle Burner, regulating Qi and relieving depression.

Application

• For Damp obstructing the Middle Burner with distension in the chest, loss of appetite or diarrhea and abdominal pain, take an infusion made with jasmine, tea and agastache mixed with boiling water.

Preparation

Jasmine is taken decocted or infused.

Nutritional information

Jasmine contains volatile oils, which mainly consist of benzyl acetate, linalool, linalyl acetate, benzyl alcohol and jasmone.

ROSE (BCGMSY)

Rose is the flower of *Rosa rugosa* of the Rosaceae family, found in Jiangsu, Zhejiang, Fujian, Shandong, Hebei and Sichuan and cultivated in gardens and nurseries. Gather the flowers in spring and summer for use fresh or dried.

Rosa rugosa, also known as Japanese or Kamchatkan rose, is widely used in Britain for hedging. Although the hips are strikingly large, it is *Rosa roxburghii* which is used for rosehips in this text.

Properties

Rose has a pungent, sweet flavor, a slightly Warm nature and a propensity for the Spleen and Liver channels. It has the effects of resolving Damp, harmonizing the Middle Burner, regulating Qi, relieving depression, activating Blood circulation and dispersing Blood stasis.

Application

• In the treatment of Damp Bi and stagnation of Qi, with distension in the upper abdomen, loss of appetite, nausea and vomiting, take rose infusion made together with jasmine and agastache. For abdominal pain and diarrhea, take rose infusion alone. In *Supplement to the Compendium of Materia Medica* (BCGMSY), rose is used in abdominal pain owing to disorders of Liver Qi or Stomach Qi and fasting dysentery, where rose infusion or decoction is taken orally.

• In the treatment of irregular menstruation, coughing and vomiting of blood, with Blood stasis, abscess, swelling and pain, the *Collected Recipes from the Siheting* (SHTJF) records a rose electuary where rose decoction and brown or white sugar are boiled down. The *Herbal Mirror* (BCJa) recommends rose in the treatment of acute mastitis and sores and swellings, where rose or rose powder is taken in wine.

• Rose oil (from *R. gallica, centifolia* or *damascena*) is highly prized for use in virtually all menstrual problems.

Preparation

Rose is used in decoctions, wine or water infusions or electuaries.

Nutritional information

Rose contains citronellol, geraniol, nerol and engenol. It also contains quercitol, amaroid and tannin. The volatile oils it contains have the effect of increasing the secretion of bile in rats.

SEVILLE ORANGE FLOWER (YPXC)

Seville orange flower is the flower bud of *Citrus aurantium var. amara* of the Rutiaceae family, cultivated in southern regions of China. Gather the flowers in summer to be used oven-dried or fresh.

Properties

Seville orange flower has a pungent, bitter flavor, a Neutral nature and a propensity for the Stomach and Liver channels. It has the effects of regulating the Liver, regulating Qi, harmonizing the Stomach and arresting vomiting.

Application

For disharmony of the Liver and Stomach, with

distension and pain in the upper abdomen, discomfort in the chest and the hypochondrium, nausea, vomiting and loss of appetite, take Seville orange flower infusion or in a decoction made with finger citron, citron or orange cakes.

Preparation

Seville orange flower is taken infused or decocted.

Nutritional information

Seville orange flower contains volatile oils, which mainly consist of limonene, linalool, geraniol and citronellol. It also contains neohesperidin and naringin.

GARDENIA FLOWER (DNBC)

Gardenia is the flower of *Gardenia jasminoides* of the Rubiaceae family, found in all the provinces south of the Yangtze River. Gather the flowers in spring and summer for use fresh or dried.

Properties

Gardenia has a pungent, slightly bitter flavor, a Cool nature and a propensity for the Lung and Liver channels. It has the effects of clearing Heat, dissolving Phlegm, clearing the Liver and cooling Blood.

Application

• For a cough owing to Heat in the Lungs or to Phlegm-Heat, with sticky sputum and dry throat, the *Medical Herbs in Southern Yunnan* (DNBC) recommends gardenia decoction made with honey to be taken orally. It is also used with dried or fresh persimmon.

• For a cough owing to Heat in the Lungs or to Liver Fire attacking the Lungs, coughing of blood or nasal bleeding, take gardenia by itself in an infusion or with selfheal and honey.

Preparation

Gardenia is taken infused as tea or decocted.

Nutritional information

Gardenia contains volatile oil.

TEA (XXBC)

Tea is the young leaf buds of *Camellia sinensis* of the Theaceae family, cultivated in south-west and east China, Hubei and Shannxi. Gather the leaves in spring or autumn for use fresh or processed.

Properties

Tea has a slightly bitter, sweet flavor, a Cool nature and a propensity for the Heart, Liver, Stomach, Bladder and Large Intestine channels. It has the effects of refreshing the mind and the eyes, relieving thirst, aiding digestion, inducing urination and detoxification.

There are many varieties of tea. Green China teas have a Cool nature as described above. Some black China and Indian varieties are thought to be more warming and strong tea in excess is considered to cause Phlegm.

Although described as 'refreshing the mind', habitual intake of tea can result in deficient Qi, particularly Zhong Qi. An early woodcut from China shows ladies at the royal court swooning lethargically from the effects of excessive tea consumption and varicose veins may occur in heavy users. Tea tasters provide some interesting clues to other effects of long term tea consumption. One interesting condition is known as 'tea taster's palsy'. It takes the form of partial paralysis, possibly a result of Phlegm blocking the channels. The other, due to tea damaging the Stomach Yin, is the deeply fissured 'tea taster's tongue'.

Application

• For Wind-Heat attacking upwards with faintness and aching in the head and eyes, or for somnolence, take tea infusion alone or together with other herbs. The *Daily Herbal* (RYBC) recommends tea in the treatment of headache due to exogenous Wind, where a tea decoction made with chuanxiong rhizome and the stalk of Chinese spring onion is taken. Chuan Qiong Cha Tiao Wan pills, used for Wind-Cold headache and other symptoms at the Wei/Tai Yang stage of colds and 'flu, are taken with strong green tea for maximum effect. The formula amplifies the ingredients given above.

• For thirst caused by summer Heat, take tea infusion on its own or with black plums. It is also used together with honeysuckle flower.

• For distension in the upper abdomen and loss of appetite owing to indigestion of fatty food, take tea by itself or in a decoction made with Chinese hawthorn.

• For scanty, difficult urination of the Heat type, take tea by itself or with lygodium spores, as in the lygodium spore powder (SJZL).

• For dysentery owing to Heat poison or diarrhea, take tea alone or decocted with black plums. *A Different Herbal* (BCBS) recommends that, for diarrhea, tea should be taken mixed with vinegar.

Preparation

Tea is steeped in boiling water for drinking, decocted or powdered.

Notes

It is not desirable for people with insomnia to drink tea.

Nutritional information

Tea contains caffeine, theophylline, theobromine, xanthine, tannin, volatile oil, triterpenoid saponin, vitamins B and C.

Tea has the effects of exciting the cerebral cortex, invigorating ventricular systole and increasing heart rate, reducing the concentration of serum cholesterol and the degree of arteriosclerosis, strengthening the resistance of the capillaries, inducing urination, increasing the secretion of gastric juice, exciting the metabolism and inhibiting *Shigella shigae*, *Staphylococcus aureus*, streptococcus and *Pseudomonas aeruginosa*.

Part Three

Diet recipes and diet prohibitions for common illnesses

Internal illnesses 13

Traditional Chinese Medicine differentiates internal illnesses carefully, supplementing deficiency, reducing excess and regulating the function of the Vital Organs, and in diet therapy this differentiation is equally important. Since the Spleen and Stomach are the foundation of Postnatal Qi (i.e. the Qi necessary to sustain life after birth), it is important to regulate and protect their function during illness and to avoid dietary items which could damage them.

For the purposes of this book, internal illnesses include externally originating fevers including epidemics.

Epidemic exterior diseases may penetrate through the various levels into the interior of the body as Heat or Fire to damage the Yin and generate Wind, which in turn can cause the Blood to flow recklessly.

Dietary Therapy in these instances should therefore focus on clearing Heat, cooling Blood and nourishing and protecting the Yin. Generally foods with a Warm or Dry nature, a fragrant smell or a pungent spicy taste should be avoided in these situations as they could increase the Heat and further damage the Yin. Light and cool foods are preferred. Damp may also be present, particularly in lingering conditions. If it is, it should be resolved or relieved through dietary measures.

THE COMMON COLD

The common cold is caused by Wind invading the human body. It is a common disease characterized by headache, nasal obstruction, running nose, sneezing, fever and chills.

The common cold is due to abnormal extremes of temperature or fatigue, causing the striae of skin and muscles to become loosely open and Wei Qi to become weak. When the weather changes radically, pathogenic factors invade the Lungs and cause the disease.

Generally there are two types of common cold, the Wind- Cold type and the Wind-Heat type. When seasonal factors are involved, these may induce Cold-Damp or summer Heat (an epidemic occurring specifically in summer and sometimes combining with Damp). People in good physical condition will mainly manifest diseases with superficial symptoms which are more easily relieved; the aged and the fragile have a weaker defence against pathogens, which will enter into the inner parts of the body and aggravate the condition. In patients in poor health there may be Yang or Yin deficiency.

Recommended foods

It is desirable for patients with the common cold to have soft and liquid food, e.g. thin porridge, noodles, lotus rhizome powder and fresh vegetables. According to the patient's condition, foods that can promote the dispersing of Cold by means of inducing perspiration should be used, e.g. ginger, spring onion, coriander, chillies; or foods that can help disperse Wind-Heat and clear Heat, e.g. fresh mulberry leaves, Chinese cabbage, mung beans, turnips and pears.

Foods to avoid

Generally, greasy food, seafood and tonifying foods are to be avoided.

Diet recipes

Cold of the Wind-Cold type

Symptoms are nasal obstruction, sneezing, running nose, itching in the throat, coughing, profuse liquid sputum or, in more serious cases, chills and fever, headache and body aching, lack of sweating, tongue coating thin and white, pulse floating or floating and tense. Dietary Therapy should be directed at relieving the exterior syndrome by means of dispersing Cold.

The recommended diet is a ginger and brown sugar infusion, made with 10 g of ginger mixed with a suitable amount of brown sugar in boiling water. Fresh ginger is more effective for exterior symptoms such as this, but dried ginger may be used. Drink the liquid as tea.

Ginger can help relieve the exterior syndrome by inducing perspiration. In cases with chills and lack of sweating, 6 g of perilla leaves can be added to the infusion.

Alternatively ginger and the stalk of spring onion, 12 g each, with 50–100 g of unpolished non-glutinous rice can be made into a gruel to be taken orally according to *The Verified Records of Diet* (YSBL). For those who have Yang-Qi deficiency, this recipe can be adapted by adding milkvetch root and dates, 15 g each, to the ginger and brown sugar infusion.

Cold of the Wind-Heat type

Symptoms are fever, slight intolerance to cold and wind, sweating, headache and faintness, nasal obstruction, running nose, dry mouth and thirst, sore throat, coughing, yellow and sticky sputum, tongue coating thin and yellow, pulse floating and rapid. Dietary Therapy should be directed at relieving the Wind and Heat syndrome.

The recommended diet is mulberry leaves and chrysanthemum, 6 g each, and 3 g of peppermint mixed with a suitable amount of white sugar in boiling water to be taken as tea.

The mulberry leaves, chrysanthemum and peppermint are both foods and medicines, which can disperse Wind-Heat and clear the head and eyes; white sugar is a condiment and can promote the production of Body Fluids to moisten the Dryness. For patients with deficiency of Yin, the recipe can be modified by adding dwarf lilyturf root and the stem of dendrobium, 12 g each, to nourish Yin by promoting the production of Body Fluids.

Cold with damp

Symptoms are fever, chills, heaviness in the head, pain and weakness in the limbs, general fatigue, loss of appetite, white tongue coating, soft pulse. Dietary Therapy should be directed at relieving the exterior syndrome and removing Damp.

The recommended diet is a decoction made with 10 g of purple perilla (wrapped in cloth) and 30 g of coix seeds. Boil the latter in water and add the purple perilla when the coix seeds are cooked and soft. Boil for a few minutes, then take out the purple perilla. Add some brown sugar for flavor. Drink the decoction and eat the coix seeds.

Purple perilla can relieve exterior syndrome, disperse Cold and regulate the Stomach. Coix seeds can remove Damp and promote urination.

Cold with summer-Heat and Damp

Symptoms are fever, intolerance to wind, sweating, dizziness and heaviness in the head, pain and weakness all over, great thirst, scanty dark urine, red tongue with yellow greasy coating, soft and rapid pulse. Dietary Therapy should be directed at removing the summer-Heat, resolving Damp and relieving exterior syndrome.

The recommended diet is a decoction of honeysuckle flower 10 g, lotus leaf 15 g, peppermint 6 g, and skin of watermelon (chopped) 60 g. Boil the watermelon skin first, then the rest. Take the strained decoction with some white sugar added for flavor.

Peppermint can relieve the Wind and exterior syndromes. Honeysuckle flowers, lotus leaves and the skin of watermelon can clear Heat and relieve the summer-Heat syndrome. The skin of watermelon can also remove Damp and promote urination.

EPIDEMIC FEBRILE DISEASES (IN THE FOUR LEVELS)

Epidemic febrile diseases are represented by Wind epidemic febrile diseases, including spring epidemic febrile disease, summer febrile disease and autumn Dryness.

Epidemics are viewed as passing from superficial to deep layers of the Qi system. The penetration may be considered in terms of :

- The Six Stages (Tai Yang, Yang Ming, Shao Yang, Tai Yin, Shao Yin, Jue Yin)
- The Four Levels (Wei (Defensive Qi), Qi, Ying (Nutritive Qi), Xue (Blood))
- The Three Burners (Upper – Pericardium and Lungs; Middle – Stomach, Colon and Spleen; Lower – Kidney and Liver)

The Four Levels framework was developed to explain the progression of Heat-induced epidemics in particular. If internal conditions predispose, the exterior pathogen may pass rapidly through the levels or directly affect one of the deeper levels.

This group of epidemic febrile diseases is characterized by fever without Damp; clinical symptoms are marked feverish symptoms and unusually high fever, which is often accompanied by great thirst and a red tongue with yellow coating. When the disease has entered the phase of Ying/Blood, there can be a dark red tongue, macular eruption, even delirium and convulsion.

Epidemic febrile diseases are caused by exposure to Yang pathogens such as Wind-Heat, summer-Heat or Dry-Heat. The disease first invades the Lung defence system and causes disease in the external defence of the body; then it spreads rapidly into the Lung and the Stomach, which means the disease has reached the Qi level. Symptoms will indicate which level is affected. Because of the different causes and the different physical conditions of the patients, clinical manifestations are inevitably varied.

Recommended foods

Food that is light in taste and soft and liquid in texture is recommended. Examples are lotus rhizome starch, soya bean milk, gruel and fresh vegetables. Depending on the patient's condition, different foods should be used. For patients with pathogens invading the Lung defence mechanism, use infusions which disperse Wind-Heat, such as chrysanthemum, mulberry leaves and peppermint. For patients with pathogens reaching the Qi phase, use foods which will clear Heat or promote the production of Body Fluids, such as Chinese cabbage, turnips, balsam pears, watermelon, lotus rhizome and sugarcane. For patients with pathogens entering into Ying/Blood, use foods that can help clear Heat and cool Blood, such as young bamboo leaves, lotus plumule, tomatoes, capsella and purslane. For patients with Heat impairing the genuine Yin, use foods that will nourish and nurture Yin, such as mussels, tortoise meat, turtle or cuttlefish.

Foods to avoid

Generally, foods that have a pungent taste, fragrant smell and Warm or Hot nature should be avoided or taken with care. Examples are ginger, garlic, chillies, fermented glutinous rice, wine, mutton, fried or roasted food. Moreover, it is important not to eat too much.

Diet recipes

Pathogens invading the Wei and Qi

Symptoms include fever, slight intolerance to wind and cold, absent or little sweating, faintness or headache, coughing, slight thirst, red tongue with a thin and white coating, floating and rapid pulse. Dietary Therapy should be directed at relieving the exterior syndrome by using drugs that have a pungent taste and a Cool nature, which can purge Heat from the Lungs.

The recommended diet is an infusion of mulberry leaves, chrysanthemum and crushed almonds, 6 g each, 3 g of peppermint and 250 g of turnip. Chop up the turnip and crush it to obtain the juice. Steep the other items in boiling water for two or three changes of water, i.e. they may be used to make three batches of infusion before being discarded (see Introduction). Strain and take the infusion mixed with turnip juice, adding suitable amounts of white sugar for flavor.

Mulberry leaves, chrysanthemum and peppermint are pungent in taste and Cool in nature and have the effect of relieving the exterior syndrome. Peppermint and almond can move and regulate the Lung Qi and turnip is used to clear Heat and promote the production of Body Fluids.

Pathogens at the Qi level

Symptoms are high fever, profuse perspiration, red face and great thirst, a yellow and dry tongue coating, and a full and rapid pulse. Dietary Therapy should be administered to clear Heat and protect the Body Fluids, using gypsum and reed rhizome gruel (SYXJa).

The recommended diet is fresh reed rhizome 30 g, gypsum 60 g, decocted and strained. Put in 100 g of non-glutinous rice and add some more water to make a liquid gruel to be taken with some white sugar added for flavor.

Fresh reed rhizome and gypsum can both clear full Heat in the Qi phase and protect Body Fluids. Non-glutinous rice can nourish Stomach Qi.

Heat at the Ying/Blood level

Symptoms are fever, dry mouth, restlessness, semiconsciousness or delirium, macular eruption, nasal bleeding, vomiting of blood, a dark red tongue and rapid pulse. Dietary Therapy should be administered to clear Heat and cool the Blood by using, for example, the modified Ying clearing decoction of honeysuckle flower and rehmannia root, 15 g each, lilyturf root 12 g, young bamboo leaves 6 g, cogongrass rhizome 30 g.

First put the rehmannia root and lilyturf root in water and bring to the boil. Then put the other ingredients in and simmer. Strain the decoction, add honey or white sugar for flavor and take regularly.

This recipe is an adaptation from a decoction for clearing up Ying Heat (WBTB). Honeysuckle and young unfolded bamboo leaves can clear the Mind and purge Heat; rehmannia and lilyturf root clear Heat and nourish Yin, and rehmannia and cogongrass rhizome can cool the Blood and arrest bleeding.

Yin impairment of the Lungs and Stomach

Symptoms are slight fever or no fever, dry coughing, little or no sputum, dry mouth, thirst, red tongue with little coating and a thready pulse. Dietary Therapy should be administered to nourish Yin and promote the production of Body Fluids by using, for example, the five-juice mix, as follows.

Fresh lotus rhizome, pears, waterchestnuts, reed rhizome and lilyturf root in suitable amounts (lilyturf root about 60 g, other items not less than 200 g) are cut up and crushed to obtain the juice, which should be taken cold or warm.

All these items can nourish Yin and promote the production of Body Fluids, while reed rhizome, pears and waterchestnuts can also clear up Heat. The recipe can also be adapted by using rehmannia, fresh dendrobium, fresh reed rhizome, pears and sugarcane, which is the new five-juice mix formulated in the *Revised General*

Treatise on Febrile Diseases (CDGWRL), which has the same actions.

Excessive Heat agitating Wind

Symptoms are high fever, thirst, faintness and headache, hot sensation in the hands and feet, possible clonic convulsion, red tongue with yellow coating, a taut and rapid pulse. Dietary Therapy should be administered to clear the Liver and relieve Wind syndrome by using, for example, hooked uncaria and rehmannia root, 15 g each decocted and strained, mixed with celery and turnip 250 g each, chopped up and crushed to obtain the juice. Add white sugar for flavor. To be taken in 3–4 servings.

Hooked uncaria and celery can relieve Liver Wind, rehmannia root can nourish Yin and regulate the Liver and turnip can clear up Heat and promote the production of Body Fluids.

Impairment of Liver and Kidney Yin

Symptoms are slight fever, hot sensation in the palms and soles, dry throat and tongue, lassitude or clonic convulsion, a dry and dark red tongue with scanty tongue coating, a threadxy and rapid pulse or an empty and large pulse. Dietary Therapy should be administered to nourish Yin and nurture Body Fluids.

The recommended diet is the minor wind-calming pearl (WBTB), comprising the yolk of one fresh chicken egg, E Jiao 6 g, tortoise plastron 18 g, shelled mussels 9 g and a suitable amount of water. First boil the tortoise plastron and mussels. Remove the residue, add the E Jiao and heat until the gelatin melts. Put in the yolk mix well and take in one dose.

Egg yolk and E Jiao can nourish Yin and nurture Body Fluids; mussels and tortoise plastron can nourish Yin and suppress rising Yang.

DAMP-HEAT SYNDROME

This term refers to the Damp type of epidemic febrile diseases, including summer-Damp and latent summer- Heat. This group of diseases is characterized by the combination of Damp and Heat syndrome; clinically, there is an excessive Heat as well as stagnation of Damp.

The illness has a relatively slow evolution and tends to be protracted. At first, the major symptoms are afternoon fever, heaviness and aching in the body, stuffness in the chest and in the upper abdomen, yellow and greasy tongue coating and a slow pulse. The Damp-Heat syndrome is mostly seen in summer and autumn when the weather is wet and in persons who are prone to Damp-Heat or who have internal Damp. The external factors and the internal factors interact to cause this group of diseases.

Although the aetiology and development of the illness involve the Wei Qi and Ying/Blood, it mainly lingers in the Qi phase and affects mainly the Spleen and Stomach. The condition of the Central Qi is the key to the proportion of Damp and Heat. In the later stages, there can be Dryness with hemofecia, pathogenic factor remaining and Cold impairing Yang.

Recommended foods

It is desirable for patients with this group of diseases to have diets that are light in taste, liquid and soft in texture. It is best to use foods with a pungent taste, that have the effects of removing Damp and clearing up Heat, e.g. peppermint, fresh agastache, lotus leaves, tsaoko, coix seeds, soya bean sprouts, fresh bamboo leaves, wax gourd and jasmine.

Foods to avoid

Patients should avoid foods that are fatty and rich in taste, fried or sauced, foods that can increase Heat and aggravate Damp or foods that tend to be too sweet and are not easy to digest.

Diet recipes

Obstruction of Wei Qi by pathogenic factors

Symptoms are chills, recessive fever that is

higher in the afternoon, severe headache, heaviness and pain in the body, fullness in the chest and the upper abdomen, no desire to drink, white and greasy tongue coating, and a soft and slow pulse. Dietary Therapy should employ fragrant and pungent foods to disperse and absorb Damp. A recommended gruel uses fresh agastache 10 g, half of a fresh lotus leaf, fresh reed rhizome 30 g, coix seeds and non-glutinous rice, 50 g each, decocted in a suitable amount of water and strained. Put the coix seeds and non-glutinous rice in the liquid and make a gruel. Meanwhile, soak the agastache and lotus leaf in hot water and obtain the juice. Add this to the gruel when it is ready and bring to the boil. The gruel is to be taken twice a day. White sugar may be added for flavor if desired.

The fragrant and pungent agastache can disperse Damp in the exterior of the body and purify turbidity; lotus leaf can raise the clear Yang Qi in the Spleen and Stomach to help absorb Damp and turbidity; reed rhizome and coix seeds can clear up Heat and remove Damp.

Stagnation of Damp in the Middle Burner

Symptoms are afternoon fever, distension in the upper abdomen, vomiting, loss of appetite and thirst, loose and difficult stool, scanty urine, tongue coating that is pale white or turbid and greasy. Diet therapy should be directed at relieving Damp and regulating Qi.

Make a gruel with coix seeds 60 g, flat beans 60 g and non-glutinous rice 50 g in water; infuse the shells of cardamon seeds and orange peel, 3 g each, and strain the liquid, which is then added to the cooked gruel and brought to the boil. To be taken twice a day. White sugar may be added for flavor if desired.

Coix seeds and flat beans can reinforce the Spleen and remove Damp, the shells of cardamon seeds and orange peel can regulate Qi and absorb Damp. For cases with high fever, omit flat beans and orange peel and add the liquid from a reed rhizome and bamboo leaf decoction. The adapted recipe is more effective in clearing up and purging Heat pathogens.

Dryness and hemofecia

Symptoms are feverishness, blood in the stool and a dark red tongue. Dietary Therapy should be directed at cooling the Blood and arresting bleeding.

A recommended recipe is rehmannia root 30 g and fresh honeysuckle flowers 15 g, infused in boiling water or boiled slightly, then strained. Liquidize 120 g of fresh purslane and strain it. Mix the two juices thoroughly and take cold. White sugar may be added for flavor if necessary.

The three items are all effective in clearing up Heat, cooling the Blood and arresting bleeding. In addition, rehmannia root can nourish Yin and moisten Dryness.

Pathogenic factor remaining

Symptoms include slight stuffiness in the chest and upper abdomen, poor appetite, thin and greasy tongue coating. Diet therapy should be directed at resolving and purging the pathogen by using drugs that are light and clear in nature and fragrant in smell. A recommended diet is a decoction of reed rhizome and the five leaves (WRJW). Take 10 g each of the leaves of eupatorium, agastache, peppermint, lotus and loquat and 30 g of reed rhizome. Boil the items (for not more than 10 min) in a suitable amount of water, strain the liquid and take with a little bit of white sugar added for flavor.

Reed rhizome, loquat leaves and peppermint leaves can clear up remaining Heat, while the leaves of eupatorium, agastache and lotus can disperse Damp and turbidity, invigorate the Spleen and regulate the Stomach.

Pathogens turning to Cold and impairing Yang

Symptoms are a pale complexion, feeling cold, lassitude, cold limbs, scanty urine, a pale tongue with a white and greasy or slippery tongue coating, a deep and thready pulse. Dietary Therapy should warm the Middle Burner and the Kidney.

A recommended diet is a thick soup made with sliced giant typhonium tuber 10 g boiled in a suitable amount of water to remove the disagreeable taste. Add 250 g of diced mutton to the liquid and boil on a low heat till the meat is cooked. Add ginger and orange peel, 6 g each and cook till the meat is well done. Add salt and spring onion for flavor. Take the meat and soup at mealtimes.

Sliced giant typhonium tuber and mutton can warm and nourish the Kidney Yang. Ginger and orange peel can warm and reinforce the Stomach and alleviate Damp.

COUGH

Cough is a common symptom in diseases of the respiratory system. It may be attributed to external invasion or internal impairment of the Lungs which fail to ventilate and send down the Counterflow Qi.

Exogenous cough is caused by the invasion of external pathogens into the Lungs, which obstruct the Lung Qi. Cough due to internal impairment is due to both excessive pathogens and deficiency of the body's resistance. The pathogenic factors are mainly Phlegm and Fire.

Recommended foods

For patients with a cough, it is desirable to have food with a light flavor or food that will help dissolve Phlegm and arrest coughing. For the Cold syndrome, ginger and leaf mustard are advisable; for a Heat syndrome, such foods as Chinese cabbage, crown daisy chrysanthemum, turnip, bamboo shoots and persimmons are recommended. For patients with a deficient cough, use foods that have the property of reinforcing and moistening the Lungs or nourishing Yin, such as loquats, oranges, pears, persimmons, lily bulb, walnuts and honey.

Foods to avoid

Do not take seafood, greasy, sweet or hot, spicy food, such as fish, prawns, fatty meat, pepper, chillies or garlic. Food should not be too salty or too sweet. Alcohol and tobacco are also to be avoided.

Diet recipes

Cough due to Wind-Cold invading the Lungs

Symptoms include loud coughing, shortness of breath, itching throat, liquid and white sputum, often with nasal obstruction, running nose, headache, soreness and weakness all over, chills, fever, lack of sweating, tongue coating thin and white, pulse floating or floating and tense. Diet therapy should be directed at arresting cough by means of expelling Wind and Cold pathogens.

The recommended diet is ginger 10 g, cut up into strips, infused in boiling water and strained. Take the infusion with some maltose (about 15–30 g) regularly instead of tea.

Fresh ginger can expel Wind and Cold and arrest cough and maltose can moderate cough.

Cough due to Wind-Heat invading the Lungs

Symptoms are a cough, coughing up sputum with difficulty, thirst, fever or headache, intolerance to wind, sweating, thin and yellow tongue coating, and a floating and rapid pulse. Dietary Therapy should be directed at expelling the Wind, clearing up Heat and ventilating the Lungs.

The recommended diet is the leaves of mulberry and chrysanthemum, 6 g each, crushed almond 9 g, cogongrass rhizome 30 g and peppermint 3 g infused in boiling water, to be taken from time to time.

Almond can ventilate the Lungs and relieve the cough, the leaves of mulberry, chrysanthemum and peppermint can expel Wind and Heat and cogongrass rhizome can clear up Heat and promote the production of Body Fluids. Turnip juice may be added, which helps to clear up Heat and dissolve Phlegm.

Cough caused by Dryness and Heat

Symptoms include a dry cough with none, or only little sputum, which is sticky and difficult to cough up, itching, dry, sore throat, dry lips, nose and mouth, fever and slight intolerance to cold, tongue red at the tip, with a thin and yellow coating, and a small and rapid pulse. Dietary Therapy should be directed at arresting the cough by moistening the Lungs. A juice of pears and lotus rhizome is recommended (JBDC); chop up the pears and the lotus rhizome in equal amounts, liquidize and strain. Take the juice liberally.

This recipe has the effect of clearing up Heat, moistening Dryness and arresting cough. Snow pear juice can also be used.

Cough caused by accumulation of Phlegm and Damp in the Lungs

Symptoms are a cough with a lot of white and sticky sputum, stuffiness in the chest, fullness in the stomach, sickness, poor appetite, a white and greasy tongue coating and a soft and slippery pulse. Dietary Therapy should be directed at reinforcing the Spleen, expelling the Damp and dissolving Phlegm.

Orange peel 3–6 g with 30–60 g of unpolished non-glutinous rice, to be taken liberally. Alternatively, grind the orange peel into a fine powder, add 3 g of it to the gruel and bring to the boil. White sugar may be added for flavor if necessary.

This recipe has the effect of reinforcing the Spleen and Stomach, expelling Damp and dissolving Phlegm.

Cough caused by accumulation of Phlegm-Heat in the Lungs

Symptoms are a cough, shortness of breath, profuse yellow and thick sputum which is difficult to cough up, chest pain when coughing, fever, dry mouth and thirst, a red tongue with a thin and yellow coating, and a slippery and rapid pulse. Dietary Therapy should be administered to cleanse the Lungs and dissolve Phlegm. The reed rhizome gruel is recommended (SYXJa).

Use fresh reed rhizome 100 g, zhuru (a Chinese medicine made from bamboo) 15 g, polished roundgrained non-glutinous rice 60 g, and ginger 6 g. Decoct the reed rhizome and zhuru and strain the liquid. Cook the rice in the liquid and add ginger when the gruel is about cooked. The gruel should be liquid in texture and taken twice a day.

The reed rhizome and zhuru can cleanse the Lungs and dissolve Phlegm.

Liver Fire invading the Lungs

Symptoms are a cough characterized by the rising of Counterflow Qi, a red face, dry throat, little scanty sputum that is sticky and difficult to cough up, chest distress and pain when coughing, a bitter taste in the mouth, a thin and yellow tongue coating with little moisture, taut and rapid pulse. Dietary Therapy should be directed at cleansing the Liver and purging the Lungs. An infusion made with gardenia 15 g and dried persimmon 60 g is recommended, to be taken regularly.

Fresh gardenia flowers can clear Heat in the Liver and Lungs and dried persimmon can moisten the Lungs and dissolve Phlegm.

Dryness of the Lungs due to Yin deficiency

Symptoms include a dry cough with absent or little sputum which is sticky or bloodstained, a dry mouth and throat, a red tongue with little coating, and a thready and rapid pulse. Dietary Therapy should be directed at nourishing the Yin and moistening the Lungs. A thick soup made with tremella 15 g, soaked in advance, lily bulbs 10 g and crystal sugar should be cooked on a low heat. The combination of tremella and lily bulbs is much more effective in nourishing Lung Yin than if they were used separately.

DIFFICULT BREATHING

In TCM this category includes all types of dyspnea, including asthma. The differentiation of difficult breathing consists of assessing the relative balance between external pathogens and deficiency of the body's resistance.

When the difficult breathing is caused by the invasion of external pathogens, or the obstruction of Lung Qi by the accumulation of Phlegm and turbidity, the illness is Full in nature; when it is due to internal deficiency of the body's resistance and the disorder of the Qi's functions of lifting, sending down, exhalation and inhalation, the illness is Deficient in nature. For Full disease, the Lungs and the Spleen are where the problem lies; and for Deficient disease, the Lung and the Kidney are at the root.

Recommended foods

Recommended foods for the disease are those with a mild and light taste which have the effects of dissolving Phlegm and reinforcing the Spleen. Examples are tangerine, kumquat, persimmons, turnips, mustard greens, lotus rhizome, lotus seeds, Chinese yam and flat beans.

Foods to avoid

Raw or cold food, fatty and greasy food or foods with a pungent taste are to be avoided, as are foods that tend to produce Phlegm, such as wine, fish, prawns and strong tea.

Diet recipes

Wind-Cold invading the Lungs

Symptoms are shortness of breath, stuffiness in the chest, a cough with liquid, white sputum and, at the onset of the disease, intolerance to cold, headache and lack of sweating, a thin, white tongue coating, and a floating and tense pulse. Dietary Therapy should be directed at dispersing Cold, regulating the Lungs and relieving difficult breathing.

Take ginger and purple perilla leaves, 6 g each, almonds 9 g and some brown sugar, steeped in boiling water.

Ginger and purple perilla leaves can disperse Cold and regulate the Lungs and almond can relieve cough and difficult breathing.

Wind-Heat invading the Lungs

Symptoms include shortness of breath or gasping, a cough with yellow sticky sputum, thirst, stuffiness in the chest, restlessness, sweating, or fever, flushing, a red tongue with yellow coating, and a floating and rapid pulse. Dietary Therapy should be directed at expelling Wind and clearing up Heat, regulating the Lungs and relieving difficult breathing.

The flowers of towel gourd 10 g, infused in boiling water for 10 minutes, should be taken while still hot, with honey added for flavor, two or three times a day.

The flowers of towel gourd have the effect of clearing up Heat and relieving difficult breathing. An infusion of mulberry leaves, chrysanthemum, peppermint leaves and almond is also recommended for this disease.

Phlegm obstructing the Lungs

Symptoms are difficult breathing and a cough, profuse and thick sputum which is difficult to cough up, sounds of sputum in the throat, stuffiness in the chest or even chest pain when coughing, together with vomiting, lack of taste in the mouth, a white and greasy tongue coating and a slippery pulse. Dietary Therapy should be directed at drying the Damp, dissolving Phlegm, sending down the Counterflow Qi and relieving difficult breathing.

An infusion of orange peel and almonds is recommended, made of orange peel (chopped into strips) and almonds (crushed), 6 g each, soaked in boiling water, to be taken with white sugar added for flavor. The items also make a gruel.

The orange peel can dry the Damp and dissolve Phlegm and the almonds can send down Counterflow Qi and relieve difficult breathing.

Difficult breathing due to deficiency of the Lungs

Symptoms are shortness of breath, thin voice, coughing with a low and thin sound, spontaneous perspiration, intolerance to wind, a light red tongue, and a soft and weak pulse. Dietary Therapy should be directed at reinforcing the Lung Qi and relieving difficult breathing. The following recipe is recommended (SJZL).

Decoct and strain baked milkvetch root 30 g and pilose asiabell root 15 g. The decoction is to be used in two equal parts, one in the morning and the other in the evening. Make a gruel with the decoction by adding 12 g of sweet almonds and 60 g of non-glutinous rice and some more water, with white sugar added for flavor when the gruel is ready.

Pilose asiabell root and milkvetch root can reinforce Lung Qi, while sweet almonds can relieve difficult breathing.

Difficult breathing due to deficiency in the Kidney

Symptoms include protracted breathing with difficult inhalation, the condition being aggravated on exertion, perspiration, cold limbs, dark complexion and lips, emaciation and fatigue, a pale tongue and a deep and weak pulse. Dietary Therapy should be directed at reinforcing the Lungs and the Kidney and relieving breathing. The following recipe is recommended (YSJCF).

Sweet almonds and walnut kernels, 250 g of each, are boiled in a suitable amount of water and condensed. When the concoction is about to dry up, add 500 g honey. Stir well and bring to the boil.

Walnuts reinforce the Kidney, while sweet almonds reinforce the Lungs. Both have the effects of arresting cough and relieving difficult breathing.

PULMONARY ABSCESS

Clinical symptoms are coughing, chest pain, fever, spitting up foul sputum, or even blood and pus in the sputum.

The mechanism of this disease is pathogenic Heat stagnated in the Lungs turning the Body Fluids into Phlegm, and pathogens obstructing the collaterals in the Lungs, where Blood stasis forms. When the Phlegm-Heat and Blood stasis accumulate and become entangled in the Lungs, abscess develops. Furthermore, when the tissues and Blood go bad and pus forms, the abscess will discharge

During the recovery period, there can be a state in which the pathogens have gone but the body's resistance is still weak, with Yin impaired and Qi exhausted.

Recommended foods

Patients with this disease should have light and mild foods, that have the effects of clearing up Heat, dissolving Phlegm and moistening the Lungs. Examples are wax gourd, purslane, lotus rhizome, bamboo shoots, oranges, pears, loquats, turnips, water chestnuts and arhat fruit.

Foods to avoid

Fatty and rich foods and foods that are pungent and irritating. Tobacco and alcohol are also to be avoided.

Diet recipes

In the first stage

The patient may have fever and chills, a cough with scanty sticky sputum, chest pain which is aggravated by coughing, difficult breathing, a dry mouth, a thin and yellow or white tongue coating and a floating, rapid and slippery pulse. Dietary Therapy should be directed at clearing up the Lungs and relieving the exterior symptoms. A tea made with houttuynia, reed rhizome and cogongrass rhizome, 30 g each, and 6 g of peppermint is decocted for drinking liberally.

In the developing stage

Symptoms are aggravated fever in the body followed by perspiration, restlessness, coughing, shortness of breath, stuffiness and pain in the chest which prevent the person turning over, coughing with turbid and foul sputum, a dry mouth and throat, a yellow and greasy tongue coating, and a slippery and rapid pulse. Dietary Therapy should be directed at clearing up Heat, removing toxins and dissolving Blood stasis.

A salad made with 60 g each of fresh dandelion and houttuynia, blanched in boiling water and drained, should be taken with soy sauce, salt and vinegar added for flavor.

This recipe has the effects of clearing up Heat and removing toxins. The recipe will work better when it is used with peach kernel gruel, which has the effects of dissolving Phlegm and removing Blood stasis.

In the ulceration stage

Symptoms include coughing with blood and pus in the sputum, or porridge-like sputum with a very foul odor, stuffiness and pain in the chest, or even gasping and inability to lie down, fever and redness in the body, thirst, yellow greasy tongue coating and a slippery and rapid pulse. Dietary Therapy should be directed at removing pus and toxins.

The recommended recipe is a decoction of reed rhizome, coix seeds and kernels of wax gourd, 30 g each, boiled in water. Add 60 g houttyunia and boil a little further, then discard the residue. The decoction is to be taken with honey added for flavor, three times a day.

Houttyunia and reed rhizome can clear up Heat and remove toxins and the other items can ease the discharge of pus.

The recovery period

Symptoms are subsiding fever, the cough being alleviated (coughing up less pus and blood, sputum becoming liquid and clear), or dull pain in the chest, inability to lie for long, shortness of breath, spontaneous perspiration and night sweats, afternoon fever, a hot sensation in the chest, dry mouth and throat, emaciation, a red tongue, and a thready and rapid or thready and weak pulse. Dietary Therapy should be directed at nourishing Yin and reinforcing the Lungs. Glehnia root gruel is recommended (ZP), made with glehnia root 30 g, non-glutinous rice 60 g and a suitable amount of crystal sugar. First decoct the glehnia root and strain. Add the non-glutinous rice to make a gruel, season with crystal sugar when the gruel is cooked and boil until the sugar melts. The gruel is to be taken as a meal twice a day.

This recipe has the effect of nourishing the Lungs, nurturing Yin, dissolving Phlegm and arresting coughing.

PULMONARY TUBERCULOSIS

Pulmonary tuberculosis is a kind of infectious consumptive disease caused by the invasion of the tuberculosis pathogen into the Lungs. Clinical symptoms are a cough, coughing up blood, hectic fever, night sweats, chest pain and emaciation. By nature, the disease is Yin deficiency which would in turn cause impairment to the five Zang organs.

The condition of the body's resistance is not only the key to the onset of the disease, but also the decisive factor for its development and con-

sequence. Generally, the disease first impairs the Lungs. When the Yin of the Lungs is impaired and has lost its nourishment and moisture, the major manifestation will be lack of Lung Yin; then Kidney Yin will be marred and the Heart and Liver will also become involved. When the disease is in both the Lungs and the Spleen, there is impairment of both Qi and Yin; in the later stages, the Lungs, Spleen and Kidney are all deficient. Deficiency of Yin will cause impairment to the Yang, leading to deficiency of both Yin and Yang, which is a grave situation.

Recommended foods

Pulmonary tuberculosis greatly impairs the body's resistance. Therefore patients should eat more nourishing food, according to the individual condition. For example, for nourishing Yin and reinforcing the Lungs, one should eat such foods as chickens, cow or goat's milk and honey. For reinforcing the Lungs and moistening Dryness, such foods as tremella, lily bulbs, pears, lotus rhizome and loquats are to be used. For reinforcing the Spleen and Stomach, Chinese yam, lotus seeds coix seeds and dates are to be used.

Foods to avoid

Foods that are pungent in taste, Dry and Hot in nature, which can impair Yin Body Fluids, such as chillies and ginger, are prohibited. Tobacco and alcohol should also be avoided.

Diet recipes

Impairment of Lung Yin

Symptoms are a dry cough with little sputum, sometimes stained with fresh blood, or hectic fever, hot sensations in the palms and soles, a dry mouth and throat, dull pain in the chest. Tongue is red at the tip and the edges with a thin coating and the pulse is thready and rapid. Dietary Therapy should be directed at nourishing Yin and moistening the Lungs.

A gruel made with asparagus cochinchinensis 15–30 g, non-glutinous rice 30–60 g and some crystal sugar is recommended. First the asparagus is boiled and strained. Add non-glutinous rice to make a gruel and a little crystal sugar when the gruel is cooked.

Asparagus can moisten Dryness and nourish Yin, clear up the Lungs and send down Lung Fire, and non-glutinous rice can reinforce the Stomach.

Hyperactivity of Fire due to Yin deficiency

Symptoms include coughing, choking with little sputum, coughing up profuse yellow, sticky sputum, coughing up fresh blood from time to time, hectic fever, flushing, night sweats, restlessness and insomnia, fidgetiness, pain in the chest and hypochondrium, a dark red tongue, and a thready and rapid pulse. Diet therapy should be directed at nourishing Yin and sending down Fire.

The recommended diet is rehmannia root and asparagus cochinchinensis, 30 g each, washed clean, decocted and strained. Cook 100 g of rice in the decoction to make a thin gruel, to be taken several times a day.

Rehmannia root nourishes Yin and clears up Heat, while asparagus cleanses the Lungs and sends down Fire.

Impairment of Qi and Yin

Symptoms are coughing, general weakness, thin voice, shortness of breath, occasional bloodstained sputum (the blood is pale in colour), hectic fever, pale complexion and flushing. Tongue is tender and red with a thin coating and the pulse is thready, weak and rapid. Dietary Therapy should be administered to replenish Qi and nourish Yin.

The recommended diet is fragrant solomonseal 30 g, decocted and strained. Cook 60 g of non-glutinous rice in the decoction and add a suitable amount of white sugar when the gruel is ready.

This recipe is effective in reinforcing the Spleen and moistening the Lungs, enriching Qi and nourishing Yin. The recipe can be adapted by adding pilose asiabell root and glehnia root, 10 g each, boiled together to enhance the effects.

Deficiency of both Yin and Yang

Symptoms are a cough, difficult breathing, short-ness of breath, occasional bloodstained sputum, hectic fever, cold sensation, intolerance to wind, spontaneous perspiration, night sweats, coarse voice, loss of comprehension, edema in the face and body, loss of appetite, loose stool or diarrhea, oral ulcer and lack of Body Fluids. Tongue is smooth and red, or pale and enlarged and the pulse is thready or empty, large and weak. Dietary Therapy should be directed at reinforcing the Essence and the Blood, nourishing Yin and assisting Yang.

The recommended diet is duck steamed with cordyceps (BCGMSY). Put 10 g cordyceps inside the duck and secure the duck with string. Add a suitable amount of soy sauce and rice wine. The duck is to be taken steamed.

Cordyceps reinforces the Kidney Yang and replenishes the Vital Qi; duck meat nourishes Yin and redresses the deficiency.

COUGHING UP BLOOD

Coughing up blood is also known as hemoptysis. Blood is coughed up from the respiratory tract, often with sputum. Sometimes there is only fresh blood, with some foam. This disease is mainly due to external pathogens invading the Lungs, Liver Fire burning upwards; or due to the hyperactivity of Fire due to Yin deficiency, leading to impairment of collaterals of the Lungs. When this happens, Blood will go astray and come out from the respiratory tract.

Recommended foods

It is desirable for patients with this disease to have foods that are effective in clearing Fire and moistening Dryness. Examples are pears, loquats, persimmon and lotus rhizome.

Foods to avoid

Foods that are pungent in taste and have the effects of irritating the Fire are to be avoided. Such foods include ginger, chillies, pepper and wine.

Diet recipes

Wind-Heat invading the Lungs

Symptoms are itching in the throat, coughing, blood in the sputum, dry mouth and nose, or fever in the body, a red tongue with thin yellow coating and rapid pulse. Dietary Therapy should be administered to clear Heat, moisten the Lungs and arrest bleeding. An electuary made with autumn pears and cogongrass rhizome is recommended.

Autumn pears (or pears), fresh lotus rhizome, fresh cogongrass rhizome, 150 g each, are cut up and squeezed to obtain the juice. The residue is decocted to obtain further juice. Put all of the juice together and condense by boiling. Add honey to make an electuary, to be taken orally.

Autumn pears, lotus and honey can clear Heat and moisten the Lungs, cogongrass rhizome can clear Heat and arrest bleeding.

Another recommended recipe is a kind of sweet to be taken orally, made with puffball and sugar. Puffball is effective in clearing Heat and arresting bleeding.

Liver Fire invading the Lungs

Symptoms are coughing, blood in the sputum, or coughing up solely fresh blood, pain in the chest and hypochondrium, a bitter taste in the mouth, a red restless tongue with yellow thin coating and a taut and rapid pulse. Dietary Therapy should be directed at cooling and clearing the Liver, purging the Lungs, cooling the Blood and arresting bleeding by using, for example, a gruel made with gardenia seeds (PJF).

Raw gardenia seeds and roasted gardenia seeds, 6 g each, are ground into powder, mixed and divided into four equal parts. Non-glutinous rice 120 g is made into a gruel by boiling in water. Add one part of the powder when the gruel is about cooked. Mix it well and boil further till the gruel is cooked.

Raw gardenia seeds can cleanse the Liver and purge the Lungs, while roasted gardenia seeds can cool the Blood and arrest bleeding.

Heat in the Lungs due to Lung deficiency

Symptoms include coughing with little sputum, which is bloodstained, or coughing up fresh blood from time to time, dry mouth and throat, a hot sensation in the face, restlessness, a red tongue and a thready and rapid pulse. Dietary Therapy should be directed at nourishing Yin, moistening the Lungs and arresting bleeding.

The recommended diet is a thick soup made with tremella and wood-ears, 30 g each or in suitable amounts, softened by soaking in water and stewed with crystal sugar.

Tremella and wood-ears used together can enhance the effects of nourishing Yin, moistening the Lungs and arresting bleeding.

APHONIA

Aphonia is characterized by a weak, thin voice or even total loss of voice. The disease lies mainly in the Lungs, but also involves the Kidney. The major cause of the disease is the invasion of external pathogens, causing obstruction to the Lungs and the respiratory tract, or it may be attributable to Dryness of the Lungs owing to impairment of Body Fluids which fail to moisten the air tract.

Recommended foods

For aphonia caused by invasion of Wind-Cold, treatment should be directed at ventilating and dispersing the exogenous pathogens by using ginger and spring onions; for aphonia caused by the entanglement of Phlegm and Heat, or by Dryness of the Lungs due to impairment of Yin fluids, recommended foods are pears, persimmon, oranges, loquats, Chinese olive and tremella. For cases with deficiency in both the Lungs and the Kidney, almonds and walnuts can be used.

Diet recipes

Aphonia due to Wind-Cold

Symptoms are sudden loss of voice or hoarse voice, together with coughing, nasal obstruction, stuffiness in the chest, headache and intolerance to cold, thin, white tongue coating, and a floating pulse. Dietary Therapy should be directed at dispersing Wind and Cold, regulating and easing Lung Qi by using, for example, a drink of ginger and purple perilla leaves (BCHY).

Ginger and purple perilla leaves, 3 g each, and brown sugar 15 g are infused in boiling water for 10 minutes and taken while the liquid is still hot.

Ginger can disperse Wind and Cold, while purple perilla leaves can also disperse Wind and Cold and at the same time will regulate and ease the Lung Qi.

Aphonia due to Phlegm-Heat

Symptoms include low and unclear voice, coughing with sticky sputum, dry mouth, dryness and pain in the throat, yellow and greasy tongue coating and a slippery and rapid pulse. Diet therapy should be directed at clearing up and dissolving Phlegm-Heat by using, for example, a persimmon calyx sugar (SXJYSP).

Persimmon calyx and white sugar in equal amounts are boiled in a little water on a low heat and mixed well before turning off the heat. Pour the syrup into a well-greased baking tin while still hot. Smooth it flat and let it cool down, then cut it in to small pieces.

Persimmon calyx is effective in clearing Heat, dissolving Phlegm and moistening Dryness.

Dryness of the Lungs due to impairment of Body Fluids

Symptoms are hoarse voice, dryness in the throat and mouth, together with coughing and Counterflow Qi, red tongue with a thin coating, and a thready and rapid pulse. Diet therapy should be directed at cleansing the Lungs and moistening the Dryness.

Take liquorice 25 g, decocted and strained. Add 100 g honey and 250 g olives, boiled on a low heat till the liquid is about to dry. Take the syrup orally.

Aphonia due to Yin deficiency of the Lung and Kidney

Symptoms include persistent hoarse voice and dry throat, together with dry cough, tinnitus, dizziness, hot sensation in the palms and soles, soreness and weakness in the back and knees, a red tongue with little coating, and a thready and rapid pulse. Dietary Therapy should be administered to nourish Yin and send down Fire by using, for example, a gruel of asparagus and rehmannia (see Pulmonary Tuberculosis).

PALPITATION

Palpitation is a subjective feeling of rapid beating of the heart. It includes alarmed palpitation (Jing ji) and severe palpitation (Zheng chong).

The symptom is related to poor health, mental irritation, excessive fatigue and repeated invasion of external pathogens. The mechanisms of the disease are deficiency of Heart Qi and Blood, exhaustion of Heart Yang, stagnation of fluids in the interior, or obstruction of the collaterals by Blood stasis, leading to malnourishment of the Heart or agitation of the Heart and Mind, culminating in unrest of the Heart and Mind. The disease lies in the Heart, but it is also closely related to the Liver, Spleen and Kidney.

Recommended foods

Diets recommended for patients with palpitation should vary with the different types of the disease. For cases of the deficient type, it is desirable to have foods that are effective in nourishing the Heart and tranquilizing the Mind, such as pig's heart, eggs, longan, litchi, mulberry, magnolia vine fruit and grapes. For cases with deficiency of Heart Blood, use foods that can replenish Blood and Qi, such as chicken, pigeon and dates. For patients with hyperactivity of Fire due to Yin deficiency, use foods that can nourish Yin and send down Fire, such as pears, lily bulb, wheat, oyster and duck. For patients with deficiency of Heart Yang, it is desirable to have foods that can warm and reinforce the Heart Yang, such as goat's milk, lamb's heart, cinnamon and dried ginger. For patients with obstruction of Heart Blood, use foods that can activate Blood circulation and disperse stasis, such as roses, Chinese hawthorn and brown sugar.

Foods to avoid

Generally, pungent, irritating, fatty and rich foods are to be avoided. Examples are wines, strong tea and coffee.

Diet recipes

Deficiency of Qi and Blood

Symptoms include palpitations, shortness of breath, dizziness, dull complexion, fatigue, loss of appetite, spontaneous perspiration, a pale tongue, and a thready and weak pulse. Dietary Therapy should be directed at replenishing Qi and Blood, nourishing the Heart and tranquilizing the Mind by using, for example, pig's heart stewed with Chinese angelica root (ZZYJ).

One pig's heart is cut open, stuffed with 30 g of pilose asiabell root and 15 g of Chinese angelica root and steamed in a stewing pot, with the pig's heart not touching the water. Season with salt when the heart is cooked. Drink the soup and eat the heart.

Pilose asiabell root enriches Qi, Chinese angelica root nourishes Blood, while pig's heart reinforces the Heart and nourishes Blood. Longans can be added to the recipe to reinforce the Heart and Spleen, nourish the Blood and tranquilize the Mind.

Hyperactivity of Fire due to Yin deficiency

Symptoms include palpitations, restlessness, insomnia, dizziness, hot sensations in the palms and soles, tinnitus, soreness in the back, a red tongue with little or no coating, and a thready and rapid pulse. Dietary Therapy should be administered to nourish Yin and tranquilize the Mind by using a soup made with lily bulb and egg yolk (JGYL).

Take lily bulb 60 g, washed clean and boiled in three bowls of water, till there are two bowls of water left. Put two well-beaten egg yolks into the lily bulb decoction, adding some white sugar or crystal sugar for flavor. To be taken twice a day.

Lily bulb cleanses the Heart and tranquilizes the Mind, egg yolk nourishes Yin and nurtures Blood. The recipe can be used in combination with mulberries, magnolia vine fruit and lotus seeds.

Sluggish Heart Yang

Symptoms are palpitations, restlessness, stuffiness in the chest, shortness of breath, pale complexion, cold feeling in the body, cold limbs, a pale tongue, and a weak or deep, thready and rapid pulse. Dietary Therapy should be directed at warming and reinforcing the Heart Yang, tranquilizing the Mind and relieving palpitation by using lamb's heart steamed with cinnamon bark and ginseng.

Cinnamon bark and ginseng, 5 g each, are powdered and put into a lamb's or pig's heart, to be taken steamed.

Ginseng greatly tonifies the Vital Qi, cinnamon bark warms and activates the Heart Yang while the lamb's heart nourishes the Heart and tranquilizes the Mind.

Retention of Fluids invading the Heart

Symptoms include palpitation, dizziness, fullness in the chest and the upper abdomen, cold feeling in the body and limbs, scanty urine, or edema in the lower limbs, thirst without desire to drink, nausea and vomiting up saliva, white slippery tongue coating, and a taut and slippery pulse. Dietary Therapy should be directed at warming and dissolving the retained Body Fluids by using, for example, cinnamon bark gruel (SYXJa).

Cinnamon bark 3 g, poria 15 g and mulberry bark 10 g are decocted and strained. Add 50 g of non-glutinous rice to the liquid to make a gruel to be taken orally.

Cinnamon bark warms and invigorates the Heart Yang to dissolve Fluid retention, poria helps by absorbing Damp, mulberry bark induces urination, while non-glutinous rice reinforces the Spleen and nourishes the Stomach.

The recipe can also be used in combination with ginger and onion to enhance the effects of invigorating Yang and dissolving Fluid retention.

Obstruction of the Heart Blood

Symptoms are palpitation and restlessness, stuffiness in the chest, paroxysmal pericardiac pain, or livid lips and finger nails, a dark tongue, sometimes with blood in the tissues, and an uneven or knotted and intermittent pulse. Dietary Therapy should be directed at activating Blood circulation, dissolving Blood stasis, unblocking channels and relieving pain.

The recommended diet is safflower 6 g and one lamb's heart steamed in a stewing pot, with the heart not touching the water, seasoned with salt.

Safflower activates Blood circulation and unblocks the channels, removes stasis and relieves pain, while the lamb's heart nourishes the Mind and relieves palpitation. The recipe can also be used in combination with suitable amounts of onion and Chinese hawthorn to enhance the effects of activating Blood circulation and relieving pain.

CARDIAC PAIN (ANGINA)

Cardiac pain is a disease characterized by stuffiness and pain in the area of the Heart and the chest. It is marked by paroxysmal pain, which extends to the neck, the arms and the upper abdomen, or is accompanied by palpitation and shortness of breath. In grave cases, there may be cold limbs, perspiration and a faint pulse, which are the signs of sudden exhaustion of Yang Qi. The more serious cases will not be discussed in this chapter.

Cardiac pain is often triggered off by exposure to cold, fatigue or emotional factors. It may be the result of congenital deficiency, deficiency in the Heart, the Spleen and Kidney, disharmony of the Vital Organs. Other causes could be emotional disturbances or intemperance of diet, leading to stagnation of Qi, stasis of Blood or obstruction by Phlegm culminating in the obstruction of the vessels of the Heart and malfunction of the collaterals. The disease lies in the Heart, but is also linked to deficiency of Yin, Yang, Qi and Blood or disturbance in such internal organs as the Liver, Spleen and Kidney.

Recommended foods

Patients with cardiac pain should eat foods with a clear nature and light taste, for example, kelp, laver, seaweeds, bean shoots and other bean products, green vegetables, lean pork, vegetable oil and Chinese hawthorn.

Foods to avoid

Foods that are rich, fatty or irritating should be avoided, for example, animal kidneys, shellfish (crabs, snails, clams) and wine. Tea and coffee should be taken in moderation.

Diet recipes

Obstruction of Heart Blood

Symptoms include stabbing pain in the chest, which has a fixed location and extends to the shoulders and the back, stuffiness and shortness of breath, occasional palpitations, a dark tongue with spots at the tip or edges, a deep and uneven or knotted pulse. Dietary Therapy should be directed at activating Blood circulation, dissolving Blood stasis and unblocking the collaterals. One recommended recipe is lamb's heart stewed with safflower (see Palpitation).

Stagnation of Yin Cold

Symptoms are chest pain extending to the back, which is aggravated when encountering cold, stuffiness in the chest, shortness of breath and palpitations. In grave cases, there may be difficult breathing, inability to lie flat, pale complexion, cold limbs, pale tongue coating, and a deep and thready pulse. In the treatment of these illnesses, Dietary Therapy should be directed at relieving obstruction and activating Yang.

The recommended recipe is a decoction made with snakegourd fruit 12 g, onion 9 g, and a suitable amount of millet or rice wine, decocted together and strained, to be taken in a few sessions.

Snakegourd fruit eases Qi, dissolves hard masses and Phlegm, onion activates Qi and relieves pain, activates Yang and dissolves knotted tissues. Millet or rice wine is used for the purpose of relieving obstruction, activating Yang and assisting the effects of the other herbs.

Deficiency of both Qi and Blood

Symptoms are stuffiness in the chest, cardiac pain, palpitations, dizziness, fatigue, dull complexion, pale or dark red tongue, and a knotted and intermittent or thready and weak pulse. Dietary Therapy should be directed at replenishing Qi and Blood.

The recommended recipe is a thick soup made with Chinese angelica root and pilose asiabell root, 10 g each (wrapped in a cloth bag), and eel 500 g (cut into small pieces). Cook them together for one hour. The fish and the soup are to be taken at meals after seasoning, with the bag of medicine removed.

Chinese angelica root and pilose asiabell root can replenish Qi and Blood. Eel can redress deficiency, make up for the impairment, and enrich Qi and Blood.

Exhaustion of Heart and Kidney Yang

Symptoms include cardiac pain, palpitations, shortness of breath, spontaneous perspiration, cold feeling in the body and limbs, soreness in the back and knees, diarrhea and loose stool, a pale tongue with white coating, and a weak or knotted and intermittent pulse. Dietary Therapy should be directed at warming and reinforcing the Heart and the Kidney.

The recommended recipe is gruel made with cinnamon bark 6 g, decocted and strained. Add 50 g of non-glutinous rice to the liquid to make a gruel, to be taken orally. Cinnamon bark can warm Yang.

This recipe can be used in combination with longans to reinforce the Heart and nourish the Mind. When the recipe is used together with Chinese chives sauteed with walnuts, the effect of warming and tonifying the Kidney Yang is enhanced.

INSOMNIA

Clinical symptoms of insomnia are varied, from difficulty in getting to sleep, waking easily, intermittent sleep, to total sleeplessness throughout the night. The disease is usually due to overanxiety impairing the Heart and the Spleen; hyperactivity of Yang due to deficiency of Yin and loss of coordination between the Heart and the Kidney; deficiency of the Heart and Gallbladder with timidity and restless Mind; depression of the Liver turning into Fire and irritating the Mind; undigested food turning into Phlegm-Heat, causing discomfort in the Stomach, leading to mental derangement.

Recommended foods

It is desirable for patients with insomnia to have plain and light foods.

More specifically, for cases with deficiency of both the Heart and the Spleen, patients should have foods that can reinforce the Heart and the Spleen, such as wheat, lotus seeds, dates, longan. For cases with hyperactivity of Fire due to deficiency of Yin, it is desirable to have foods that can help nourish the Yin and send down the Fire, such as lily bulb, chicken eggs, oysters, mussels and turtle meat. For cases due to depression of the Liver turning into Fire, use foods that tend to cleanse the Liver and regulate Qi, such as celery, mung beans, plums, and oranges. For cases caused by disharmony in the Stomach, patients should have foods that can assist digestion and remove stagnation of foods, such as Chinese hawthorn, turnips and water chestnuts.

Foods to avoid

Rich, fatty or irritating foods such as strong tea and coffee, and pungent, spicy foods such as chillies and ginger should not be taken. Patients should also eat smaller meals than usual.

Diet recipes

Deficiency of both the Heart and the Kidney

Symptoms include frequent dreams, being very easy to wake, palpitations, amnesia, dizziness, fatigue, loss of appetite, a dull complexion, a pale tongue with thin coating and a thready pulse. Dietary Therapy should be directed at reinforcing the Heart and the Spleen, nourishing Blood and tranquilizing the Mind.

The recommended recipe is a decoction for reinforcing both the Heart and the Spleen. Decoct longan, lotus seeds and dates, 15 g each. Drink the liquid and eat the longan, lotus seeds and dates.

Longan nourishes the Heart and the Spleen, nurtures Blood and tranquilizes the mind. Dates replenish Blood and Qi, while lotus seeds nourish the Heart and tranquilize the Mind.

Deficiency of the Heart and Gallbladder Qi

Symptoms are insomnia, dreamfilled sleep, being easy to wake, timidity and palpitations, being easily alarmed, shortness of breath, fatigue, a pale tongue, and a taut and thready pulse. Dietary Therapy should be directed at reinforcing Qi, nourishing the Heart and calming the Mind.

The recommended recipe is rice cooked with pilose asiabell root and dates (XYL). Pilose asiabell root 10 g and dates 30 g are cooked for about 30 minutes. Take out the pilose asiabell root and dates and add 50 g white sugar to the liquid. Boil the mixture down to a thick sauce and set aside. Steam the dates and 250 g rice until well cooked and place them onto a dish. Pour the sauce onto the rice with the dates.

Pilose asiabell root replenishes Qi, dates replenish Blood and reinforce the Spleen, nourish the Heart and tranquilize the Mind. Glutinous rice reinforces the Middle Burner and replenishes Qi.

Hyperactivity of Fire due to Yin deficiency

Symptoms include restlessness, insomnia, palpitations, dizziness, tinnitus, amnesia, soreness in the back, spermatorrhea, hot sensations in the chest, palms and soles; dry mouth, a red tongue, and a thready and rapid pulse. Dietary Therapy should be directed at nourishing Yin and sending down the pathogenic Fire.

The recommended recipe is mulberry electuary (BCYY) made with fresh mulberry 1000 g or dried mulberry 500 g, washed clean, boiled in a suitable amount of water and strained. Boil further on a low heat until the juice is condensed. Add 300 g of honey to make an electuary, to be taken twice a day, one tablespoonful at a time, mixed with boiling water.

Mulberry is effective in nourishing Yin and replenishing Blood. When the Yin fluids are replenished, the deficient Fire dies down by itself and all the symptoms will be relieved.

Disharmony in the Stomach

Symptoms include insomnia, heaviness in the head, loss of appetite, distension in the abdomen, profuse sputum, belching, nausea, a greasy and yellow tongue coating and a slippery and rapid pulse. Dietary Therapy should be directed at assisting digestion, dissolving sputum, harmonizing the Stomach and tranquilizing the Mind.

The recommended recipe is a gruel made with pinellia tuber 6 g, decocted and strained with the residue removed. Add 100 g sorghum to make a gruel and 150 g chopped turnip when the gruel is half cooked. Eat the gruel in two meals.

Pinellia tuber dries up Damp and dissolves Phlegm. When the disease involves Phlegm-Heat, turnip can be replaced with zhuru. Turnip is especially good for sending down Qi and assisting digestion, dissolving Phlegm and harmonizing the Middle Burner. Sorghum can reinforce the Spleen, absorb Damp and harmonize the Stomach.

EXCESSIVE SWEATING

Excessive sweating (hyperhidrosis) refers to a disease caused by incoordination of the Yin and Yang, disharmony of Ying and Wei, and irregularity of the striae of the skin and muscles in opening and closing the pores, leading to the outflow of Body Fluids, resulting in the abnormal perspiration of the whole or parts of the body. Here we only discuss spontaneous perspiration and night sweating.

Spontaneous perspiration is sweating in the daytime which is not related to environmental factors. The symptom is aggravated by physical exertion. The most common causes of day sweats are deficient Lung Qi leading to instability of the Defensive Qi which leaves the pores flaccid, and disharmony of Ying and Wei leading to malfunction of the Wei defensive system.

Night sweats involve sweating at night during

sleep, which will stop once awake. The most common causes are Heat in the interior due to Yin deficiency and irritation of Body Fluids which flow out as sweat.

Recommended foods

Patients with hyperhidrosis should have foods that are light in taste and nutritious in content, such as wheat, glutinous rice, spinach, tomatoes, carrot, beancurd and soy milk. For patients with night sweats, it is desirable to have foods that can help nourish and nurture Yin, such as lily bulb, tremella, duck, turtle meat and cuttlefish. For spontaneous perspiration with deficiency of Qi, use foods that can replenish Qi and reinforce the Spleen, such as lotus seeds, longan, dates, Chinese yam and chicken.

Foods to avoid

These include foods that are pungent in taste and can irritate Fire, such as Chinese spring onion, garlic, Chinese chives, chillies and wine.

Diet recipes

Disharmony of Lung defence

Symptoms are sweating, intolerance to wind which is aggravated by physical exertion; susceptibility to catching cold, fatigue and weakness, a dull complexion, a thready pulse and a thin white tongue coating. Dietary Therapy should be directed at replenishing Qi and consolidating the exterior defence.

The recommended food is chicken cooked with milkvetch root (SYSD). Stuff one prepared chicken with 30 g milkvetch root, some ginger and Chinese spring onion, Shaoxing wine and salt to season. Tie the chicken with string and steam it until cooked.

Chicken can replenish Qi and Blood, while milkvetch root reinforces Qi and consolidates the exterior defence.

Disharmony of the Ying and Wei

Symptoms are sweating, intolerance to wind,

soreness all over the body, alternating chills and fever, sweating in half of the body or parts of the body, thin white tongue coating and a slow pulse. Diet therapy should be directed at harmonizing Ying and Wei.

A recommended food is a soup made with ginger and dates (stoned), 500 g each, liquorice 60 g, dried and powdered together, mixed with 10 g of salt. Take 10 g of the powder mixed with boiling water before a meal every morning.

Ginger used together with dates can harmonize the Spleen and the Stomach and coordinate the Ying and Wei. The recipe can also be used in the form of a decoction made with ginger and dates.

Hyperactivity of Fire due to Yin deficiency

Symptoms include night sweating, spontaneous perspiration, hot sensations in the chest, palms and soles, or afternoon fever, flushing, thirst, a red tongue with little coating and a thready and rapid pulse. Dietary Therapy should be directed at nourishing Yin and clearing up Fire.

A recommended recipe uses one blackboned chicken, with 250 g rehmannia root cut up, mixed with maltose and stuffed into the chicken, which is then steamed. Eat the chicken only, discarding the stuffing.

Blackboned chicken can reinforce the Yin, rehmannia root can nourish Yin and clear Heat, maltose can replenish Qi and moisten Dryness. The recipe can also be used in combination with magnolia vine fruit and dogwood fruit to nurture Yin and arrest sweating.

INDIGESTION

Indigestion is marked by poor appetite, fullness in the abdomen, eructation with fetid odor and acid regurgitation. It is mostly due to poor diet or overeating of rich, fatty foods or raw and cold foods, causing malfunction of the Spleen and Stomach which fail to digest and absorb, resulting in retention of food in the Middle Burner. It can be due to weakness in the Spleen and Stomach which fail to perform their functions, causing stagnation of food.

Recommended foods

It is important for patients with indigestion to take meals properly and moderately. It is desirable for them to have soft, liquid foods that are easy to digest, such as porridge, lotus rhizome powder and soy milk. For cases due to stagnation of foods from intemperance of diet, use foods that assist digestion and dissolve stagnation, such as Chinese yam, flat beans, lotus seeds, coix seeds, euryale seeds and pig's trotter.

Foods to avoid

Oily, greasy, dry and indigestible foods, such as muesli, are to be avoided.

Diet recipes

Intemperance of diet

Symptoms include fullness, pain and tenderness in the abdomen, loss of appetite, eructation with fetid odor and regurgitation, together with vomiting up of undigested food, passing loose, foul stools, alleviation of pain after vomiting or diarrhea, or constipation, a thick and greasy tongue coating and a slippery and rapid pulse. Dietary Therapy should be directed at assisting digestion and dissolving stagnation.

A recommended food is a soup made with Chinese hawthorn and baked germinated barley, 30 g each, and turnip 250 g, decocted together. Add a suitable amount of white sugar for flavor. Drink the soup and eat the turnip.

Chinese hawthorn helps dissolve stagnation of meats, germinated barley helps dissolve stagnation of cereals, while turnip assists digestion and sends down the Central Qi.

Another recommended food is Chinese hawthorn balls.

Weak Spleen

Symptoms are lethargy, loss of appetite, fullness in the abdomen, belching, nausea, undigested food in loose stools, a pale tongue with white coating and a slow and weak pulse. Dietary Therapy should be directed at replenishing Qi

and reinforcing the Spleen, assisting digestion and dissolving food stagnation.

A recommended food is Spleen-reinforcing cakes (YXZZCXL) made with dates 250 g, rhizome of largeheaded atractylodes 30 g wrapped in gauze, and dried ginger 15 g, boiled in a suitable amount of water for about an hour. Take out the dates and mash. Add 15 g of the powder of chicken's gizzard membrane and 500 g of flour to the mashed dates to make thin pancakes.

Rhizome of largeheaded atractylodes and dates can replenish Qi and reinforce the Spleen, dried ginger can warm and invigorate the Spleen Yang, while chicken's gizzard membrane can assist digestion and dissolve food stagnation. When there are no cold symptoms in the Middle Burner, the dried ginger may be omitted.

VOMITING

Vomiting is caused by Counterflow Qi as a result of the failure of the Stomach to perform its function of harmonizing and sending down the Qi.

The Spleen and the Stomach have an interior and exterior relationship. In normal physical conditions, the Stomach is in charge of receiving while the Spleen is in charge of digesting and transformation. The Spleen Qi and the Stomach Qi, one going up and the other going down, maintain the Qi in performing its functions, so that the essence from foods and drinks can be absorbed and transported around the whole body. When the Stomach Qi rises instead of going down, vomiting is likely to occur. There are two kinds of vomiting, Full and Deficient. Full vomiting is due to the invasion of the stomach by pathogenic factors, causing turbid Qi to rise adversely; Deficient vomiting is due to sluggish Stomach Yang or deficiency of Stomach Yin, which is no longer in harmony and fails to perform its function of sending down.

Recommended foods

For serious cases of vomiting, temporary fasting is to be employed. But for general cases, it is best to have foods with a plain light taste, which are easily digested or have the effect of arresting vomiting. Examples are thin porridge, lotus rhizome powder, soy milk, fresh ginger, flat beans, red bay berries and Seville orange flower.

Foods to avoid

Irritating foods such as wine, Chinese spring onion and garlic or greasy, fishy or smelly foods are to be avoided.

Diet recipes

External pathogens invading the Stomach

Symptoms include sudden onset of vomiting, intolerance to cold, fever, aching in the head and body, fullness in the chest and upper abdomen, a white and greasy tongue coating, and a soft and slow or floating pulse. Dietary Therapy should be directed at dispersing the pathogens, relieving exterior syndrome and harmonizing the Stomach to arrest vomiting.

The recommended food is ginger (sliced) and purple perilla leaves, 3 g each, and a suitable amount of brown sugar, infused in boiling water for 5 minutes and covered with a lid. Drink the infusion in one session while it is still hot.

Fresh ginger and purple perilla leaves can relieve the exterior syndrome and disperse Cold, harmonize the Stomach and arrest vomiting. Brown sugar, which is used for flavor, has the effect of dispersing Cold and warming the Stomach.

Another recommended food is ginger prepared with sugar and vinegar. The latter has a stronger effect of harmonizing the Stomach and arresting vomiting.

Stagnation of Foods

Symptoms include vomiting up sour Stomach contents, fullness in the upper abdomen, weight loss, belching aggravated after eating but alleviated after vomiting, passing foul, loose stool, constipation, a thick and greasy tongue coating, and a slippery and full pulse. Dietary Therapy should be directed at assisting digestion and dissolving stagnation.

The recommended food is a soup made with Chinese hawthorn and turnip (see indigestion).

Obstruction of the interior by Phlegm retention

Symptoms are vomiting clear liquid, phlegm and saliva, fullness in the upper abdomen, loss of appetite, dizziness, palpitation, a white and greasy tongue coating and a slippery pulse. Dietary Therapy should be directed at warming and dissolving Phlegm retention, harmonizing the Stomach in order to send down the Counterflow Qi.

The recommended food is a tea made with ginger 9 g and dried orange 100 g, sliced and mixed with boiling water for drinking liberally.

Fresh ginger is pungent in taste and Warm in nature. It has the effects of harmonizing the Stomach, dispersing fluid retention and arresting vomiting. Dried orange has a sweet taste and a slightly Warm nature. It has the effect of reinforcing the Spleen, sending down the Central Qi and dissolving Phlegm. The two used together can disperse the retention of Phlegm, harmonize the Stomach, send down the Counterflow Qi and arrest vomiting. Dried orange can also be eaten by itself.

Liver Qi invading the Stomach

Symptoms include vomiting, regurgitation of acid, frequent belching, stuffiness and pain in the chest and the hypochondrium, a tongue that is red at the edges with thin greasy coating and a taut pulse. Dietary Therapy should be administered to regulate Qi, harmonize the Stomach, send down the Counterflow Qi and arrest vomiting.

The recommended food is a drink made with orange peel, zhuru and dried persimmon 30 g each, with ginger 3 g, boiled in water twice over. Filter the decoction and add a suitable amount of white sugar.

Orange peel can regulate Qi, send down Counterflow Qi and arrest vomiting. Zhuru can clear up Heat and arrest vomiting. Fresh ginger warms the Stomach and arrests vomiting. The combination of Cold and Hot drugs is especially effective in arresting vomiting. Dried persimmon nourishes the Stomach.

The recipe can be used in conjunction with

Seville orange flower and plums to enhance the effects of easing the Liver and regulating Qi.

Deficient Cold in the Spleen and Stomach

Symptoms are vomiting which is easily triggered off by any immoderate diet, pale complexion, fatigue, dry mouth without desire for drinking, cold limbs, loose stool, a pale tongue and a soft and weak pulse. Dietary Therapy should be directed at warming the Middle Burner, reinforcing the Spleen, harmonizing the Stomach and arresting vomiting.

The recommended food is thick mutton soup (YSZY) made with mutton (or lean pork) 250 g, diced, tsaoko, dried mandarin peel, galangal rhizome, pepper and ginger, 3 g each, wrapped in a cloth bag and tied. Boil all the ingredients and add one sliced turnip when the mutton is about cooked. Boil further till the mutton is well cooked. Remove the cloth bag and add seasoning.

Mutton can replenish Qi, warm the Middle Burner and tonify deficiency. Turnip assists digestion, sends down the Central Qi and harmonizes the Middle Burner. Tsaoko and dried mandarin peel can invigorate the Spleen and reinforce the Stomach. Pepper, galangal rhizome and fresh ginger can warm the Middle Burner, disperse Cold, send down the Counterflow Qi and arrest vomiting.

Deficiency of Stomach Yin

Symptoms include repeated vomiting, occasional dry vomiting, dry mouth and throat, poor appetite, a red tongue with little moisture and a thready and rapid pulse. Dietary Therapy should be administered to nurture Yin and harmonize the Stomach, send down the Counterflow Qi and arrest vomiting.

For the recommended recipe, take one snow pear (peeled). Insert five cloves into the pear. Steam the pear in a pan which is sealed with a lid. Remove the cloves. Melt 30 g of crystal sugar with water and pour the syrup onto the pear.

The snow pear is Cold in nature. It has the effects of reinforcing the Stomach and nurturing the Yin. Cloves activate Qi and harmonize the Stomach, send down Counterflow Qi and arrest

vomiting. Crystal sugar nourishes Yin and harmonizes the Stomach.

HICCUPS

Hiccups are due to accumulation of Cold Qi; excessive Dryness and Heat inside the body; stagnation of Qi and obstruction by Phlegm, or due to deficiency of Qi and Blood. These lead to malfunction of the vital organs and disturbance of Qi, culminating in Counterflow Stomach Qi rushing up to irritate the diaphragm.

Recommended foods

Diets recommended for patients with hiccups should vary with different types of symptoms. For cases due to Cold in the Stomach or deficient Cold in the Spleen and Stomach, it is desirable to have foods that are effective in warming the Middle Burner, dispersing Cold or reinforcing the Spleen and Stomach, such as fresh ginger, pepper, broad beans, crucian carp and mutton. For cases due to Heat in the Stomach or deficiency of Stomach Yin, use foods that can cleanse the Stomach, send down Fire or nourish Stomach Yin, such as loquats, red bay berries, pears, sugarcane and crystal sugar. For cases due to Liver Qi invading the Stomach, patients should eat foods that can assist the circulation of Qi and harmonize the Stomach, such as finger citron, broad bean and oranges.

Foods to avoid

Foods that tend to cause stagnation of Qi, such as sweet potatoes, beans and taro, should be avoided, as should raw fruits and melons, and foods that are pungent and Dry.

Diet recipes

Coldness in the Stomach

Symptoms include hiccups with a deep and vigorous sound, discomfort in the diaphragm and the upper abdomen which is alleviated by warmth but aggravated by cold, loss of taste and thirst, white and damp tongue coating and a slow pulse. Dietary Therapy should be administered to warm the Middle Burner and send down the Counterflow Qi.

The recommended food is brown sugar 250 g, boiled in a little water till the liquid is condensed. Then add fresh ginger (chopped up) 30 g, and clove powder 5 g, and mix well. Boil further till the mixture makes filaments when picked up and is no longer sticky and then pour it out into a flat tin and let it cool a bit before cutting it into small pieces. Take 3–4 pieces at a time.

Cloves warm the Middle Burner, send down Counterflow Qi and arrest hiccups, Fresh ginger warms the Stomach and disperses Cold and brown sugar warms the Stomach as well as being a condiment. When the three are used together, the effects are enhanced.

Uprushing of Stomach Qi

Symptoms are vigorous hiccups, foul breath, thirst, scanty dark urine, constipation, yellow tongue coating and slippery and rapid pulse. Dietary Therapy should be directed at clearing Heat and arresting hiccups.

The recommended food is a gruel of fresh reed rhizome 30 g with persimmon calyx 10 g, decocted and strained. Make a thin gruel with non-glutinous rice in the decoction and add a suitable amount of crystal sugar for flavor.

Reed rhizome clears up Heat in the Stomach, persimmon calyx sends down Counterflow Qi and arrests hiccups while non-glutinous rice can reinforce the Stomach and harmonize the Middle Burner.

Liver Qi invading the Stomach

Symptoms include frequent hiccups which are triggered off or aggravated by emotional disturbance, accompanied by stuffiness in the chest, loss of appetite, fullness in the upper abdomen and hypochondrium, excessive bowel sounds, a white, thin tongue coating and a taut pulse. Dietary Therapy should be directed at regulating Qi and the Liver and sending down the Counterflow Qi.

The recommended food is a decoction of persimmon calyx 10 g and white plum blossom 5 g.

After it comes to the boil, remove the residue, add a suitable amount of crystal sugar for flavor and take from time to time.

Persimmon calyx sends down Counterflow Qi and arrests hiccups while white plum blossoms can regulate the Liver, relieve depression of the Liver, regulate Qi and harmonize the Stomach.

Deficiency of Spleen and Stomach Yang

Symptoms include hiccups with low and thin sounds, shortness of breath, pale complexion, cold hands and feet, loss of appetite, fatigue, a pale tongue with white coating, and a deep, thready and weak pulse. Dietary Therapy should be directed at warming and reinforcing the Spleen and Stomach, harmonizing the Middle Burner and sending down Counterflow Qi.

The recommended food is a soup made with one sizable crucian carp, gutted and scaled, stuffed with a suitable amount of ginger, garlic, pepper, orange peel and amomum fruit, stewed with salt. Drink the soup and eat the fish.

Crucian carp can warm and reinforce the Spleen and the Stomach to relieve hiccups. Ginger and garlic can enhance the effects of warming the Middle Burner and harmonizing the Stomach.

Deficiency of Stomach Yin

Symptoms are hiccups with a short sound, dry mouth and tongue, restlessness, a red tongue with little moisture, and a thready and rapid pulse. Dietary Therapy should be directed at reinforcing the Stomach, promoting the production of Body Fluids and arresting hiccups.

The recommended recipe is a Stomach reinforcing decoction (WBTB) made with amomum fruit, lilyturf root, fragrant solomonseal and rehmannia root, 10 g each, decocted and strained. Add a suitable amount of crystal sugar for drinking as a tea.

By using amomum fruit, lilyturf root, fragrant solomonseal, rehmannia root and crystal sugar together, this recipe is effective in reinforcing the Stomach, promoting the production of Body Fluids and relieving hiccups. A suitable amount of persimmon calyx can be added to send down the Counterflow Qi and arrest the hiccups.

DIFFICULTY IN SWALLOWING

Difficulty in swallowing is a disease characterized by obstruction of swallowing, inability to swallow and vomiting on attempting to swallow. In minor cases, there is only difficulty in swallowing but in serious cases, there is obstruction of food on swallowing.

The disease can be due to mental depression, excessive drinking, impairment by immoderate meals, fatigue or deficiency of Qi and Blood. The major mechanisms are stagnation of Qi, obstruction by Phlegm, Blood stasis and exhaustion of Body Fluids. Stagnation of Qi and obstruction by Phlegm often interact and lead to entanglement of Phlegm and Qi, or entanglement of Phlegm with stasis, which narrows the esophagus and causes obstruction.

Recommended foods

It is desirable for these patients to have foods that are rich in nutrition or have the effects of reinforcing the Stomach, nourishing Yin and dissolving stasis, such as cow's milk, soy milk, lotus rhizome juice, juice of sugarcane and juice of Chinese chives.

Foods to avoid

Pungent, spicy and irritating foods are to be avoided. It is also undesirable to have smelly, fishy or dry, hard foods.

Diet recipes

Exhaustion of Body Fluids and Blood stasis

Symptoms include difficulty and pain on swallowing, dry mouth and throat, hot sensations and emaciation, dry stool which tends to be very hard like goat's droppings, dry skin, a red, dry or livid tongue and a thready and uneven pulse. Dietary Therapy should be directed at nourishing the Stomach, promoting the production of Body Fluids, activating the circulation of Blood and dissolving stasis.

The recommended food is a Middle Burner calming drink of five juices (ZYNKX) made with pear juice and lotus rhizome juice 15 g each, the juice of Chinese chives and the juice of ginger 5 g each and cow's milk 250 g, mixed well and heated for drinking.

Pear juice, lotus rhizome juice and cow's milk can nourish the Stomach and promote the production of Body Fluids. The juice of Chinese chives can activate Blood circulation and dissolve stasis, while fresh ginger can harmonize the Stomach and send down Counterflow Qi.

Impairment of both Qi and Yin

Symptoms are difficulty in swallowing food, fatigue, emaciation, shortness of breath, hard dry stools, pale and barely moistened tongue and a thready and weak pulse. Dietary Therapy should be directed at replenishing Qi and Yin and promoting the production of Body Fluids to moisten Dryness.

The recommended food is the recipe for an electuary (LLYH) using cow's milk, juice of reed rhizome, ginseng, longan, juice of sugarcane and pear juice in equal amounts, plus a little juice of fresh ginger and some honey, boiled together into an electuary to be taken from time to time.

Cow's milk, ginseng and longan can replenish Qi and Blood and harmonize the Stomach, while the juice of reed rhizome, pear juice and the juice of sugarcane can clear up Heat, nourish Yin and promote the production of Body Fluids. Fresh ginger is used to harmonize the Stomach and send down Counterflow Qi. Honey is used for flavor, but it also has the effect of reinforcing the Middle Burner and moistening Dryness.

As for cases due to accumulation of Blood stasis or to Qi deficiency and Yang exhaustion, diet therapy is not so effective, so their treatment is not discussed here.

RETENTION OF DAMP (IN THE STOMACH AND SPLEEN)

Retention of Damp in the Spleen and Stomach is characterized by a general heaviness, fatigue, stuffiness in the chest and fullness in the upper abdomen, loss of taste and appetite, with a greasy tongue coating.

Illnesses caused by Damp are classified into external Damp and internal Damp. The former is caused by the invasion of the Damp pathogen from outside, resulting in obstruction of the Middle Burner, while the latter is caused by malfunction of the Spleen and Stomach which fail to digest and absorb the essence of food, resulting in retention of fluids inside the body. The two types are also interrelated. When the external Damp causes disease, it manifests in the Spleen and Stomach; when the Spleen and Stomach fail to function normally, retention of Damp is more likely to occur.

After the Damp pathogen obstructs the Spleen and Stomach, in patients with constitutional Deficient Cold in the Spleen and Stomach the pathogen is more likely to turn into Coldness; in patients with accumulation of Heat in the Stomach and the Intestines or with hyperactivity of Fire due to Yin deficiency, the pathogen is more likely to turn into Heat. But Damp is a Yin pathogen with a sticky and sluggish nature. When Damp is excessive , Yang is weakened and the pathogen is more likely to turn into Coldness. Therefore, clinically, there are more cases of Damp retention turning into Coldness than turning into Heat.

Recommended foods

For patients with Damp retention, it is desirable to eat foods that are light in taste and have the effects of removing Damp. Examples are wax gourd, soya bean sprouts, cowpeas, red beans, water spinach, coix seeds, flat beans, fresh agastache and jasmine.

Foods to avoid

It is undesirable to have raw, cold, sweet, greasy foods and things that are not easy to digest. Alcohol is to be avoided.

Diet recipes

Damp obstructing the Spleen

Symptoms include fatigue in the limbs and the body, severe headache, stuffiness in the chest and fullness in the upper abdomen, loss of appetite, stickiness or sweetness in the mouth, loss of taste, a white and greasy tongue coating and a soft and slippery pulse. Dietary Therapy should be administered to dissolve turbidity and relieve Damp.

The recommended food is a gruel made with flat beans 50 g and red beans 100 g, decocted by boiling in water. Add fresh leaves of agastache 6 g and round cardamon seeds 3 g. Boil twice over. Remove the agastache and round cardamon seeds and season with salt. Eat the beans and drink the soup.

Flat beans and red beans can dissolve Damp. Round cardamon seeds and agastache can dissolve Damp and harmonize the Middle Burner.

Damp and Heat obstructing the Middle Burner

Symptoms are a bitter taste and stickiness in the mouth, poor appetite, stuffiness in the chest and fullness in the abdomen, thirst without desire to drink, dark urine, or low fever, yellow greasy tongue coating and a soft rapid pulse. Dietary Therapy should be directed at clearing up Heat and relieving Damp.

The recommended recipe is a soup made with soya bean sprouts, 150 g, and a little ginger, adding 250 g sliced wax gourd when the soya beans are cooked. Boil further till the wax gourd is cooked and season with salt. Drink the soup and eat the soya bean sprouts and the wax gourd.

Soya bean sprouts and wax gourd can clear Heat and relieve Damp to remove the Damp-Heat which obstructs the Middle Burner. Fresh ginger can harmonize the Stomach. When the disease occurs in the summer a gruel made with lotus leaves is also effective.

Deficiency in the Spleen and obstruction of Damp

Symptoms are fatigue, lethargy, heaviness in the limbs, discomfort in the upper abdomen, loss of appetite, reluctance to eat oily or greasy foods, loose stool or diarrhea, pale and enlarged tongue with a thin and greasy coating, and a soft and slow pulse. Dietary Therapy should be directed at reinforcing the Spleen and dissolving Damp.

The recommended recipe is an eight-ingredient gruel (FMZZ) using euryale seed, Chinese yam, poria, lotus seeds, coix seeds, white flat beans, pilose asiabell root and rhizome of large-headed atractylodes, 6 g each. Wrap the last two items in cloth. Boil everything in water, remove the bag of herbs after boiling and add 150 g of rice to the decoction to make a gruel to be taken in several servings.

The herbs used are effective in reinforcing and nourishing the Spleen, while poria, coix seeds and flat beans can also relieve and dissolve Damp.

EPIGASTRIC PAIN

Epigastric pain refers to pain in the upper abdomen around the xiphoid process. The pain is often accompanied by belching, regurgitation of acid and vomiting.

Epigastric pain is mostly due to intemperance of diet, Liver Qi invading the Stomach, a weak Spleen and Stomach, or invasion of the Stomach by external pathogens leading to stagnation and obstruction of Stomach Qi, malfunction of the Stomach in digesting and sending down, or even stasis, obstruction or malnutrition of collaterals in the Stomach, i.e. the Stomach organ itself may eventually be affected. The disease lies in the Stomach, but it is closely linked to the Liver and the Spleen.

Recommended foods

For patients with epigastric pain it is desirable to have foods that are fine, soft in texture and have the effects of reinforcing the Spleen and the Stomach, such as thin gruel, noodles, lotus rhizome powder, soya milk, cow's milk and oranges.

Foods to avoid

It is undesirable to have raw, cold, dry and hard foods. Alcohol and strong tea are also to be avoided. Persons with profuse gastric acid should not have foods that are too sour in taste. Examples are vinegar, lemons and plums. Meals should be taken at regular times and helpings should be moderate.

Diet recipes

Impairment due to food stagnation

Symptoms include pain in the Stomach, Fullness in the upper abdomen, eructation with fetid odor and acid regurgitation, anorexia and loss of appetite, or vomiting up undigested foods with the pain being alleviated after vomiting or passing wind; difficult stools, a thick and greasy tongue coating and a slippery deficient pulse. Dietary Therapy should be directed at assisting digestion and dissolving Stagnation of Food.

The recommended food is spiced betel nuts (LKZS) made with betel nuts 200 g, dried mandarin peel 20 g, cloves and katsumadai seeds, 10 g each, boiled in water with some salt till the liquid is about to dry up. After it cools down, cut up the mixture into lumps roughly the size of soya beans. Take 5–10 lumps after meals and chew them well.

Betel nuts have the effects of assisting digestion and dissolving stagnation. Being cooked with dried mandarin peel, cloves and katsumadai seeds, they have a stronger effect in reinforcing the Stomach, activating the circulation of Qi and relieving pain.

Another recipe is a gruel made with onion, which has the effects of reinforcing the Stomach, assisting digestion, sending down the Central Qi and dissolving stagnation.

Liver Qi invading the Stomach

Symptoms are abdominal fullness, pain in the upper abdomen extending to the hypochondrium, frequent belching, difficult defecation with the pain being aggravated by emotional disturbance; a thin white tongue coating and a taut pulse. Dietary Therapy should be directed at regulating the Liver Qi, harmonizing the Stomach and relieving pain.

The recommended recipe is an infusion made with finger citron (chopped) 5 g and roses 6–10 g, mixed with boiling water to be drunk as a tea.

Both items have the effects of easing the Liver, relieving depression, regulating Qi and relieving pain.

Accumulation of Heat in the Liver and the Stomach

Symptoms include burning heat and pain in the

upper abdomen, restlessness, discomfort in the stomach and acid regurgitation, a dry mouth, a bitter taste, a red tongue with yellow coating, a taut and rapid pulse. Dietary Therapy should be directed at purging Heat and harmonizing the Stomach.

The recommended recipe is balsam pear 150 g, cut into large chunks and marinated in salt water, Chinese olives 50 g and one pig's tripe. Boil them together till the tripe is well cooked. Eat the tripe and drink the soup.

Balsam pear and Chinese olives can purge Heat, while pig's tripe can reinforce the Spleen and Stomach. When the three are cooked together, they have the effect of purging Heat without impairing the Spleen and Stomach.

Cold invading the Stomach

Symptoms are sudden onset of pain in the upper abdomen, intolerance to cold with the pain being alleviated by warmth. Or there can be intolerance to cold, fever, pain in the head and the body. Tongue coating is white, and the pulse is taut and tense. Dietary Therapy should be directed at warming the Stomach, dispersing Cold and relieving pain.

The recommended recipe is a decoction of seven grains of pepper and ten dates (stoned), with a suitable amount of brown sugar added for flavor. Drink the decoction and eat the dates.

Dates can reinforce the Spleen and warm the Stomach, pepper can warm the Stomach, disperse Cold and relieve pain. Brown sugar can help warm the Stomach besides being a condiment. For cases that have such exterior symptoms as intolerance to cold, fever, aching in the head and the whole body, a drink of ginger, sugar and purple perilla can be used.

Stasis of Blood

Symptoms include stabbing pain in the upper abdomen at a fixed spot, a dark red tongue and an uneven pulse. Dietary Therapy should be directed at activating Blood circulation, dissolving stasis and relieving pain.

The recommended recipe is a gruel (SHF) made with peach kernels (skin and tip removed) 10 g and rehmannia root 10 g, decocted and strained, adding 100 g of non-glutinous rice to make a gruel. When the gruel is cooked, add 2 g of cinnamon bark powder and 50 g of brown sugar. Take in two servings, one in the morning, the other in the afternoon.

Peach kernels and brown sugar can activate Blood circulation and dissolve Blood stasis. Cinnamon bark can warm and activate Blood Vessels and relieve pain. Rehmannia root can nourish Yin and replenish Blood. The addition of rehmannia allows the other ingredients to clear stagnation and move Blood without damaging the Blood or Yin.

Deficient Cold in the Spleen and Stomach

Symptoms are a dull pain in the Stomach, alleviated by warmth or massage; regurgitation of clear liquid, loss of appetite, fatigue, or loose stool, cold limbs, a pale tongue and a weak pulse. Dietary Therapy should be directed at warming the Middle Burner and reinforcing the Spleen.

The recommended recipe is soup (YSZY) made with barley 200 g. Mutton 500 g and five tsaoko fruits are boiled till the mutton is cooked. Take out the mutton and tsaoko. Mix the decoction with the barley soup and boil further till the barley is well cooked. Cut the mutton into small pieces, put them into the soup and season with salt. Take in several servings.

Mutton can reinforce deficiency and warm the Middle Burner, barley can replenish Qi and nourish the Stomach, while tsaoko can warm the Middle Burner and activate the Spleen.

Deficiency of Stomach Yin

Symptoms are a dull pain in the Stomach, a hot sensation – like being hungry, a dry mouth and throat, dry stools, a red tongue with little moisture, and a thready and taut pulse. Dietary Therapy should be directed at nourishing the Yin and reinforcing the Stomach.

The recommended recipe is the Stomach nourishing soup (see Hiccups).

ABDOMINAL PAIN

Abdominal pain refers to the symptom of pain in

the lower abdomen, below the Stomach. The causes of abdominal pain are varied. Here we only discuss abdominal pain involving exposure to Cold, intemperance of diet, emotional disturbance and constitutional deficiency in Yang, leading to stagnation of Qi, obstruction of the Vessels and Collaterals and malfunction of the Channels.

Recommended foods

Different food recipes should be prescribed according to the patient's specific conditions. For cases caused by accumulation of Cold, use foods that can help warm the Middle Burner and disperse Cold, such as dried ginger, pepper and brown sugar. For cases involving deficient Cold, take foods that are warm and tonifying, such as mutton and maltose. For cases involving stagnation of Qi and Blood stasis, it is desirable to have foods which ease and activate the Qi, activate the circulation of Blood and dissolve stasis, such as mustard greens, egg, Chinese hawthorn and brown sugar. For cases due to Retention of Food or indigestion, it is desirable to control the amount of food intake and to eat foods that assist digestion and help dissolve Food Stagnation, such as onion, turnip, acanthaceous indigo, Chinese hawthorn and water chestnuts.

Foods to avoid

Persons with deficient Cold should not take Cool or Cold foods such as melons and raw fruits. Those with stagnation of Qi and Blood stasis should avoid foods such as beans and taro, while those with indigestion should not eat greasy, indigestible foods.

Diet recipes

Accumulation of Cold

Symptoms are acute abdominal pain alleviated by warmth but aggravated by cold; loss of appetite, no thirst, clear and copious urine, normal or loose stools, tongue coating that is thin and white, a deep and tense pulse. Dietary Therapy should be directed at dispersing Cold and relieving pain.

The recommended diet is common fennel gruel

(BCGM) made with non-glutinous rice 50 g. Add a suitable amount of common fennel shoots when the gruel is nearly cooked. Add salt and lard to season and take orally.

Another recommended diet is dumplings stuffed with common fennel shoots and pork or mutton.

Deficient Cold

Symptoms include dull and intermittent pain in the abdomen alleviated by warmth but aggravated by cold, hunger or fatigue, with the symptoms being alleviated after meals or rest, loose stool, lethargy, shortness of breath and intolerance to cold, a pale tongue with white coating, and a deep and thready pulse. Dietary Therapy should be directed at warming the Middle Burner and tonifying the deficiency, relieving the pain and spasm.

The recommended diet is the Middle Burner Reinforcing Chicken. Take one chicken thoroughly cleaned and stuff it with cinnamon twigs and fresh ginger, 9 g each, common peony root 12 g, seven dates, liquorice 6 g or maltose 100 g. The chicken should be steamed.

Cinnamon twig, common peony root, fresh ginger, dates, maltose and liquorice are ingredients of the Minor Decoction for Strengthening the Middle Burner as recorded in the *Revised General Treatise on Febrile Diseases*, which is effective in warming the Middle Burner, tonifying the deficiency, relieving pain and spasm. Chicken can warm the Middle Burner, replenish Qi and tonify deficiency.

Stagnation of Qi

Symptoms are fullness in the abdomen, a migratory pain extending to the hypochondrium and the lower abdomen, stuffiness in the chest, belching, thin and white tongue coating, and a taut pulse. Dietary Therapy should be directed at regulating the Liver Qi.

The recommended diet is Xiang-Sha Tang (BJFY) which is made by boiling white sugar 500 g, in water till the liquid is thickened. Add 15 g citron fruit powder and 10 g amomum fruit powder, well mixed. Boil further till the sugar makes filaments when picked up. Cool down and cut into small pieces. To be taken twice a day, three pieces a time.

Citron fruit and amomum fruit can regulate the Liver and relieve stagnation, regulate Qi and relieve pain.

Blood Stasis

Symptoms are protracted abdominal pain which is severe and has a fixed location, a dark and livid tongue, and a uneven and sticky pulse. Dietary Therapy should be directed at activating Blood circulation and dissolving Blood stasis.

The recommended recipe is peach kernel gruel (see Epigastric pain).

Indigestion or Food Stagnation

Symptoms include fullness, pain and tenderness in the abdomen, eructation with fetid odor and acid regurgitation, nausea and vomiting, constipation or diarrhea, a greasy tongue coating and a slippery pulse. Dietary Therapy should be directed at assisting digestion and harmonizing the Middle Burner.

The recommended diet is turnip gruel (BCGM) made with 100 g non-glutinous rice. When the gruel is half cooked, put in 150 g chopped turnips. Boil further till the gruel is well cooked. Add salt and some lard to season.

Turnip can assist digestion and send down the Central Qi. When eaten in a gruel, it is good for harmonizing the Stomach. Turnip and onion decoction is also an effective cure.

DIARRHEA

Diarrhea is a disease marked by frequent defecation of loose or watery stools. The disease is mainly due to exposure to external pathogens, intemperance of diet, emotional disturbance and weakness in the Vital Organs, leading to deficiency of the Spleen and excessive Damp and malfunction in absorbing and transforming. The disease lies in the Spleen, the Stomach, the Small Intestines and the Large Intestines and is also closely linked to the Liver and the Kidney.

Recommended foods

For patients with diarrhea, it is desirable to have foods that are easy to digest, such as liquid gruel, noodles and lotus rhizome powder. For serious cases, it is important to have sugar and salt water frequently (see recipe under 'Table Salt', p. 128). For cases with Heat syndrome, strong tea can be prescribed.

Foods to avoid

It is undesirable to have foods that contain crude fibers or greasy, raw and Cold foods that are difficult to digest. Examples are celery, Chinese chives, soya bean shoots, fatty meat, cold drinks and baked foods.

Diet recipes

Cold-Damp

Symptoms are loose or watery stools, abdominal pain and excessive bowel sounds, distension in the upper abdomen, loss of appetite; or fever and intolerance to cold, headache, nasal obstruction, soreness in the limbs and body, thin and white or white and greasy tongue coating, and a soft and slow pulse. Dietary Therapy should be directed at dispersing Cold and dissolving Damp.

The recommended diet is a drink made with fresh ginger 10 g, tsaoko 5 g and a suitable amount of brown sugar, decocted for drinking regularly.

Fresh ginger can disperse Cold and relieve an exterior syndrome, tsaoko can dissolve Damp while brown sugar can warm the Middle Burner besides being a condiment.

Damp-Heat

Symptoms include diarrhea, abdominal pain, urgent defecation or difficult stools which are yellowish brown and foul, a sensation of heat in the anus, thirst, scanty yellow urine, yellow and greasy tongue coating and a soft and rapid or slippery and rapid pulse. Dietary Therapy should be directed at clearing Heat and dissolving Damp.

The recommended diet is purslane gruel (SYXJa) made with 60 g of non-glutinous rice. When the gruel is nearly cooked, put in 30–60 g of purslane and bring to the boil. It may be eaten with salt or white sugar for flavor.

Purslane can clear Heat and remove toxins to arrest diarrhea. Non-glutinous rice reinforces the Stomach and harmonizes the Middle Burner. Purslane used as a vegetable is also an effective cure.

Stagnation of Food in the Stomach and Intestines

Symptoms are abdominal pain alleviated after passing stools; excessive bowel sounds, foul stool with the odor of bad eggs, fullness in the abdomen, a foul breath and eructation, loss of appetite, a turbid tongue coating, and a slippery and full pulse. Dietary Therapy should be directed at assisting digestion and dissolving stagnation.

The recommended diet is a drink made with rice crust 60 g and Chinese hawthorn 15 g, decocted together, adding a suitable amount of brown sugar to season for drinking.

Rice crust can reinforce the Spleen, assist digestion and arrest diarrhea, Chinese hawthorn can aid digestion and dissolve stagnation.

Deficiency of the Stomach

Symptoms include loose stool with undigested food in it, loss of appetite, fullness in the abdomen, lethargy and general weakness, a dry yellow complexion, a pale tongue with white coating, and a slow and weak pulse. Dietary Therapy should be directed at reinforcing the Spleen and removing Damp.

The recommended diet is lotus seed cakes (SCSS) made with roasted lotus seeds and glutinous (or non-glutinous) rice 200 g each, poria 100 g, ground together into powder. Add to the powder a suitable amount of white sugar, mix well and add some water to make a dough for steaming. Cut the cooked cake into small pieces when it has cooled down.

Lotus seeds can reinforce the Spleen and strengthen the Intestines and poria can reinforce the Spleen and remove Damp.

Deficiency or exhaustion of Kidney Yang

Symptoms are pain below the navel in the early morning, excessive bowel sounds, diarrhea, symptoms being slightly alleviated after passing stools, intolerance to cold in the abdominal area, cold lower limbs, soreness in the back and knees, a pale tongue with a white coating, and a deep and thready pulse. Dietary Therapy should be aimed at reinforcing the Kidney to arrest diarrhea.

The recommended diet is psoralea fruit 15 g and one pig's kidney, washed clean and chopped, boiled together in water. Add some salt to season. Eat the kidney and drink the soup. Take the preparation once or twice a day.

Psoralea fruit warms and reinforces the Spleen and the Kidney and thus arrests diarrhea. Pig's kidney reinforces the Kidney.

DYSENTERY

Dysentery is a disease occurring mostly in the summer and autumn, marked by abdominal pain, a strong urge to defecate or urinate, red and white stools. The disease is due to exposure to Damp-Heat and epidemic toxic Qi from the outside, or due to a raw and cold diet affecting the Vital Organs from the inside. Damp-Heat, epidemic toxins and Cold-Damp may stagnate and accumulate in the Intestines, preventing the Intestines from transforming food, leading to stagnation of Qi and Blood, resulting in pus and bad Blood.

Of the different types of dysentery, the one caused by epidemic toxins is called toxic dysentery. It has sudden onset and dangerous symptoms and here we omit this type. When the disease is prolonged, there can be deficiency in both the Spleen and the Kidney.

Recommended foods

Patients with dysentery should have foods that are light in taste, easy to digest and contain little fibre. Examples are liquid gruel, lotus rhizome powder and noodles. For cases of frequent stools, it is desirable to have sugar and salt water (boiled) (see recipe under 'Table Salt', p. 128). Foods that have the effects of clearing Heat, removing toxins and relieving the dysentery include purslane, houttuynia, onion, garlic, balsam pears, Chinese hawthorn, honeysuckle flower and tea. For cases of protracted dysentery with weakness in the Spleen and Kidney, foods that can reinforce the Spleen and Kidney and consolidate the Intestines include Chinese yam, lotus seeds, euryale seeds, crucian carp and plums.

Foods to avoid

It is undesirable to take foods that are greasy, raw and Cold and not easy to digest. For cases of the Damp-Heat type, foods that have a Warm and tonifying nature, such as cow's milk, chicken eggs and Chinese chives, are to be avoided.

Diet recipes

Dysentery of the Damp-Heat type

Symptoms include abdominal pain, a strong urge to defecate or urinate, pus and blood in the stools, frequent defecation amounting to some ten or more times a day, a hot sensation in the anus, dark and scanty urine, possibly a fever, a yellow and greasy tongue coating, and a slippery and rapid pulse. Dietary Therapy should be directed at clearing Heat and removing toxins. The recommended diet is purslane gruel (see Diarrhea).

Dysentery of the Cold-Damp type

Symptoms are a jellylike stool more white than red, accompanied by abdominal pain, a strong urge to defecate or urinate, loss of appetite, fullness in the abdomen, heaviness in the head and body, a pale tongue with white and greasy coating, a soft and weak pulse. Dietary Therapy should be directed at warming and dissolving Cold-Damp, removing the toxins and arresting dysentery.

The recommended diet is a soup made with dried ginger 6 g, garlic 15 g and a suitable amount of brown sugar, decocted till the garlic is cooked. Drink the decoction and eat the garlic.

Dried ginger can warm the Middle Burner and disperse Cold and Damp, garlic can warm the Middle Burner and reinforce the Stomach and at the same time remove the toxins and arrest dysentery, while brown sugar adds flavor to the soup and warms the Stomach.

Another recipe is garlic soaked in sugar and vinegar.

Deficiency of both the Spleen and Kidney

Symptoms include protracted dysentery or recurrent episodes of the disease, with heaviness and distension in the anus, loose stool with pus and blood, a sallow complexion, emaciation, a pale tongue with white coating, and a deep and thready pulse. Dietary Therapy should be directed at reinforcing the Spleen, tonifying the Kidney and consolidating the Intestines.

The recommended diet is the immortals' gruel (SSBY) made with Chinese yam and euryale seeds, 50 g each, and non-glutinous rice 100 g, cooked together into a gruel with water, adding brown sugar or salt to season. Eat the gruel in two servings, one in the morning, the other in the afternoon.

Chinese yam and euryale seeds can reinforce the Spleen and tonify the Kidney, consolidate the Intestines and arrest diarrhea, while non-glutinous rice nourishes the Stomach Qi. For cases with persistent toxins, the recipe can be used alternately with purslane gruel.

CONSTIPATION

Constipation is a disease marked by obstruction of stools, prolonged intervals between stools, or difficulty in passing stools.

The disease is attributable mainly to Dryness and Heat accumulated internally, stagnation of Qi, deficiency of Qi failing to circulate, Blood deficiency causing a dryness of the Intestines, or to accumulation of Yin Cold, resulting in malfunction of the Intestines.

Recommended foods

Patients with constipation should have fresh and soft vegetables, such as spinach, carrot, tremella and wood-ears, fresh fruits such as peach, persimmon, bananas and figs; and foods that have the effects of moistening the Intestines and aiding bowel motions, such as sesame, honey, walnut, sweet almond and pine nuts.

Foods to avoid

Foods that are pungent and spicy, Hot and irritating, such as garlic, chillies and peppers, should not be eaten.

Diet recipes

Accumulation of Heat

Symptoms are obstruction of stools for days, a red face, fever in the body, distension or pain in the abdomen, a dry mouth, a bitter taste, a red tongue with yellow coating or yellow and dry coating, and a slippery and rapid pulse. Dietary Therapy should be directed at clearing Heat and moistening the Intestines.

The recommended diet is a soup made with water spinach and cluster mallow, 250 g each, decocted together, adding 50 g of sesame seed oil and some salt to season. Eat the vegetables and drink the soup.

Water spinach and cluster mallow can clear Heat and aid bowel motions. Sesame can moisten the Intestines and help ease the bowels.

Another recipe uses water spinach by itself. Blanch it with boiling water, then add sesame seed oil and other condiments, and eaten as a salad.

Deficiency of Blood

Symptoms are constipation, dull complexion, dizziness, palpitation, pale lips and tongue, and a thready and uneven pulse. Dietary Therapy should be directed at nourishing Blood and moistening Dryness.

The recommended diet is a gruel (BCGM) made with spinach and glutinous rice, 200 g each. Blanch the spinach in boiling water and cook the glutinous rice in the spinach water to make a gruel. Add the spinach to the gruel and bring to the boil. Take the gruel over a few days with honey added for flavor.

Spinach can nourish Yin and replenish Blood, moisten the Intestines and aid bowel motions.

Knotweed 30 g can be added to the gruel during cooking, which can enhance its effects.

Another way of using spinach is to blanch it with boiling water, add sesame seed oil and eat as a salad.

Qi deficiency

Symptoms include difficulty in passing stools, spontaneous perspiration, shortness of breath, a pale complexion, fatigue, a pale tongue with white coating, and an empty pulse. Dietary Therapy should be directed at replenishing Qi and moistening the Intestines.

The recommended recipe is a milkvetch root decoction (JGY) made with milkvetch root 15 g, dried mandarin peel 5 g and hemp seeds 10 g, decocted together. Add 100 g of honey to the decoction, which should be drunk in one day.

Milkvetch root enriches Qi, hemp seeds and honey moisten the Intestines and ease the bowels, while dried mandarin peel regulates Qi.

Yang deficiency

Symptoms are difficulty in passing stools (which are very hard), clear and profuse urine, a pale complexion, cold limbs, intolerance to cold, coldness and pain in the abdomen or soreness and coldness in the spine and back, a pale tongue with a white coating, and a deep and slow pulse. Dietary Therapy should be directed at warming the Yang and aiding bowel motions.

The recommended recipe is a gruel made with desert cistanche 15 g, mutton and non-glutinous rice 100 g each, a little salt, two stalks of Chinese spring onion and three slices of fresh ginger. First boil the desert cistanche and ginger to obtain the juice. Add mutton (finely sliced) and non-glutinous rice to make a gruel. When the gruel is ready with the mutton cooked, add the Chinese spring onion and salt to season. Take the gruel in the early morning and late afternoon.

Desert cistanche warms the Kidney and aids bowel motions, mutton enriches Qi and Blood and warms the Lower Burner, while non-glutinous rice nourishes the Stomach. The non-glutinous rice can be omitted so that the recipe becomes a mutton soup.

VOMITING BLOOD

Hematemesis is vomiting of blood from the stomach. The blood is bright or dark red like coffee granules, containing the remains of food.

The problem is mainly due to accumulation of Heat in the Stomach which burns the collaterals of the Stomach, Liver Fire invading the Stomach and impairing the vessels in the Stomach, improper diet or fatigue impairing the Stomach from inside, or deficiency of Qi failing to control Blood.

Recommended foods

There are Full and Deficient syndromes in the disease. For Full cases, diet should be plain and light in taste. It is best to have foods that are effective in cooling Blood and arresting bleeding, such as liquid gruel, capsella, wood-ears, tremella, day lily, houttuynia and lotus rhizome. For deficient cases, it is desirable to have foods that reinforce the Spleen and replenish Qi, such as cow's milk, eggs, Chinese yam and lotus seeds.

Foods to avoid

In either case, foods that are dry, hard, pungent and spicy and tend to agitate pathogenic Fire should be avoided. Examples are wine, chillies, pepper and roasted foods.

Diet recipes

Full syndrome

Symptoms are profuse hematemesis, with bright red or dark red blood containing the remains of food, a bitter taste, foul breath, distension and pain in the abdomen and the hypochondrium, constipation or dark stools, a red tongue with yellow and greasy coating, and a slippery and rapid pulse. Dietary Therapy should be aimed at clearing Heat, cooling the Blood and arresting bleeding.

The recommended diet is a drink (YXZZCXL) made with fresh lotus rhizome 120 g (sliced) and fresh cogongrass rhizome 120 g (roughly chopped), decocted together for drinking as tea from time to time.

Fresh lotus rhizome cools Blood and arrests bleeding, while cogongrass rhizome clears up Heat, cools Blood and arrests bleeding.

Deficient syndrome

Symptoms include recurrent hematemesis which comes and goes but fails to be cured, with dark red or light red blood, poor appetite, fatigue, palpitations, a pale complexion, a pale tongue and a thready, weak pulse. Dietary Therapy should be directed at replenishing Blood and arresting bleeding.

The recommended diet is a thick soup (TSL) made with one cup of fresh lotus rhizome juice, boiled with some water, 5 g of notoginseng and one chicken egg mixed together and put into the boiling decoction. Salt and cooking oil may be added to season the soup. Take twice a day with meals.

The juices of lotus rhizome and notoginseng can arrest bleeding, dissolve stasis and promote the regeneration of new tissues, while chicken eggs can enrich the Blood. If 5 g of ginseng powder is added, the soup will be more effective in enriching Qi and controlling Blood.

Chicken stewed with milkvetch root and noto-ginseng is also an effective treatment.

BLOODY STOOLS

This disease is mainly due to accumulation of Damp-Heat in the Intestines, which burns the vessels, or to deficiency of the Central Qi which fails to control the Blood.

Recommended foods

For cases owing to Damp-Heat in the Intestines, use fresh vegetables such as lotus rhizome, day lily, water spinach, egg plant, cluster mallow, wood-ears, purslane and houttuynia and fresh fruits such as banana, water chestnuts and per-simmon. For cases owing to deficient Cold in the Spleen and Stomach, take the above mentioned items plus eggs, chicken and finless eel, which are tonifying in nature.

Foods to avoid

Generally, foods that are pungent, spicy and irritating are to be avoided. Examples are chillies, fresh ginger and wine.

Diet recipes

Damp-Heat in the Intestines

Symptoms include fresh blood in the stools, difficult or loose stools, together with abdominal pain, a bitter taste, yellow and greasy tongue coating, and a soft and rapid pulse. Dietary Therapy should be directed at clearing and dissolving Damp-Heat, cooling the Blood and arresting bleeding.

The recommended diet is 10 g pagoda tree flower and 250 g large intestines of pig (SXJYSP). Stuff the flower into the intestines before stewing and add some salt to season. Drink the soup and eat the intestine.

Pagoda tree flower can cool the Blood and arrest bleeding, clear up Heat and remove Damp while large intestines of pig can consolidate the Large Intestines.

Deficient Cold in the Spleen and Stomach

Symptoms are dark red or even black blood in the stools, dull pain in the abdomen, desire for warm drinks, a dull complexion, fatigue, loose stool, a pale tongue and a thready pulse. Dietary Therapy should be directed at reinforcing the Spleen, warming the Middle Burner and arresting bleeding.

The recommended diet is chicken, stewed with notoginseng and preserved ginger, 10 g each, and Chinese yam 50 g. Stuff the herbs into the chicken before stewing and add salt to season when the chicken is cooked. Eat the chicken and drink the soup.

Chicken warms and enriches Qi and Blood, notoginseng can arrest bleeding and promote the generation of Blood, preserved ginger can warm the Middle Burner and arrest bleeding, and Chinese yam can reinforce the Spleen.

JAUNDICE

Jaundice is a disease marked mainly by yellowness in the body, the eyes and the urine. Its major characteristic is yellowing of the sclerae.

Jaundice has external and internal causes. External causes include exposure to external pathogens and intemperance of diet; internal causes are mainly deficient Cold in the Spleen and Stomach and internal deficiency from impairment. External causes and internal causes usually interact to result in the disease. The key to the onset of the disease is Damp, which tends to obstruct the Middle Burner and cause malfunction of the Spleen and the Stomach in lifting and sending down, and affects the functions of the Liver and the Gallbladder in dispersing and discharging. When the bile leaves its normal route, it will infiltrate into the skin through the Blood. Yang jaundice is mainly due to the accumulation of Damp-Heat, which burns the bile and drives it to flow out to the skin; Yin jaundice is mainly due to obstruction by Cold-Damp, causing sluggish Spleen Yang which results in the outflow of bile.

Recommended foods

Patients with jaundice should have foods that are light in taste and nutritious, such as cow's milk, lean pork, chicken eggs and bean products, and foods that have the effects of inducing urination and removing Damp, such as water spinach, capsella, young shoots of Zizania aquatica, mountain rorippa, acanthaceous indigo, coix seeds, red beans, wax gourd, loach and river snails. It is important to take some sugar.

Foods to avoid

Fatty, rich food and foods that are pungent, spicy and irritating are to be avoided.

Diet recipes

Yang jaundice

Symptoms include yellowness of the body and the eyes, fever and thirst, fullness in the chest and upper abdomen, loss of appetite, nausea, difficult urination, dull pain or hard mass in the right hypochondrium, constipation or loose stool, yellow and greasy or thick, greasy and slightly yellow tongue coating, and a taut, slippery and rapid or soft and slow pulse. Dietary Therapy should be directed at clearing Heat and removing Damp.

The recommended diet is fresh mountain rorippa 250 g, washed, cut up and sauteed in cooking oil with salt added for flavor, to be eaten as a vegetable.

Alternatively mountain rorippa and acanthaceous indigo blanched in boiling water are made into a salad with seasoning, or made into a soup, which can increase the effects of clearing Heat, removing Damp and relieving the jaundice.

Yin jaundice

Symptoms are a dark or ashen yellowness in the body and the eyes, loss of appetite, distension in the abdomen, loose stools, lassitude, intolerance to cold, loss of taste, no thirst, a pale tongue with a greasy coating, and a soft and slow or deep and slow pulse. Dietary Therapy should be directed at warming the Middle Burner, reinforcing the Spleen and dissolving Damp.

The recommended diet is a gruel made with oriental wormwood 10 g and dried ginger 6 g, decocted and strained. Add 60 g coix seeds to the decoction to make a gruel with some brown sugar for flavor.

Oriental wormwood can remove Damp and relieve jaundice, coix seeds can reinforce the Spleen and remove Damp, while dried ginger warms the Middle Burner and disperses Cold.

HYPOCHONDRIAC PAIN

Hypochondriac pain occurs on one or both sides of the body, just below the ribs. It is a common subjective symptom clinically.

The Liver is located under the hypochondrium over which its channels are distributed. The Gallbladder is attached to the Liver and its channels also run along the hypochondrium. Therefore, the two organs are held responsible for hypochondriac pain. The disease is due to emotional disturbance, depression of the Liver

Qi, protracted depression of Qi leading to stagnation of Qi and Blood stasis, exhaustion of Essence and Blood leading to deficiency of Liver Yin, resulting in malnutrition of the collaterals or to malfunction of the Spleen leading to stagnation of Damp-Heat.

Recommended foods

For patients with hypochondriac pain, use foods that are fresh and easy to digest that have the effects of regulating and reinforcing the Liver, such as finger citron, white plum blossom, roses, pig's liver, lean pork, eggs and beancurd.

Foods to avoid

It is undesirable to have fatty, pungent or fishy foods. For cases with deficiency of the Liver, foods that are Warm and tonifying, such as mutton, should be avoided.

Diet recipes

Depression of Liver Qi

Symptoms include distension and a migratory pain under the hypochondrium, which is affected by emotional factors; stuffiness in the chest, shortness of breath, loss of appetite, frequent belching, a thin tongue coating and a taut pulse. Dietary Therapy should be directed at regulating the Liver Qi.

The recommended diet is plum blossom tea made with white plum blossoms 6 g and finger citron 10 g, infused in boiling water. Add a suitable amount of white sugar or honey for flavor. To be drunk as a tea.

Plum blossoms can regulate the Liver and harmonize the Stomach, while finger citron can regulate the Liver Qi and relieve depressed Qi.

Stagnation of Blood

Symptoms are occasional masses under the hypochondrium, a dark red tongue, and a deep and uneven pulse. Dietary Therapy should be directed at activating the Blood circulation and dissolving stasis.

The recommended diet is a drink made with curcuma root 10 g, decocted; add roses 6 g and bring to the boil. Add a suitable amount of brown sugar and drink as tea.

Curcuma root can regulate the Liver Qi, activate Blood and relieve pain, while roses can regulate Qi and relieve depression, activate Blood circulation and disperse Blood stasis. Brown sugar can help to activate Blood circulation, besides being a condiment.

Damp-Heat in the Liver and Gallbladder

Symptoms include hypochondriac pain, a bitter taste, stuffiness, loss of appetite, nausea and vomiting, red eyes or yellowness in the eyes, the body and the urine, a yellow and greasy tongue coating, and a taut, slippery and rapid pulse. Dietary Therapy should be aimed at clearing Heat and removing Damp.

The recommended diet is a soup (TPSHF) made with river snails 300 g and river clams (shelled) 150 g. Keep the snails for one or two days in clear water (changed regularly) to clean them. Boil slightly after cleansing. Pick out the meat and add to the clams, which are then boiled in water. Add oil and salt for flavor. Drink the soup and eat the meat.

River snails can clear Damp-Heat and induce urination, while clams can clear Heat. The recipe can be used in conjunction with mountain rorippa and acanthaceous indigo, which will enhance the effects of clearing Heat and removing Damp.

Deficiency of Liver Yin

Symptoms include dull pain under the hypochondrium, which is aggravated by physical exertion, a dry mouth and throat, a hot sensation in the chest, dizziness, a red tongue with little coating, and a thready, taut and rapid pulse. Dietary Therapy should be directed at nourishing Yin and reinforcing the Liver.

The recommended diet is an electuary made with common peony root 50 g, liquorice 10 g and mulberry 500 g, boiled together in water and strained. Condense the liquid on a low heat, add 200 g of honey and boil further to make an electuary, to be taken twice a day, one spoonful at a time mixed with boiling water.

Common peony root and liquorice can nourish and regulate the Liver and relieve pain and spasm, while mulberries can nourish Yin.

VERTIGO

Vertigo is a disease marked by faintness and a sense of the head spinning. In mild cases, the symptom can be alleviated by shutting the eyes for a little while, but in grave cases patients have the feeling of being in a moving boat or vehicle and cannot stand still or have other symptoms such as nausea, vomiting and perspiration.

The disease is mostly deficient in nature. When there is deficiency of Yin, there will be hyperactivity of Liver Yang; when there is deficiency of Blood, there will be malnutrition of the brain; when there is deficiency of Qi, the clear Yang cannot rise; and when there is exhaustion of the Essence, there will be insufficiency of the Sea of Marrow (the brain). All of these may cause vertigo. In addition, the disease may be caused by Phlegm obstructing the Middle Burner, turbid Yin failing to descend, or clear Yang failing to rise.

Recommended foods

Diets should be prescribed according to the patient's condition. For cases owing to hyperactivity of Liver Yang or obstruction of the Middle Burner by Phlegm, use foods that are light in taste and can help send down the pathogenic Fire, expel the Phlegm and clear the head and the eyes. Examples are celery, turnips, Chinese cabbage and chrysanthemum. For cases owing to deficiency of Qi and Blood, it is desirable to have foods that can reinforce Qi and Blood, such as chicken, eggs, dates, longan. For cases owing to exhaustion of Kidney Essence, take foods that can help replenish Essence, nourish Yin and suppress hyperactivity of Yang. Examples are sesame, black beans and mussels.

Foods to avoid

With hyperactivity of Liver Yang or obstruction by Phlegm, salty, fatty or very sweet foods and offal should be avoided. For deficiency of Qi and Blood, do not eat melon or other raw and cold fruits. For exhaustion of Kidney Essence, avoid foods that irritate Fire and lift Yang, such as hot peppers, ginger and fermented glutinous rice.

Diet recipes

Hyperactivity of Liver Yang

Symptoms are dizziness and tinnitus which are aggravated by mental depression, restlessness, distension and pain in the head, paroxysmal feverish sensation in the head and face, lack of sleep and dreaminess, a red tongue with a yellow coating, and a taut pulse. Dietary Therapy should be directed at calming the Liver and suppressing hyperactivity of Liver Yang.

The recommended diet is celery gruel (BCGM) made with 30 g celery, washed and chopped, and 50–100 g non-glutinous rice boiled together to make a gruel for drinking twice a day.

Celery has the effects of dissolving Phlegm, expelling pathogenic Wind, calming the Liver and promoting acuity of vision. Celery is also used in salads.

Deficiency of Qi and Blood

Symptoms include vertigo aggravated by movement of the body and triggered off by fatigue, pale complexion, finger nails looking dull, shallow breathing, reluctance of speech, palpitations, insomnia, a pale tongue with a thin and white coating, and a thready and weak pulse. Dietary Therapy should be directed at replenishing Qi and Blood.

The recommended diet is one chicken, gutted and thoroughly cleaned, stuffed with 15 g of Chinese angelica root and 15 g of pilose asiabell root (QKSY). Stew the chicken with Chinese spring onion and ginger in a suitable amount of water till it is well cooked. Discard the herbs and season with salt; eat the meat and drink the soup.

Pilose asiabell root reinforces the Middle Burner and replenishes Qi, Chinese angelica enriches and regulates Blood, while chicken replenishes Qi and Blood.

Deficiency of the Liver and Kidney

Symptoms are dizziness, tinnitus, soreness and weakness in the back and knees, seminal emission and leukorrhea. In cases with more Yang deficiency, there will be cold limbs and profuse urination at night and in cases with more Yin deficiency, there will be hot sensations in the chest, palms and soles, night sweats, a red tongue with little coating, and a deep and thready pulse. Dietary Therapy should be directed at reinforcing the Liver and the Kidney.

The recommended diet is prepared black soya bean (JYQS) made with dogwood fruit, poria, Chinese angelica root, mulberry, prepared rehmannia root, psoralea fruit, dodder seed, eclipta, magnolia vine fruit, Chinese wolfberry, wolfberry bark and black sesame, 10 g each, decocted four times. Put in 500 g black soya beans (soaked in warm water overnight), boil till the liquid dries up and then roast the beans. They may be taken as often as necessary.

Black beans can reinforce the Spleen and the Stomach. With the combined benefits from all the drugs used in the preparation, it is effective in reinforcing the Liver and the Kidney.

Obstruction of turbid Phlegm

Symptoms include dizziness, heaviness in the head, stuffiness in the chest, nausea, loss of appetite, somnolence, a greasy tongue coating, and a taut and slippery pulse. Dietary Therapy should be directed at reinforcing the Spleen and removing the Damp.

The recommended diet is 10 g immature bitter orange and 30 g rhizome of largeheaded atractylodes, decocted three times (PWL). Discard the residue. Cook non-glutinous rice in the decoction. Cover the rice with a lotus leaf when it is nearly ready and heat further till it is well cooked. Eat the rice for breakfast and supper.

Immature bitter orange regulates Qi, dissolves Phlegm and food retention, largeheaded atractylodes rhizome reinforces the Spleen and dissolves Damp, while lotus leaf lifts and nourishes the Stomach Qi and helps the other drugs in reinforcing the Spleen and replenishing Qi.

WIND-STROKE

Wind-stroke is a disease whose major symptoms are; a sudden collapse from loss of consciousness, wry mouth and eyes, difficult speech and semiparalysis. There are also cases with only facial paralysis.

The disease is due to deficiency of Qi and Blood, plus emotional disturbance or impairment from improper diet or fatigue, leading to deficiency of Yin in the lower parts of the body and excessive Fire in the upper parts. When Qi and Blood leave their normal courses and Liver Wind rushes up with Phlegm to obscure the clear orifices and goes transversely into the collaterals; or when there is deficiency of Qi and stasis of Blood leading to malnutrition of channels and collaterals, Wind-Stroke is likely to occur.

Recommended foods

Wind-Stroke is classified into cases involving the Vital Organs and those involving the Channels and Collaterals. The acute symptoms involve the Vital Organs, while the sequelae are related to the Channels. For those cases involving the Vital Organs, during the period of coma, oral feeding is prohibited and patients should be fed nasogastrically with liquid foods that are nutritious and easy to digest, such as cow's milk, soy milk, lotus rhizome powder and fruit juice. During the recovery period, foods should be prescribed according to the different condition of the patient. Recommended foods are those that can reinforce the Liver and the Kidney, replenish Qi and Blood, dissolve Phlegm or remove stasis. Examples are mulberry, Chinese wolfberry, pears, wax gourd, water chestnuts, black beans, chicken, ox's bone marrow and sea cucumber.

Foods to avoid

Intially, avoid foods that are fatty, greasy, Warm and Dry, such as pork soup, mutton or beef juice. In the recovery period, foods that are fatty, sweet and cause Phlegm should not be taken. Examples are pig's fat, wine, strong tea, ginger and chillies.

Diet recipes

Wind-Stroke involving the Vital Organs

Yang stroke

Symptoms are suddenly falling to the ground, loss of consciousness, clenched hands, lockjaw, a red face, gasping, a red tongue with yellow and greasy coating, and a taut, slippery and rapid pulse. Dietary Therapy should be directed at clearing up Heat, dissolving Phlegm and regaining consciousness.

The recommended diet is hemp seed gruel (SJZL) made with fresh peppermint leaves and fresh ears of schizonepeta, 30 g each, washed and chopped, decocted and strained. Put in roasted hemp seeds 30 g and non-glutinous rice 50–100 g to make a thin gruel, which is then filtered for nasogastric feeding. Hemp seeds can tonify the deficiency and relieve the Wind syndrome in the five Vital Organs; schizonepeta and peppermint can clear up Heat and ease the throat to dissolve Phlegm. When made into a gruel, they are effective in the treatment of Wind-stroke with Phlegm-Heat obscuring the clear orifices. Bamboo juice can also be added to the recipe to dissolve Phlegm and promote consciousness.

Yin stroke

Symptoms include suddenly falling to the ground, a relaxed jaw and hands, quietness, a pale complexion, dark lips, excessive saliva, white and greasy tongue coating, and a deep and slippery or slow pulse. Dietary Therapy should be aimed at regaining consciousness by using pungent and Warm foods and at dissolving Phlegm and calming the pathogenic Wind.

The recommended diet is a thick soup (SJZL) made with sweet sedge 10 g and a pair of pig's kidneys (chopped, boiled and strained). Add 150 g of non-glutinous rice and 10 g of the stalks of Chinese spring onion to the decoction to make a gruel, which is then filtered for nasogastric feeding.

The stalks of Chinese spring onion can activate

Yang, sweet sedge can dissolve turbidity, while non-glutinous rice and pig's kidney can enrich Qi and help to nourish the body.

Exhaustion

Symptoms are suddenly falling to the ground, loss of consciousness, closed eyes and open mouth, snoring and thin breathing, extended hands, cold limbs, cold sweat all over the body, incontinence of feces and urine, paralysis of the limbs, flaccidity of the tongue, and a tracing pulse. Dietary Therapy should be directed at enriching Qi and restoring consciousness.

The recommended diet is ginseng gruel (SJBC) made with ginseng 3 g (powdered), a suitable amount of crystal sugar and 50–100 g of non-glutinous rice, made into a thin gruel. When the gruel is cooked, filter it for nasogastric feeding.

Ginseng can reinforce the five Zang Organs and tonify the Vital Qi, non-glutinous rice can reinforce the Spleen and nourish the Stomach and crystal sugar can reinforce the Middle Burner and the Stomach.

Wind-Stroke involving the Channels and Collaterals

Deficiency of the Collaterals combines with a Wind pathogen entering the internal organs. Symptoms are numbness in the hands, feet, muscles and skin, or sudden onset of facial paralysis, difficult speech, hemiplegia, thin and white tongue coating, and a floating and taut or taut and thready pulse. Dietary Therapy should be directed at nourishing Blood, reinforcing Yin and activating the Collaterals.

The recommended diet is a wine made with rehmannia root 50 g and low alcohol wine 2500 ml. Put the two into a large bottle. Then roast 500 g black beans and add to the bottle while still hot. Seal the bottle and store it for 7 days before drinking.

Rehmannia root nourishes Blood, the beans reinforce Kidney Yin while wine warms the channels and activates the Collaterals.

Deficiency of Qi, Blood stasis and obstruction of channels and collaterals

Symptoms include hemiplegia, facial paralysis, difficult speech, saliva running from the corner of the mouth, fatigue and weakness, frequent urination, a pale or spotted tongue and a deep and weak pulse. Dietary Therapy should be directed at replenishing Qi and activating the Collaterals.

The recommended diet is a gruel (SJBC) made with one ox's tripe, washed, chopped and boiled till the tripe is almost cooked. Add non-glutinous rice 100 g, a suitable amount of spring onion stalk, ginger, fermented soya beans and Sichuan pepper to make a gruel. Add some salt to season before eating. Ox's tripe and non-glutinous rice can reinforce the Middle Burner and enrich Qi; spring onion, ginger and Sichuan pepper can activate the Collaterals besides being condiments.

HEADACHE

A headache is seen in a number of acute and chronic conditions. In terms of Chinese medicine, a headache is often due to exposure to external Wind, Cold, Damp and Heat pathogens which tend to cover up the clear Yang; or due to turbid Phlegm or Blood stasis obstructing the channels and collaterals; or to accumulated anger turning into pathogenic Fire, leading to deficiency of Yin and hyperactivity of Yang which tends to go upwards and irritate the clear Qi; or to deficiency of Qi and Blood with insufficiency of the Liver and the Kidney, leading to malnutrition of the brains.

Recommended foods

For cases of exogenous headache, use foods that can help disperse the pathogenic Wind, such as spring onion, ginger, agastache, celery and chrysanthemum. For cases owing to deficiency in the Liver and insufficiency of Qi and Blood, it is desirable to have foods that can nourish the Liver and the Kidney, replenish and nurture Qi and Blood. Such foods include dates, black bean, litchi, longan, chicken, beef. For cases due to Phlegm and Blood stasis, take foods that can help reinforce the Spleen, remove Damp, activate Blood circulation and dissolve stasis. Examples are Chinese yam, coix seeds, oranges, Chinese hawthorn and brown sugar.

Foods to avoid

With exogenous headache, avoid rich fatty foods such as pork, chicken or sea cucumber. For deficiency of Liver, Qi and Blood, foods that are Warm and Dry, such as ginger and garlic, or Cold, such as melon, should not be eaten. For Phlegm and Blood stasis, do not eat fatty foods and those that cause Damp.

Diet recipes

Headache owing to pathogenic Wind-Cold

Symptoms are a headache extending to the neck and back, intolerance to wind and cold often accompanied by coughing and sneezing, thin and white tongue coating, and a floating pulse. Dietary Therapy should be directed at dispersing Wind and Cold.

The recommended diet is a gruel made with spring onion and fermented soya beans (BCGM). Make a gruel with 50–100 g non-glutinous rice. Put in the stalks of spring onion and fermented soya beans after the gruel is cooked. More water may be added and the gruel reheated, to provide several servings.

The recipe has the effects of relieving the exterior syndrome, expelling Wind pathogens and dispersing Cold pathogens. Slices of fresh ginger can be added to the gruel during cooking.

Headache due to pathogenic Wind-Heat

Symptoms include distension and aching in the head, fever and intolerance to wind, thirst and a sore throat, dark urine, a red tongue with yellow coating, a floating and rapid pulse. Dietary Therapy should be directed at dispersing pathogenic Wind and clearing up Heat.

The recommended diet is a tea made with mulberry leaves and peppermint, 20 g each, with dog thorn 10 g, infused in boiling water. Add a suitable amount of white sugar for drinking as tea.

The items used in the recipe are effective in dispersing Wind and clearing Heat, clearing and soothing the head and the eyes.

Headache owing to disorder of Liver Yang

Symptoms are a headache and dizziness, restlessness, insomnia, red face and eyes, a bitter taste, a red tongue with a thin and yellow coating, and a taut and vigorous pulse. Dietary Therapy should be aimed at calming the Liver and suppressing hyperactivity of Yang.

The recommended diet is chrysanthemum gruel (LLHY) made with non-glutinous rice 50–100 g and 10 g of chrysanthemum added when the gruel is cooked. Bring it to the boil for a while.

This recipe can disperse Wind and Heat, clear up Liver Fire, and is applicable to a headache of the Wind-Heat and the Liver Yang types. The effects of clearing Heat and calming down the Liver will be enhanced by adding hooked uncaria.

Kidney deficiency

Symptoms are pain in the head, dizziness and tinnitus, soreness and weakness in the back and knees, a red tongue with little coating, and a thready and rapid pulse. Dietary Therapy should be directed at replenishing the Essence and tonifying the Kidney.

The recommended diet is fermented mulberry rice (SJBC) made with fresh mulberries 1000 g, washed and squeezed to obtain the juice. Add 500 g of glutinous rice to the juice to make a gruel. When the gruel is cooked, mix in brewer's yeast. Cover it with a lid and and keep it warm. A few days later, the gruel will ferment and can then be taken.

Mulberries can reinforce the Liver and the Kidney and calm down deficient Wind.

Deficiency of Qi and Blood

Symptoms include a headache and dizziness aggravated by physical exertion, a dull complexion, palpitations, a pale tongue with thin white coating, and a thready and weak pulse. Dietary Therapy should be directed at replenishing Qi and Blood.

The recommended diet is bean soup with milkvetch root (YXCZL) made with milkvetch root 30 g (wrapped in cloth) and black beans

100 g, boiled together in water seasoned with salt. Eat the beans and drink the soup.

Milkvetch root and black beans used together can replenish Qi and nourish Blood.

Phlegm

Symptoms are headache and faintness, stuffiness in the chest and the upper abdomen, nausea and vomiting of phlegm and saliva, a white and greasy tongue coating, and a taut pulse. Dietary Therapy should be directed at dissolving Phlegm and expelling pathogenic Wind.

The recommended diet is Yuhumian (HJJF) made with preserved arisaema tuber, preserved pinellia tuber, 10 g each, and gastrodia tuber 15 g, decocted together and strained. Make a dough with the decoction and 1000 g of wheat flour and turn it into noodles. Cook the noodles in several sessions, adding cooking oil, spring onion, ginger juice and table salt to season.

Preserved arisaema tuber and pinellia tuber can dry Damp and dissolve Phlegm. Gastrodia tuber can expel pathogenic Wind and relieve pain.

Blood Stasis

Symptoms are prostration, with a stabbing headache which has a fixed location, a dark red tongue, and a thready and uneven pulse. Dietary Therapy should be directed at activating Blood circulation and dissolving Blood stasis.

The recommended diet is Ox's Brain Wine Infusion (SJBC) made with one brain of ox (sliced), dahurian angelica root and chuanxiong rhizome, 10 g each, boiled together in wine, to be taken while still warm, before sleep.

Chuanxiong rhizome and dahurian angelica can activate Blood circulation and dissolve Blood stasis, expel pathogenic Wind and relieve pain. Ox's brain can reinforce the brain. Therefore the recipe has the effects of both purging and reinforcing.

PAINFUL URINATION SYNDROME (LIN ZHENG)

'Lin' is a Chinese classification for problems involving frequent, short, dripping, painful and difficult urination or urination with pain reaching the lumbar area. The keynotes are discomfort and difficulty.

The disease is usually caused by accumulation of Damp-Heat in the Lower Burner. In cases where Damp-Heat flows downwards and leads to malfunction of the Bladder in absorbing fluids, it will cause pain and burning when passing water and is classed as Damp-Heat in the Bladder. (Strictly speaking this syndrome is usually considered separately from the Lin diseases, with another type (Qi Lin) making up the five classes of Lin.) When the Heat burns up the urine and causes the formation of bladder stones, it is called Stone Lin. When the Heat burns the Blood Vessels and causes Blood to come out with urine, it is called Blood Lin. When there is disturbance of the function of absorbing fluids and dividing the clear from the turbid, it is called Damp Lin. When the disease is prolonged and causes deficiency in the Spleen and the Kidney, it is called Fatigue Lin.

Recommended foods

There are Full and Deficient cases of Painful Urination. For the Full cases, it is desirable to have foods that help remove Damp and relieve the symptoms. Examples are red beans, flat beans, mung beans, cluster mallow, water spinach, wax gourd, pears and grapes. For the Deficient cases, use foods that reinforce the Spleen and the Kidney, such as wheat, maize, soya beans, sesame, walnuts, sturgeon and pig's kidney.

Foods to avoid

In Full cases, avoid foods that are Dry and Hot and cause Damp, such as fried food, chillies and fermented glutinous rice. In deficient cases, raw and Cold foods should not be eaten.

Diet recipes

Damp-Heat in the Bladder

Symptoms are a burning pain in the urinary tract, heaviness and pain in the lower abdomen, fever and intolerance to cold, thirst, a red tongue with a yellow coating, and a slippery and rapid pulse. Dietary Therapy should be directed at clearing Heat and relieving pain and stagnation.

The recommended diet is a soup made with rush pith and spring onion stalk, 10 g each, and towel gourd 500 g (cut up), boiled together in water (DPBC). When the gourd is cooked, season it with some salt for eating and drinking at meals. Rush pith and towel gourd used together can clear the Heat and ease urination, while the stalk of spring onion is effective in easing the urethra.

Stone Lin

Symptoms include heat, difficulty and pain on urination, grains of stone in the urine, interrupted urination, contracture in the lower abdomen, severe colicky pain in the back and the abdomen, or even blood in the urine, a thin and white tongue coating, and a taut or rapid pulse. Dietary Therapy should be directed at removing urinary stones.

The recommended diet is candied turnip (PJF) made with fresh turnip 500 g, washed and cut into strips before boiling in water. When cooked, add 150 g of honey and boil further on a low heat until the liquid is condensed.

Blood Lin

Symptoms are heat, difficulty and stabbing pain on urination, dark red urine or urine with blood clots, fullness and tightness in the lower abdomen, a red tongue and a rapid pulse. Dietary Therapy should be directed at cooling the Blood and easing the pain.

The recommended diet is a decoction (TPSHF) of fresh grapes and fresh lotus rhizome, squeezed to obtain 100 ml of juice from each, and fresh rehmannia root squeezed to obtain 50 ml of juice. Boil the juices together and add some honey, to be drunk after mixing with boiling water.

The combination of grapes and lotus rhizome can clear Heat, cool down Blood, induce urination and relieve stagnation.

Damp Lin

Symptoms are turbid urine which is like the water left after rice is washed or urine containing slippery and greasy matter, heat and pain in the urinary tract, a red tongue with a greasy coating, and a rapid pulse. Dietary Therapy should be directed at removing Damp and relieving stagnation.

The recommended diet is river snails cooked in wine (FSJF).

Use river snails 500 g. Remove the dirt by keeping them alive in clear water for one or two days, with the water changed regularly. Cut off the tips of the snails. Add some cooking wine and a suitable amount of water and stew until done. Pick out the meat with a needle and eat the snails with seasoning added.

River snails can clear up Heat and relieve Damp.

Fatigue Lin

Symptoms include slight redness and difficulty of urination, dripping urine, the symptoms coming and going and being aggravated by physical exertion, lethargy, soreness and weakness in the back and knees, a pale tongue and a weak pulse. Dietary Therapy should be directed at reinforcing the Spleen and tonifying the Kidney.

The recommended diet is a soup (SJBC) made with black beans 250 g, liquorice and fresh ginger, 10 g each, with a suitable amount of salt and water. Boil them together till the beans are cooked. Eat the beans at meals and drink the soup.

The black bean is used for its effects of reinforcing the Spleen and the Kidney. The recipe can be used in combination with euryale seeds and lotus seeds, which will be more effective in reinforcing the Spleen and consolidating the Kidney.

BLOOD IN THE URINE (HEMATURIA)

Hematuria is marked by blood or blood clots in the urine, without obvious difficulty, dripping or pain during urination.

The disease is caused mainly by excessive Heat

in the Lower Burner which impairs the minute blood vessels, causing the Blood to come out with urine, or by deficiency in the Spleen and the Kidney, which fail to control Blood.

Recommended foods

For full cases with Fire and Heat, it is desirable to have foods that help clear up Heat, cool down Blood, arrest bleeding and nourish Yin. Examples are grapes, sugarcane, persimmon, towel gourd, capsella and lotus rhizome. For deficient cases owing to deficiency of the Spleen and Kidney, take foods that can replenish Qi and tonify the Kidney, such as peanuts, dates, persimmon, lotus seeds, black beans and Chinese chives.

Foods to avoid

In deficient cases foods that are raw and Cold and will not arrest bleeding, such as melon and fruits, are to be taken with care as they might impair the Yang Qi. For full cases, pungent, Dry foods that irritate the Blood, such as garlic, spring onion, chives and fried foods, should not be taken.

Diet recipes

Excessive Heat in the Lower Burner

Symptoms are hot and dark urine which is stained with fresh blood, thirst, restless sleep at night, red tongue and rapid pulse. Diet therapy should be directed at cooling down Blood and arresting bleeding.

The recommended diet is a gruel (BQZHF) made with cogongrass rhizome 30 g, decocted and strained. Add 50 g of red beans and 50–100 g of non-glutinous rice to the decoction to make a gruel.

Red beans can clear up Heat and remove toxins, induce urination and disperse bad Blood, while cogongrass rhizome can clear up Heat, induce urination, cool off the Blood and arrest bleeding.

Hyperactivity of Fire due to deficiency of Yin

Symptoms are frequent urination which is

stained with blood, dizziness, tinnitus, hectic fever, hot sensation in the chest, soreness in the back and knees, a red tongue, and a thready and rapid pulse. Dietary Therapy should be directed at nourishing Yin and cooling down Blood.

The recommended diet is rehmannia root gruel (TPSHF) made with juice of raw rehmannia root 50 ml, honey 50 g, non-glutinous rice 100 g and the leaves of plantain 30 g.

Rehmannia root can nourish Yin and send down pathogenic Fire, while the leaves of plantain and honey can clear Heat and remove toxins.

Disharmony of the Spleen and the Kidney

Symptoms include protracted hematuria in which the blood is light red, pale complexion, lethargy, fatigue, loss of appetite, dizziness, tinnitus, soreness and weakness in the back and knees, a pale tongue, and a deep and weak pulse. Dietary Therapy should be directed at enriching Qi and tonifying the Kidney.

The recommended diet is mutton soup (QJYF) made with Chinese angelica root 10 g, rehmannia root and preserved ginger, 15 g each (all wrapped in cloth), and mutton 500 g (chopped), boiled together till the mutton is well cooked. Remove the wrapped medicines and season with salt.

Mutton, rehmannia root and Chinese angelica root can enrich Qi and reinforce the deficiency, while preserved ginger can warm the channels and help control Blood.

URINARY RETENTION

Urinary retention refers to difficult, dripping urination or total obstruction of urination, often without pain.

The disease is often due to exposure to external pathogens, Heat and stagnation of Qi in the Lungs which fail to regulate and clear the Water Channels; or to accumulation of Damp-Heat, causing malfunction of the Three Burners. It could also be due to mental depression leading to malfunction of the Liver in discharging and dispersing; to clear Qi failing to rise and turbid Qi failing to descend; or to exhaustion of the Fire at the Life Gate (Ming Men), leading to malfunction of the Bladder in absorbing liquids.

Recommended foods

For cases owing to obstruction of Qi by exogenous pathogens, it is desirable to have foods that are light in taste and effective in clearing the Water Channel. Examples are cluster mallow, capsella, bamboo shoots, wax gourd, towel gourd, watermelon, grapes, dried persimmon, mung beans, red beans, coix seeds and river snails. For cases owing to deficiency or exhaustion of the Spleen and the Kidney, use foods that can reinforce the Spleen and the Kidney, replenish Qi and warm Yang. Examples are walnuts, peanuts, dates, lotus seeds, chicken, beef and mutton.

Foods to avoid

Foods that are raw and Cold and tend to impair Yang Qi are to be avoided in cases of deficiency or exhaustion of the Spleen and Kidney. In cases of Qi obstruction, avoid fatty, pungent, sweet foods that cause Damp-Heat, such as pork, spring onion, garlic and longan.

Diet recipes

Heat and stagnation of Qi in the Lungs

Symptoms are difficult urination or total obstruction of urination, thirst, shortness of breath, in some cases with coughing, a yellow tongue coating, and a rapid pulse. Dietary Therapy should be directed at clearing Heat and clearing the Water Channels.

The recommended diet is a soup (ZSJYF) made with rush pith 6 g and two dried persimmons, boiled in water. Add some white sugar for flavor. Drink the soup and eat the persimmon.

Rush pith clears the Heat and removes Damp, while dried persimmon moistens the Lungs and clears Heat.

Accumulation of Damp and Heat

Symptoms include total obstruction of urination or scanty urine which is very dark and hot, distention and pain in the lower abdomen, thirst without desire for drinking, a red tongue with yellow greasy coating, and a soft and rapid pulse. Dietary Therapy should be directed at clearing and removing Damp-Heat and easing urination.

The recommended diet is talc gruel (SJZL) made with talc 30 g and pinks 15 g, decocted and strained. Add 100 g of non-glutinous rice to make a gruel. Season it with salt and add 10 g of spring onion stalk when the gruel is nearly cooked. Boil further till the gruel is well cooked.

Spring onion stalk can clear the urethra, while talc and pinks can clear up Heat and induce urination.

Depression of Central Qi

Symptoms are distension in the lower abdomen, difficult or scanty urine, fatigue, shortness of breath, a thin voice, a pale tongue with thin white coating, and a deep and weak pulse. Dietary Therapy should be directed at reinforcing the deficiency and easing urination.

The recommended diet is a thick soup made with green-headed duck (mallard) (TPSHF). Take one mallard, gutted and thoroughly cleaned, and fermented soya bean 50 g, and boil together in water. When the duck is cooked, add wax gourd (peeled) and turnip (chopped), 120 g each, and stalks of spring onion 50 g. Boil further till everything is done, season with salt and vinegar and eat before meals.

Duck reinforces deficiency, while wax gourd and turnip ease urination.

Depression of the Liver and stagnation of Qi

Symptoms include obstruction of urine or difficult urination, distension in the chest and abdomen, mental depression, restlessness, red tongue with thin and white or thin and yellow coating, and a taut pulse. Dietary Therapy should be aimed at regulating the Liver Qi and easing and inducing urination.

The recommended diet is as follows (BCSGY). To white sugar 500 g, boiled in water and reduced, add 30 g cluster mallow seeds, 50 g red tangerine peel (i.e. without the pith) and 20 g spring onion, pounded and stirred well with the syrup. Boil further till the syrup makes filaments when picked up and is no longer sticky. Pour it out on a greased flat tin and let it cool before cutting it into small pieces.

Red tangerine peel regulates Qi and relieves depression, spring onion clears the urethra, and cluster mallow seeds can ease urination.

Another diet is a cake made with the powder of red tangerine peel, toasted cluster mallow seeds and the powder of glutinous rice, where a soft dough is made with water and then steamed. Sprinkle white sugar on top and serve.

Deficiency of Kidney Qi

Symptoms are urinary obstruction or difficult urination or dripping urination, a pale complexion, lethargy, soreness and weakness in the back and the knees, cold limbs, edema, a pale tongue, and a deep, thready and weak pulse. Dietary Therapy should be directed at tonifying the Kidney and activating the discharge of water.

The recommended diet is a Kidney tonifying soup (SJZL) made with one pair of lamb's kidneys trimmed and chopped, stalks of spring onion and fresh ginger 10 g each, boiled in water till the contents are cooked. Add salt to season.

Lamb's kidney tonifies the Kidney Qi, while the stalks of spring onion and fresh ginger activate Yang. The effect of activating water discharge is enhanced with 500 g of cluster mallow added to the soup.

Obstruction of the urinary tract

Symptoms include dripping urination or intermittent obstruction of urination, distension and pain in the lower abdomen, a dark red tongue or spotted tongue and an uneven or thready and rapid pulse. Dietary Therapy should be directed at removing the stagnation and dispersing the obstruction to clear the Water Channels.

The recommended diet is walnut cookies made with 500 g of white sugar boiled in water. Condense the liquid till it makes filaments when picked up. Put in 500 g of walnuts (fried in sesame oil till crisp) while the syrup is still hot. Mix it well and pour it into a tray to cool before cutting it into small pieces.

Walnuts can tonify the Kidney and dissolve urinary stones.

EDEMA

Edema is a disease marked by swelling of the face and head, the eyelids, the limbs, the back, or even the whole body, caused by retention of fluids infiltrating to the muscles and skin.

Pathogenic Wind may invade the body from outside; fluids or Damp may infiltrate; hunger or fatigue may weaken the Kidneys or there may be Qi deficiency in the Vital Organs. This may cause malfunction of the Lungs, the Spleen and the Kidney and malfunction of the Three Burners in removing body fluids and difficulty of the Bladder in absorbing the fluids, leading to retention of fluids which rise to the superficial layers of the skin.

Recommended foods

Patients with edema should eat foods that contain little salt and foods that help reinforce the Spleen and the Kidney and activate the transportation of fluids. Examples are coix seeds, red beans, flat beans, broad beans, black beans, euryale seeds, lotus seeds, wax gourd, turnips, cluster mallow, water chestnuts, Chinese cabbage, kelp, crucian carp, snakehead mullet, carp, Pseudobagrus fuluidraco (Richardson) Kocafka, finless eels, and duck.

Foods to avoid

Raw and Cold food, melon and fruits are to be taken with care.

Diet recipes

Wind-Fluid flooding the body

Symptoms are fever, intolerance to cold, soreness in the bone joints, redness, swelling and pain in the throat, edema in the face and eyelids, the limbs and the whole body; scanty urine, a thin white tongue coating and a floating, slippery and rapid pulse. Dietary Therapy should be directed at regulating the Lungs and activating the transportation of fluids.

The recommended diet is a gruel (BCGM) made with fresh mustard greens 30 g and glutinous rice 50–100 g, to be taken regularly.

This diet can clear the flow of fluids between the upper and lower parts of the body, regulate the Lungs, dissolve the Phlegm, remove toxins and induce urination.

Damp-Fluids infiltrating the body

Symptoms are pitting edema in the whole body, scanty urine, heaviness in the body, stuffiness in the chest, loss of appetite, nausea, a white greasy tongue coating, and a deep and soft pulse. Dietary Therapy should be directed at activating the transportation of Body Fluids and relieving edema.

The recommended diet is a thick soup (SJZL) made with carp 500 g (scaled and gutted), wax gourd 500 g (chopped) and stalk of spring onion 20 g, stewed in water till the fish is well cooked and the sauce is thick.

The stalk of spring onion activates Yang, while carp and wax gourd activate the transportation of Body Fluids. This diet is especially suitable for cases with a sensation of heat and the accumulation of Damp-Heat. The carp can be replaced with snakehead mullet or crucian carp.

Deficient Yang

Symptoms include edema in the whole body, which is especially grave below the waist, distension in the abdomen, loss of appetite and loose stools, a dry yellow complexion, cold limbs, a pale tongue with white slippery coating, and a deep and slow pulse. Dietary Therapy should be directed at warming the Middle Burner, reinforcing the Spleen and relieving edema.

The recommended diet is a soup (SYXJb) made with beef 500 g, and dried ginger and vinegar 30 g each, stewed in water till the beef is well cooked. Eat the meat and drink the soup before or with a meal.

This diet has the effects of reinforcing the Spleen, warming the Middle Burner and relieving edema.

Infiltration of fluids due to deficiency of the Kidney

Symptoms are edema in the face and the whole body, especially below the waist; soreness, coldness and heaviness in the back, scanty urine, cold limbs and intolerance to cold, a pale complexion, lethargy, a pale tongue, and a deep and weak pulse. Obviously there is some overlap between this and the previous pattern (deficient Yang). Deficient Yang cases also involve the Spleen and the Lung. Dietary Therapy should be directed at tonifying the Kidney and activating the transportation of Body Fluids.

The recommended diet is a soup (QJYF) made with black beans 500 g, and low alcohol wine 50 ml. Boil the beans in the wine with water till the beans are well cooked. Eat in several servings.

This diet is effective in tonifying the Kidney, activating Yang, absorbing water and activating the transportation of Body Fluids. The diet can be adapted by adding cinnamon twigs 15 g to the soup when the beans are cooked and boiling it further, which will enhance its therapeutic effects.

ENURESIS

Enuresis is a disease marked by involuntary discharge of urine. Enuresis when the person is awake is called urinary incontinence; when the person is asleep it is called nocturnal enuresis or bedwetting.

The Bladder is in charge of holding the urine, while the Three Burners are responsible for the transportation and discharge of urine. When the Spleen and Lung Qi are insufficient and cannot control the Lower Burner and the Water Channels, or when the Kidney Qi is deficient and the Lower Burner is not solid, or when Damp-Heat flows downwards causing fluids to leave their usual course due to malfunction of the Three Burners in transporting and absorbing the water, enuresis is likely to occur.

Recommended foods

Patients with this disease should have foods that can replenish Qi, warm the Yang and consolidate the fluids. Examples are euryale seeds, lotus seeds, Chinese chives, chestnuts, ginkgo nuts, walnuts, mutton, shrimps and chicken. For cases involving Damp-Heat, use foods that are effective in clearing up Heat and relieving Damp, such as soya bean sprouts, wax gourd, watermelon and turnips.

Foods to avoid

Foods that are pungent, Warm and Dry are to be taken with care in cases involving Damp-Heat. Foods that are raw, Cold and greasy should also be avoided.

Diet recipes

Deficiency of Lung Qi and Spleen Qi

Symptoms are frequent urination which is urgent and difficult to control, dripping after passing water, a pale complexion, lethargy and shortness of breath, a pale tongue with thin white coating, and a weak and soft pulse. Dietary Therapy should be directed at reinforcing the Lungs and the Kidney.

The recommended diet is a thick soup (SJZL) made with one pig lung (finely chopped) and mutton 250 g (chopped), boiled in water on a high heat. After the first boiling, simmer over a low heat till the liquid is thickened and season it with salt and coriander. To be taken before or with a meal.

This recipe is effective in reinforcing the Lungs and the Kidney, nourishing Ying to reinforce Wei (and the body's resistance to Wind pathogens), and is suitable for patients with frequent urination and other symptoms of deficiency.

Deficiency and Cold in the Lower Burner

Symptoms include clear and profuse urine, enuresis or urinary incontinence, lethargy and fatigue, soreness and weakness in the back and the knees, intolerance to cold, a pale tongue with white coating, and a deep, thready and weak pulse. Dietary Therapy should be directed at warming and tonifying the Kidney Yang.

The recommended diet is a gruel (TPSHF)

made with one yellow hen, gutted, cleaned and chopped, milkvetch root and prepared rehmannia root, 30 g each (wrapped in cloth), boiled in water till the chicken is well cooked. Remove the wrapped herbs and the chicken bones. Use the juice and meat at different times to make gruel with 50–100 g of non-glutinous rice, seasoned with miso, to be eaten before meals.

This diet reinforces the five Zang Organs and is effective for deficient Cold in the Bladder. 10 g of cinnamon twig may be cooked together with the gruel.

Downward flow of Damp-Heat

Symptoms are frequent urination, burning urination, occasional enuresis, dark and foul urine or dripping urine, a red tongue with greasy coating, and a slippery and rapid pulse. Dietary Therapy should be aimed at clearing Damp-Heat.

The recommended diet is a soup made with red beans 250 g and fermented soya beans 30 g, boiled and seasoned with salt, to be taken orally.

This recipe is effective for clearing Heat, removing Damp and relieving the sensation of Heat.

SEMINAL EMISSION

Seminal emission is marked by the discharge of semen without sexual intercourse. When it takes place during dreams, it is called nocturnal emission; when it takes place during sleep without dreaming, or even when the person is awake (usually without an erection), it is called spermatorrhea.

The semen is housed in the Kidney, released by the Liver and commanded by the Heart. Therefore, this disease is mainly due to congenital deficiency, insufficiency and weakness of the Lower Burner, disharmony of the seminal gate, sexual intemperance, mental tiredness, hyperactivity of Fire due to Yin deficiency, incoordination of the Heart and the Kidney, or to rich food and wine causing accumulation of Damp-Heat which flows downwards to the Lower Burner and agitates the 'Sperm Palace'.

Recommended foods

For cases owing to the deficiency of the Kidney which then fails to house sperm, it is desirable to have foods that help replenish Qi, tonify the Kidney and consolidate the sperm, such as Chinese yam, lotus seeds, walnuts, ginkgo nuts, chicken, crucian carp, pig's kidney and Chinese chives. For cases owing to hyperactivity of Fire due to Yin deficiency, use foods that help nourish Yin and store sperm, such as black-boned chicken, duck, mussels, mulberries and cherries. For patients with Damp-Heat, use foods that help dissolve Damp and clear Heat, such as towel gourd, wax gourd, balsam pears, water spinach and poria.

Foods to avoid

Fatty, sweet and sour foods that are astringent are to be avoided in Damp-Heat. Examples are pork, pomegranates, cherries and plums. For hyperactivity of Fire, foods that are Hot, Dry and pungent, such as garlic and chillies, should not be eaten. In cases of deficiency of the Kidney, raw, Cold, and greasy foods such as watermelon, wax gourd and water spinach should be avoided.

Diet recipes

Hyperactivity of Fire due to Yin deficiency

Symptoms are dreaming, 'wet dreams', restless sleep, dizziness, palpitations, hot sensation in the chest, palms and soles; a red tongue with little coating, and a thready and rapid pulse. Dietary Therapy should be directed at nourishing Yin and sending down Fire, tranquilizing the Mind and consolidating sperm ('Firming the Jing').

The recommended diet (SXJYSP) is one ox's tripe, stuffed with 60 g of lotus seeds (with skin on), boiled till the contents are well cooked. Add some salt and eat the meat and drink the soup at different servings or with meals.

Lotus seeds can clear the Heat, coordinate the Heart and the Kidney and consolidate the Vital Qi, salt can induce the Fire to go downwards and ox's tripe can reinforce the deficiency and consolidate the sperm.

Deficiency in the Kidney which fails to house the sperm

Symptoms include frequent seminal emission or even spermatorrhea, a pale complexion, lethargy, soreness and weakness in the back and knees, intolerance to cold, cold limbs, a pale tongue with thin, white coating, and a deep and weak pulse. Dietary Therapy should be directed at tonifying the Kidney and consolidating the sperm.

The recommended diet is the Pan-tao-guo (Zhu Danxi's recipe, cited from CFQY) made with euryale seeds, lotus seeds (core removed), dates, walnuts (skin removed) and prepared rehmannia root, 100 g each, six pig's kidneys and powder of common fennel fruit 15 g, boiled in water and then mashed. 1 kg of glutinous rice flour and a suitable amount of white sugar are mixed with the mash and formed into a dough with some water. Make pancakes from the dough, to be eaten over a few days.

Dates can reinforce the Spleen, common fennel fruit can warm the Kidney and all the other items have the effects of tonifying the Kidney and consolidating sperm.

Downward flow of Damp-Heat

Symptoms are frequent seminal emission, a dull yellow complexion, a bitter taste, sensation of heat in the chest, red and hot urine, a yellow and greasy tongue coating, and a soft and rapid pulse. Dietary Therapy should be directed at clearing up Heat and arresting emission.

The recommended diet is Lianziliuyi Tang (RZZZF) made with lotus seeds (with core) 60 g and raw liquorice 10 g, decocted in water on a low heat till the lotus seeds are well cooked. Add some crystal sugar, eat the lotus seeds and drink the decoction.

Lotus seeds and raw liquorice used together can clear up Heat in the Heart to remove Damp, tranquilize the Mind and arrest emission.

IMPOTENCE

Impotence is the inability of young and middle-aged men to have sexual intercourse because they cannot achieve an erection or only a very weak one.

The disease is mainly deficient in nature. Most cases are due to exhaustion of Fire but occasionally there are cases which are due to excess of Fire. It is also caused by congenital deficiency, sexual intemperance, exhaustion of Fire at the Life Gate, deficiency and impairment of the Kidney Qi, or by mental depression or overanxiety impairing the Heart and the Spleen, leading to insufficiency of Qi and Blood. It is also caused by downward flow of Damp-Heat leading to flaccidity of the penis.

Recommended foods

For deficient cases, it is desirable to have foods that help replenish Qi and Blood, tonify the Kidney and strengthen Yang Qi. Examples are dates, longan, Chinese chives, walnuts, shrimps, loach and mussels.

Foods to avoid

Except for cases owing to Damp-Heat syndrome, foods that are raw, Cold and slippery should be avoided. Examples are cluster mallow, wax gourd, mussels and river snails.

Diet recipes

Exhaustion of Fire at the Life Gate

Symptoms are a flaccid penis, thin and cold semen, lethargy, dizziness, tinnitus, soreness and weakness in the back and knees, clear and profuse urine, a pale tongue with white coating, and a deep and thready pulse. Dietary Therapy should be directed at tonifying the Kidney and strengthening the masculine power.

The recommended diet (FMZZ) is walnuts 50 g, fried in sesame oil till browned. Add 500 g of Chinese chives (chopped) and stir-fry them together. Season with salt and eat at meals as often as desired.

Walnuts and Chinese chives are effective in tonifying the Kidney and strengthening the mas-

culine power. Fresh shrimps can be added to this, stir-fried to enhance the tonifying effect.

Impairment of the Heart and the Spleen

Symptoms are impotence, a dull complexion, loss of appetite, restless sleep, a pale tongue and a weak pulse. Dietary Therapy should be aimed at reinforcing the Heart and the Spleen.

The recommended diet (LLHY) is longan 15 g, five dates and non-glutinous rice 50–100 g made into a gruel.

The recipe has the effects of reinforcing the Spleen, nourishing the Heart and refreshing the Mind.

Downward flow of Damp-Heat

Symptoms include impotence, wet testicles, itching genitals with a foul odor, heaviness in the lower limbs, dark urine, a red tongue with yellow greasy coating, and a taut and rapid pulse. Dietary Therapy should be directed at clearing Heat and removing Damp.

The recommended diet is Lianziliuyi Tang (see Seminal emission).

DEFICIENCY SYNDROME

Deficiency syndrome is a general term for a group of diseases marked by a number of deficient symptoms attributable to the impairment and exhaustion of the Vital Organs and the deficiency of Yin, Yang, Qi and Blood.

This category was sometimes translated as neurasthenia–a term unpopular in the West because it was imprecise. In fact it covers many of the patterns commonly seen and successfully treated by TCM and it is possible that the unpopularity of the original term with Western medicine was due to an inability to relate it to specific treatment.

Deficiency conditions are often due to congenital deficiency, neglect leading to poor health, untreated illnesses, accumulated physical over exertion leading to internal impairment, over exhaustion of the Vital Qi, Essence and Blood and the malfunction of the viscera.

Recommended foods

Diet for patients with deficiency syndrome should vary with different types of the disease and the patient's condition. For cases with exhaustion of Yang Qi, it is desirable to have foods that help enrich Qi, warm Yang and strengthen the health as a whole. Examples are longan, litchi, dates, walnuts, potatoes, soya beans, maltose, chicken and chicken eggs, quail and quail eggs, mutton, beef, eel, crucian carp, loach and spinach. For cases owing to deficiency of Yin Blood, it is useful to eat foods that help in nourishing Blood, nurturing Yin and replenishing the Essence, such as carrot, Chinese wolfberry, wood-ears, sesame, peanuts, black beans, lotus seeds, cow's milk and goat's milk.

Foods to avoid

For exhaustion of Yang Qi, foods that are Cold or Cool should be taken with care, such as turnips, eggplant, towel gourd and mussels. In deficiency of Yin Blood, Warm, Dry foods such as spring onion, chillies, mutton and shrimps should be avoided.

Diet recipes

For cases with Qi deficiency

Deficiency of Lung Qi

Symptoms include shortness of breath, spontaneous perspiration, weak and thin voice, susceptibility to catch cold, alternating fever and chills, together with coughing, a pale complexion and a pale tongue and a weak pulse. Dietary Therapy should be directed at replenishing Lung Qi.

The recommended diet is a gruel (LLYH) made with milkvetch root 30 g, decocted and strained. Add 100 g non-glutinous rice to the decoction and some white sugar when the gruel is cooked.

This diet has the effect of enriching Lung Qi.

Deficiency of Spleen Qi

Symptoms are loss of appetite, distension in the abdomen after meals, loose stools, a dry yellow complexion, general weakness, a pale tongue with a thin white coating, and a soft and weak pulse. Dietary Therapy should be directed at reinforcing the Spleen and enriching Qi.

The recommended diet (SJZL) is pilose asiabell root 30 g, poria 15 g and ginger 6 g, decocted and strained. Add 100 g non-glutinous rice to the decoction to make a gruel. Add one chicken egg and some salt when the gruel is nearly cooked and boil further till the gruel is well cooked.

Pilose asiabell root and poria can reinforce the Spleen and enrich Qi, while fresh ginger can warm the Middle Burner.

For cases with Blood deficiency

Deficiency of Heart Blood

Symptoms are palpitations, amnesia, insomnia, dreaminess, a dull complexion, a pale tongue, and a thready or knotted and intermittent pulse. Dietary Therapy should be aimed at nourishing Blood and tranquilizing the Mind.

The recommended diet (SYXJb) is pig's heart 500 g, spring onion, ginger, fermented soya beans, soy sauce, miso (plum sauce) and yellow millet or rice wine stewed together on a low heat till the heart is cooked. When the heart is cooled, slice it for eating at meals.

This diet has the effects of replenishing Heart Blood and tranquilizing the Mind.

Another diet for the disease is Yuling electuary (made with longan and sugar steamed to reduce them).

Deficiency of Liver Blood

Symptoms include dizziness, tinnitus, night blindness, hypochondriac pain, panic, irregular menstruation, anemia, a pale complexion, a pale tongue with white coating, and a taut and thready pulse. Dietary Therapy should be directed at reinforcing and nurturing the Liver.

The recommended diet is a mutton soup (QJYF) made with Chinese angelica root, chuanxiong rhizome, rehmannia root and root of common peony, 15 g each, fresh ginger, cinnamon bark and liquorice, 10 g each, decocted and strained. Add 1000 g of mutton (diced), soy sauce, table salt, sugar and yellow millet or rice wine and stew till the meat is cooked.

This recipe contains Siwu Tang (decoction of four ingredients), which replenishes Blood and nurtures the Liver.

For cases with deficiency of Yang

Deficiency of Heart Yang

Symptoms are palpitations, spontaneous perspiration, stuffness and pain in the chest, sleepiness, cold sensation and cold limbs, a pale complexion, a pale or dull tongue, and a thready and weak, or knotted and intermittent pulse. Dietary Therapy should be directed at warming and activating the Heart Yang.

The recommended diet is a gruel (SJZL) made with non-glutinous rice 100 g. When the gruel is nearly cooked, put in one lamb's kidney (trimmed and finely chopped), onion 15 g, fresh ginger 10 g and some salt. Stir well and boil further till the meat is well cooked.

Lamb's kidney is sweet, Warm and nourishing, onion is pungent and Warm and is effective in activating the Heart Yang. Cinnamon bark can be added in the cooking to enhance the effects of warming the Heart.

Deficiency of Spleen Yang

Symptoms may show as sallow complexion, loss of appetite, cold sensation, dull spirit and fatigue, cold and pain in the abdomen, excessive bowel sounds, diarrhea with undigested food, pale tongue with white coating and a weak pulse. Dietary Therapy should be directed at warming the Middle Burner and reinforcing the Spleen.

The recommended diet (SJBC) is one ox's tripe (washed clean), stuffed with pilose asiabell root 15 g, dried ginger and walnut 10 g each, glutinous rice 250 g and seven stalks of spring onion, secured with string and boiled until soft.

Pilose asiabell root, walnuts, ox's tripe and non-glutinous rice can reinforce the Spleen and tonify deficiency, while dried ginger and stalk of spring onion warm the Middle Burner.

Deficiency of Kidney Yang

Symptoms include a pale complexion, intolerance to cold and cold limbs, profuse and clear urine, profuse urination at night, diarrhea with undigested foods in stools, soreness in the back and spine, seminal emission and impotence, a pale and enlarged tongue with white coating, and a deep and slow pulse. Dietary Therapy should be directed at warming and tonifying Kidney Yang.

The recommended diet is a gruel (YSZY) made with Chinese wolfberry shoots 100 g, one lamb's kidney (finely chopped), mutton 50 g (chopped), spring onion 30 g and non-glutinous rice 250 g seasoned with salt.

The young shoots, mutton and lamb's kidney used together can warm and tonify the Kidney Yang.

For cases with Yin deficiency

Deficiency of Lung Yin

Symptoms are a dry cough with little sputum (possibly bloodstained), dry throat, hectic fever, night sweat, flushing, a red tongue with little moisture and a scanty coating, and a thready and rapid pulse. Dietary Therapy should be directed at nourishing Yin and moistening the Lungs.

The recommended diet is an electuary (SYSS) made with one white duck (cleaned and gutted from underneath the wing), stuffed with 500 g of dates, 100 g of Stomach-regulating powder of ginseng and poria, wrapped up in cloth. Stew the duck in an earthen pot with water and some cooking wine on a low heat till the meat is cooked. Remove the bag of herbs, eat the duck and the dates.

The recipe is effective in replenishing Earth (the Spleen and Stomach) to create Metal (the Lungs), nourishing Yin and moistening the Lungs.

Deficiency of Heart Yin

Symptoms include palpitations, restlessness, insomnia, dreaming, hectic fever, night perspiration, soreness and rashes of the tongue, which is red with little moisture, and a thready and rapid pulse. Dietary Therapy should be directed at nourishing the Heart and tranquilizing the Mind.

The recommended diet is Jujuba Seed Gruel

(TPSHF) made with wild or spiny jujuba seeds 15 g, decocted and strained. Add 100 g non-glutinous rice and crystal sugar.

Wild or spiny jujuba seeds are effective in nurturing the Heart Yin and tranquilizing the Mind.

Deficiency of Stomach Yin

Symptoms are a dry mouth and lips, loss of appetite, constipation, or dry vomiting, hiccups, a bright red tongue with little coating, and a thready and rapid pulse. Dietary Therapy should be directed at nourishing the Stomach Yin.

The recommended diet is Lipi Gao (SJBC) made with lily bulb, lotus seeds, Chinese yam, coix seeds, euryale seeds and tribulus fruit, 500 g each, finely powdered. Add non-glutinous rice flour 1500 g and glutinous rice flour 500 g, thoroughly mixed. Take 250 g of the mixture at a time, add enough water to make a dough and cook cakes made from the dough in a steamer on a low heat. When they are cooked, let them cool and cut them into small pieces and sprinkle with white sugar.

Most of the medicines used in the recipe have the effect of nourishing the Stomach Yin.

Deficiency of Liver Yin

Symptoms are a headache, dizziness, tinnitus, dry eyes, light sensitivity, blurred vision, restlessness, hypochondriac pain, numbness in the body and limbs, tremor in the muscles, a dry and red tongue, taut, thready and rapid pulse. Dietary Therapy should be directed at nourishing Liver Yin.

The recommended diet is Dogwood Fruit Gruel (ZP) made with dogwood fruit 15 g, decocted and strained. Add 100 g of non-glutinous rice and some crystal sugar to the decoction to make a gruel.

Dogwood fruit is employed for its effect in reinforcing the Liver Yin.

Deficiency of Kidney Yin

Symptoms are dizziness, tinnitus or deafness, alopecia, loose teeth, soreness in the back and knees, seminal emission, abnormal erection of penis, hectic fever, flushing, a red tongue with little moisture, and a deep and thready pulse.

Dietary Therapy should be aimed at nourishing and reinforcing the Kidney Yin.

The recommended diet is a thick soup (TPSHF) made with two pig's kidneys (chopped and trimmed), Chinese wolfberry leaves (chopped), and fermented soya beans 50 g. Add salt, vinegar, pepper and spring onion to season the soup.

Pig's kidney and Chinese wolfberry leaves nourish the Kidney Yin and remove deficient Heat. In *The Essence of Diet* (YSZY), there is a recipe used in treating deficiency in the Kidney with pain in the back and spine and inability to stand for long, which can also be used in this disease. The recipe is made with rehmannia root, maltose and black-boned chicken steamed together.

DIABETES

In TCM, diabetes is known as 'thirsty-wasting disease'. It is often due to Yin deficiency, plus improper diet, overintake of fatty rich foods, emotional disturbance or mental depression leading to stagnation which turns to Fire, sexual intemperance impairing the Yin Essence leading to Heat in the Stomach and deficiency in the Kidney, exhaustion of Body Fluids and excess of Heat.

Recommended foods

For patients with diabetes, it is desirable to have foods that help clear up Heat, nourish Yin and promote the production of Body Fluids, such as spinach, turnips, balsam pears, wax gourd, fermented soya beans, millet, Chinese yam, Chinese actinidia, water chestnuts, sea cucumber, carp, river snail, blackboned chicken, duck, goose, rabbit, and cow's milk.

Foods to avoid

Foods that are pungent and irritating, such as ginger, pepper, onion and wine, are to be avoided, while foods that are high in sugar are prohibited. Examples are sweet potatoes, potatoes, sweets, biscuits and candied fruits. Intake of food in general should be moderate.

Diet recipes

Heat in the Lung impairing Body Fluids

Symptoms are thirst, a dry mouth and tongue, frequent and profuse urination, gradual emaciation, a tongue with red at the tip and the sides with a thin yellow coating, and a full and rapid pulse. Dietary Therapy should be directed at clearing up Heat and moistening the Lungs.

The recommended diet is Shenxiaozhutu Fang (TPSHF) made with one rabbit, gutted, cleaned and chopped, and mulberry bark 100 g, boiled together till the meat is well cooked. Season with salt and eat the meat and the sauce.

Rabbit meat rectifies deficiency, clears Heat and eases thirst, while mulberry bark clears Lung Heat.

Excessive Stomach Heat

Symptoms include excessive hunger, emaciation, constipation, a dry, yellow tongue coating, and a slippery, rapid and vigorous pulse. Dietary Therapy should be directed at clearing Stomach Fire, nourishing Yin and promoting the production of Body Fluids.

The recommended diet is the Five-Juice Mix (see Epidemic Febrile Disease).

Exhaustion of Kidney Yin

Symptoms include frequent and profuse urination, or turbid greasy urine, a dry mouth and tongue, emaciation, soreness in the back, tinnitus, red tongue with little coating, and a thready and rapid pulse. Dietary Therapy should be directed at nourishing Yin and consolidating the Kidney.

The recommended diet is Rehmannia Root Gruel (YZFSJ). First, rehmannia root juice 500 g and white honey 125 g are made into an electuary. Then non-glutinous rice 100 g is made into a gruel. When the gruel is cooked, put in two spoonfuls of the electuary and some butter.

This recipe has the effects of clearing Heat, nourishing Yin, moistening Dryness and promoting the production of Body Fluids. Chinese yam and euryale seeds can be added (powdered) to the gruel to help consolidate the Kidney.

Deficiency of both Yin and Yang

Symptoms are frequent urination which is turbid and greasy, copious urine, excessive thirst, a dark complexion, soreness in the back and knees, impotence, intolerance to cold, or edema in the lower limbs, a pale tongue with white coating, and a deep, thready and weak pulse. Dietary Therapy should be directed at nourishing Yin and tonifying Yang.

The recommended diet is a pancreas-nourishing drink (YXZZCXL) made with milkvetch root and Chinese yam 30 g each, rehmannia root and dogwood fruit 15 g each, decocted and strained. Boil 500 g of pig's pancreas in the decoction till cooked. Season with salt, eat the meat and drink the sauce.

Rehmannia root and dogwood fruit nourish Yin and consolidate the Kidney, while milkvetch root and Chinese yam warm and replenish Qi, and pig's pancreas moistens the Dryness and reinforces the pancreas.

BI SYNDROME

Bi syndrome is a group of diseases marked by pain, soreness, heaviness and numbness in the joints and difficulty in bending and stretching the joints.

The word 'Bi' means obstruction of Qi and Blood by pathogenic Qi. The disease is often due to poor health, overuse of muscles, or exposure to Damp, Heat, Wind and Cold, which invade the Channels and joints to obstruct Qi and Blood.

Recommended foods

Bi syndrome is classified into the Wind-Cold-Damp type and the Damp-Heat type. For cases of the Wind-Cold-Damp type, it is desirable to have foods that help expel Wind and Damp, warm the Channels and activate the Collaterals, such as chillies, spring onion, black beans, finless eel and mutton, while foods that are greasy and difficult to digest such as lard and turtle meat are to be taken with care. For cases of Damp-Heat, use foods that help clear Heat, remove Damp and relieve Bi syndrome. Examples are soya bean sprouts, red beans, coix seeds, lotus seeds, black beans, oyster mushroom, wax gourd and mung beans.

Foods to avoid

Pungent, Warm and Dry foods such as ginger, pepper, beef and mutton are to be avoided in Damp-Heat cases. In Wind-Cold-Damp cases, foods that are greasy and difficult to digest should not be eaten.

Diet recipes

Cold-Bi

Symptoms are a fixed pain with a sensation of coldness, the pain being aggravated by cold but alleviated by warmth, inability of the bone joints to bend and stretch, a white tongue coating, and a taut and tense pulse. Dietary Therapy should be directed at dispersing Cold and relieving pain.

The recommended diet is Aconite Root Gruel made with prepared aconite root slices (NB: restricted use – potentially poisonous) 10 g, dried ginger and stalk of spring onion 15 g each, decocted and strained. Add 100 g of non-glutinous rice and some honey to make a gruel.

This diet is effective in warming the Channels and dispersing Cold, relieving pain and Bi syndrome.

Wind-Bi

Symptoms are a migratory pain in the muscles and bone joints, mostly in the shoulders, back and the upper limbs, difficulty in bending and stretching the joints; together with fever and intolerance to cold, a tongue coating that is thin and white, and a floating pulse. Dietary Therapy should be directed at expelling the Wind pathogens and activating the collaterals.

The recommended diet is Weishen San (SJZL) made with milkvetch root baked after steaming, toasted tribulus fruit, notopterygium with spears removed, in equal amounts, all powdered, with two trimmed pig's kidneys. Halve each kidney,

stuff each half with 10 g of the herb powder and some salt. Wrap them in wet paper and stew till the kidneys are cooked. It is best to eat the kidneys with wine.

Pig's kidney and milkvetch tonify the Kidney and replenish Qi, while tribulus fruit and notopterygium expel pathogenic Wind and activate the Collaterals.

Damp-Bi

Symptoms include pain, heaviness and edema in the muscles and bone joints of the limbs and the whole body; difficulty in movement, with numbness in the skin and muscles, a pale tongue with white greasy coating, and a soft and slow pulse. Dietary Therapy should be aimed at removing the Damp and relieving Bi syndrome.

The recommended diet is Coix Seed Gruel (SJZL) made with hemp seeds 20 g, pounded and squeezed in gauze to obtain the juice. Add 30 g of coix seeds and 100 g non-glutinous rice to make a gruel.

According to BCSGY, for Wind-Bi in the aged, gruel made with hemp seeds should be taken with coix seeds. Then the recipe is effective in reinforcing the Middle Burner, replenishing Qi, removing Damp and edema and relieving the Bi syndrome.

Damp-Heat-Bi

Symptoms are inflammation, redness, edema and severe pain in local areas, which are alleviated by cold; difficulty in moving the bone joints, often with fever, thirst without desire to drink, stuffiness in the upper abdomen, dark urine, a red tongue with yellow greasy coating, and a slippery and rapid pulse. Dietary Therapy should be directed at clearing Heat and removing Damp.

The recommended diet is Silver Bean Soup made with red beans and coix seeds 50 g each, made into a gruel. Add 15 g of honeysuckle stem (wrapped in cloth) when the gruel is nearly cooked. Boil further till the gruel is cooked. Discard the wrapped herbs and season with salt. Eat the beans and coix seeds and drink the liquid. It can also be taken at meals.

Red beans and coix seeds clear Heat and

remove Damp, while the stem of honeysuckle clears Heat and activates the Collaterals.

ATROPHY SYNDROME (WEI ZHENG)

Atrophy syndrome is marked by emaciation, general weakness, inability to stand on the feet or hold things with the hands.

The disease is attributable to extreme Wind-Heat impairing Body Fluids, or to poor health or protracted illness leading to weakness of the Spleen and the Stomach, exhaustion of the Liver and the Kidney, which culminate in the deficiency of Essence and Blood and hence malnutrition of the muscles and tendons. It is also caused by the invasion of Damp-Heat, which leads to obstruction of Qi and Blood and flaccidity of the muscles and tendons.

Recommended foods

For patients with atrophy syndrome, it is desirable to have foods that help replenish Qi and Blood, nourish the Liver and the Kidney. Examples are dates, Chinese yam, coix seeds, chestnuts, black beans, sesame, ox marrow and cow or goat's milk. For cases due to Damp-Heat, take foods that help clear Heat and remove Damp, such as mung beans, red beans, coix seeds, Chinese yam, soya bean sprouts and mung bean sprouts.

Foods to avoid

Foods that are Warm and Dry and tend to impair the body's Yin, or those that are greasy and difficult to digest, are to be avoided.

Diet recipes

Lung Heat impairing Body Fluids

Symptoms such as initial fever or sudden onset of general weakness after febrile disease, with a hot sensation and thirst, coughing, choking and a dry throat, dark and scanty urine, a red tongue with yellow coating and a thready and rapid pulse. Dietary Therapy should be directed at clearing away Dryness and moistening the Lungs.

The recommended diet (BCGM) is non-glutinous rice 100 g, made into a gruel. Add 100 ml of cow's milk when the gruel is cooked. Bring to the boil and add some crystal sugar for flavor. According to BCJS, cow's milk 'has a sweet taste, a slightly Cold nature and is non-toxic. The sweetness and Coldness can nurture the Blood Vessels and nourish the viscera'.

Damp-Heat invading Yang Ming

Symptoms are heaviness of the body, flaccidity, distension in the chest and upper abdomen, loss of appetite, thirst without desire to drink, or recessive fever, shortness of breath, a red tongue with a yellow greasy coating, and a soft and rapid pulse. Dietary Therapy should be directed at clearing Heat and removing Damp.

The recommended diet is Chaenomeles Fruit Gruel (TPSHF) made with chaenomeles fruit 20 g, decocted and strained. Add non-glutinous rice 50–100 and some white sugar.

This recipe has the effects of harmonizing the Stomach, dissolving Damp, easing the tendons and activating the Collaterals. The therapeutic effects are enhanced if coix seeds are added and boiled with the gruel.

Weak Spleen and Stomach Qi

Symptoms include general weakness, a puffy face, lassitude, loss of appetite, distension in the abdomen, loose stool, a thin white tongue coating and a thready pulse. Dietary Therapy should be directed at enriching Qi and Blood.

The recommended diet is milkvetch root 100 g and dates 500 g, boiled in water. Discard the milkvetch root and water when the dates are soft. Add lard 50 g and glutinous rice wine 500 ml, bring to the boil and then let it cool down. Pour it into a bottle and seal it for 7 days. Eat the dates twice a day, 3–5 dates at a time.

Milkvetch root and dates can enrich Qi and Blood.

Exhaustion of the Liver and the Kidney

Symptoms are emaciation of the body, general weakness, dizziness, tinnitus, seminal emission or enuresis, irregular menstruation, a red tongue with little coating, and a thready and rapid pulse. Dietary Therapy should be directed at reinforcing the Liver and Kidney.

The recommended diet is an electuary (YSZY) made with rehmannia root 50 g, decocted and strained. Put in cooked lard and cooked beef marrow 100 g each. Condense the liquid on a low heat. Add 100 g of honey and juice of ginger 20 ml, mix it well and bring it to the boil. Pour the liquid into a bottle when cooled. Take one spoonful of the electuary at a time, mixed with boiling water.

Rehmannia root, lard, beef marrow and honey nourish the Liver and the Kidney, replenish the Essence and the Marrow. The recipe can also be made in the form of a thick soup or a gruel.

DEPRESSION

Depression is a group of diseases marked by emotional disorder and the stagnation of Qi caused by emotional disturbance.

The disease is due to accumulated anger, anxiety, sorrow and other harmful emotions which lead to disfunction of the Liver in dispersing and transmission, stagnation of Qi and disruption of the normal functioning of the Internal Organs. This culminates in the stagnation of Qi, Blood, Damp, Phlegm, Fire and Food, or even exhaustion of Yin and Yang.

Recommended foods

Patients with depression should eat foods that help regulate Qi, relieve depression, nurture the Liver and tranquilize the Heart, such as jasmine, roses, Seville orange flower, oranges, wheat, lotus seeds, lily bulb, day lily, litchi, longan, wild or spiny jujuba, mulberry, perch, and oyster.

Foods to avoid

Foods that are fatty, greasy and tend to cause Damp, or pungent, Dry foods that irritate pathogenic Fire are to be avoided.

Diet recipes

Stagnation of Liver Qi

Symptoms include emotional disorder, depression, sighing, distension and pain in the chest and hypochondrium, fullness in the upper abdomen, belching, loss of appetite or vomiting, irregular stools, irregular menstruation, thin and white tongue coating, and a taut pulse. Dietary Therapy should be directed at regulating the Liver and relieving depression.

The recommended diet is orange cakes (SJBC) made with orange 250 g (peeled and seeded), candied in 50 g of white sugar. When the orange is well soaked in the sugar, stew it on a low heat till the liquid is dried up. Pound it when cooled. Make dough with 500 g buckwheat flour and wrap the orange in the buckwheat dough with white sugar and roasted sesame seeds. Cook the cakes in a hot pan.

Orange has the effects of relieving stagnation, sending down the Counterflow Qi and harmonizing the Stomach, while buckwheat has the effects of sending down Counterflow Qi and regulating the Stomach.

Stagnation of Qi turning to Fire

Symptoms include restlessness, distension in the chest and the hypochondrium, discomfort in the Stomach and acid regurgitation, a bitter taste and a dry mouth, constipation, headaches, red eyes, tinnitus, a red tongue with yellow coating, and a taut and rapid pulse. Dietary Therapy should be directed at cleansing the Liver and purging the pathogenic Fire.

The recommended diet is pig's heart cooked with lotus seeds. Take toasted cassia seeds 15 g, decocted and strained. Add one pig's heart (chopped) and 100 g of lotus seeds with the skin on to make a thick soup. Add salt and some lard to season the soup.

Cassia seeds and lotus seeds can clear the Liver and purge pathogenic Fire.

Stagnation of Qi and Phlegm

Symptoms include sensation of obstruction in the throat ('plum-pit sensation'), stuffiness in the chest, or hypochondriac pain, a white and greasy tongue coating, and a taut and thready pulse. Dietary Therapy should be aimed at regulating Qi and dissolving Phlegm.

The recommended diet is candied kumquats (SXJYSP) made with kumquats 500 g (washed clean, seeded and flattened) candied in 250 g white sugar. When the kumquats are well candied, simmer them on a low heat till the juice is dried up. Add 250 g of white sugar when cooled.

The recipe is effective in regulating Qi, relieving depression, dissolving Phlegm and sending down Counterflow Qi.

Another recipe is a gruel made with finger citron and oranges (HYRZ).

Depression impairing the Mind

Symptoms are a dazed state, confusion, mental depression, crying, yawning, a pale tongue with thin white coating, and a taut and thready pulse. Dietary Therapy should be directed at nourishing the Heart and tranquilizing the Mind.

The recommended diet (JGYL) is liquorice and wheat 50 g each, decocted and strained. Add 500 g of dates to the decoction and boil them till the liquid is nearly dried up. Add 100 g honey, mix it well in and bring to the boil. Cool and store it for use. Take the dates from time to time.

The recipe has the effects of replenishing Blood, nourishing the Heart and tranquilizing the Mind.

Stagnation impairing the Heart and the Spleen

Symptoms include anxiety, palpitations, insomnia, amnesia, a dull complexion, dizziness, lethargy, loss of appetite, a pale tongue, and a thready and weak pulse. Dietary Therapy should be directed at reinforcing the Heart and the Spleen.

The recommended diet is date gruel (TPSHF) made with dates 50 g, poria 30 g and millet 100 g.

Dates used with millet and poria are effective in reinforcing the Heart and the Spleen and tran-

quilizing the Mind. Roses can be added to the recipe to help regulate the Liver and relieve depression.

Stagnation of Heat and deficiency of Yin

Symptoms are dizziness, palpitations, lack of sleep, restlessness, seminal emission, soreness in the back, irregular menstruation, a red tongue, and a taut, thready and rapid pulse. Dietary Therapy should be directed at nourishing Yin and clearing Heat.

The recommended diet is egg soup with lily bulb (see Palpitation).

GOITER

Goiter is a swelling on the front of the neck, which is smooth to the touch or possibly nodular.

Goiter is seen in people who live in mountainous regions and drink sandy waters. The sand in the water tends to enter the Channels with Qi and is accumulated in the neck*. The disease is also due to emotional factors which lead to stagnation of Qi, accumulation of Phlegm and Blood stasis.

Recommended foods

Patients with goiter should have foods that help remove the goiter and disperse the knotted tissues, such as oranges, persimmon, water chestnuts, kelp, sargassum, mussels, purple laver, Gracilaria, oyster, cuttlefish,

Foods to avoid

Foods that tend to cause Damp and Phlegm, Dry and Hot foods that tend to impair body Yin are to be avoided. Such foods include fermented glutinous rice, wine, chillies, ginger and fried foods.

---

* It is interesting to note that effective treatment of goiter had been recorded by Sun Si Miao by the seventh century AD, using substances such as kelp and thyroid glands. The knowledge of the relationship to deficiency of iodine was not necessary for effective treatment, as the 'river sand' theory shows.

Diet recipes

Accumulation of Phlegm and Blood stasis

Symptoms are a mass in the front of the neck as big as a walnut, often hard in texture with a pitted surface, movable with the action of swallowing, a greasy tongue coating, and a taut or taut and thready pulse. Dietary Therapy should be directed at dispersing the hard mass and removing the goiter.

The recommended diet is a soup made with three seaweeds and using dried mandarin peel 12 g, finger citron (wrapped in cloth), kelp, sargassum, cuttlefish, laver and kombu 100 g each (washed clean and chopped). Stew these in water till the meats are well cooked. Remove the wrapped herbs, add salt to season and eat the soup on its own or at meals.

Dried mandarin peel and finger citron regulate Qi and other items have the effects of dissolving Phlegm and removing goiter, while cuttlefish reinforces the Liver and the Kidney. Therefore, the recipe has the function of dispersing without impairing normal Qi or the body's resistance.

Excessive Liver Fire

Symptoms are a small or medium mass in the front of the neck, soft in texture, smooth and without nodules, and movable with the swallowing action, a hot sensation, palpitations, perspiration, trembling hands, abnormally large appetite, emaciation, protruding eyes, a red tongue, and a taut or taut and thready pulse. Dietary Therapy should be directed at nourishing Yin and dispersing masses.

The recommended diet is turtle soup with fritillary bulb and anemarrhena asphodeloides (FRLF). Tinned turtle soup, fritillary bulb 15 g, anemarrhena asphodeloides, bupleurum root, root of purple-flowered peucedanum and almonds 10 g each (wrapped in cloth) are stewed in water till the liquid is dried up. Remove the wrapped herbs and add some salt.

Turtle meat, anemarrhena asphodeloides, bupleurum root and root of purple-flowered peucedanum nourish Yin and clear up Heat; almonds nourish Dryness, while fritillary bulb and turtle shell disperse the mass and remove the goiter. Root of purple-flowered peucedanum and almonds can be omitted from the recipe.

Another diet for the disease is oyster and turtle meat stewed together.

Gynecological diseases 14

Dietary Therapy must take into account the special characteristics of women. Because they are able to menstruate, carry children, give birth and breastfeed, they have specific dietary needs.

The emphasis in Dietary Therapy is on replenishing Qi and Blood, nourishing and protecting the Liver and Kidney, strengthening the Stomach and Spleen, regulating Qi and moving Blood. This is achieved by a varied and nutritious diet and avoidance of foods which might impair Qi and Blood.

Diet should be modified to suit specific cases; for example, dysmenorrhea and amenorrhea are usually Full conditions, benefiting from foods which help to regulate Qi and move Blood and from avoidance of Cool, Cold or astringent foods. On the other hand, metrorrhagia, menorrhagia and bleeding during pregnancy are usually Deficient conditions and diet should include foods to fortify the Liver and Kidney and replenish Qi and Blood and astringent foods to hold the Blood. Foods which impair Yin, exhaust Qi or agitate Blood should be avoided.

DYSMENORRHEA

Dysmenorrhea, or abdominal pain during menstruation, is marked by aching in the lower abdomen and the lower back area around the time of menstruation, which can be accompanied by a pale complexion, profuse cold sweating over the head and face, cold extremities, nausea and vomiting.

The disease is due to emotional depression, impairment by Cold and Damp during menstruation, insufficiency of Qi and Blood, impairment or exhaustion of the Liver and the Kidney and Qi and Blood failing to flow smoothly.

Recommended foods

Patients with dysmenorrhea should have foods with a Warm nature during menstruation. Examples are brown sugar, dates, chicken eggs, Chinese chives. When the case is attributable to Qi stagnation and Blood stasis, it is desirable to have foods that can help regulate Qi and activate the circulation of Blood. Examples are rose flower, orange cakes and Chinese hawthorn.

Foods to avoid

Raw and Cold foods such as salads, cold drinks and vinegar should not be taken.

Diet recipes

Qi stagnation and Blood stasis

Symptoms are distension and pain in the lower abdomen before or during menstruation which is scanty and dribbling, with dark blood clots or fleshy membranes. The pain is alleviated after the masses are released. There is distension in the chest, hypochondrium and breasts; the tongue is dark or spotted, and the pulse is deep and taut. Dietary Therapy should be directed at activating Blood circulation and regulating Qi by using, for example, a wine made with rose flower and Chinese hawthorn.

Rose flowers 15 g, Chinese hawthorn 30 g and some crystal sugar are steeped in 500 g wine for a week, shaken once a day. Take the infusion for three days before menstruation, before going to bed.

The rose flower activates Blood and resolves stasis, regulates Qi and relieves depression, Chinese hawthorn can activate Blood circulation and resolve stasis, while wine can unblock and activate Blood circulation.

Stagnation caused by Cold-Damp

Symptoms are coldness and pain in the lower abdomen before or during menstruation. The pain tends to extend to the back and to be alleviated by warmth; the menstruation is scanty, dark in colour, with blood clots. Intolerance to cold, loose stool, white and greasy tongue coating, and a deep and taut pulse. Dietary Therapy should be directed at warming the meridians, removing the Damp and relieving pain.

The recommended diet is Atractylodes Gruel (YSZY) made with flour 1000 g, common fennel fruit, dried ginger, cinnamon bark and large-headed atractylodes, 30 g each, finely powdered. Mix the flour with the other ingredients and salt and toast them. To be taken mixed with boiling water 50 g at a time.

Common fennel fruit, dried ginger and cinna-mon bark can warm the meridians, disperse Cold, activate the stagnation and relieve pain; atractylodes can dry up the Damp, while flour can warm and nurture the Central Qi.

Weak Qi and Blood

Symptoms are a dull pain in the lower abdomen during or after menstruation, alleviated when the abdomen is massaged; pale and thin blood flow, together with a pale complexion, lassitude, a pale tongue with thin coating, and a weak and thready pulse. Dietary Therapy should be directed at reinforcing Qi and nourishing Blood.

The recommended diet is Chinese angelica root, pilose asiabell root and milkvetch root, 25 g each, sewn into a gauze bag, with mutton 500 g and some ginger, Chinese green onion and wine stewed in water till the mutton is well cooked. Remove the drugs and add salt for flavor. Eat the meat and drink the soup.

Chinese angelica nourishes the Blood and reg-ulates menstruation, pilose asiabell root and milkvetch root replenish Qi, while mutton warms the Middle Burner, replenishes Qi and fortifies the deficiency.

Impairment and exhaustion of the Liver and the Kidney

Symptoms include a dull pain in the lower abdomen after menstruation, which is pale and scanty; soreness in the back and spine, dizziness, tinnitus, a light red tongue with a thin coating, and a deep and thready pulse. Dietary Therapy should be directed at tonifying the Liver and the Kidney, replenishing the Blood and the Essence.

The recommended diet is fragrant solomonseal rhizome 150 g, rehmannia root 100 g and aspara-gus 30 g, decocted together, strained and boiled down to an electuary. Take 60 g of ox's marrow or pig's marrow from the bones after stewing and mix with the electuary. Take the mixture each morning before a meal, one tablespoon a time, mixed with warm brown rice or millet wine.

Ox's marrow tonifies the Kidney and fortifies the Essence; fragrant solomonseal rhizome, rehmannia root and asparagus tonify the Liver and Kidney and nurture Yin Blood.

AMENORRHEA

Amenorrhea is lack of menstruation in women over 18 years old, or a pause in menstruation of more than 3 months.

Deficient cases may involve deficiency of Kidney and Liver leading to exhaustion of Qi and Blood, or to weak Qi and Blood leaving the Sea of Blood empty and unable to produce menses as a surplus of Blood. The Full cases are mostly due to stagnation of Qi and Blood, Phlegm-Damp and obstruction of the Ren and Du meridians.

Recommended foods

Diet should be administered in accordance with the different types of the disease. For cases involving deficiency in the Liver and the Kidney, it is desirable to have foods that can nourish and tonify the Liver and the Kidney. Examples are animal liver, mussels, mulberries, sesame, walnuts, chestnuts, black beans. For cases due to weak Qi and Blood, use foods that can replenish Qi and nourish Blood, such as chicken, eggs, eel, grapes, litchi, longan and dates. For cases involving Qi stagnation and Blood stasis, take foods that are capable of regulating Qi and activating the circulation of Blood, such as finger citron, kumquat and Chinese hawthorn. For obstruction by Phlegm-Damp, it is desirable to have foods that can help dissolve Phlegm, such as orange cakes, grapefruit, turnips, mustard greens and ginger.

Foods to avoid

Raw and Cold foods should be avoided. For cases caused by obstruction of Phlegm, rich, fatty foods should also be avoided.

Diet recipes

Deficiency in the Liver and the Kidney

Symptoms are no menses by late puberty, or retarded menstruation which is scanty, pale and culminates in total amenorrhea, together with dizziness, tinnitus, soreness and weakness in the back and the knees, dry mouth, hot sensation in the chest, palms and soles, hectic fever with sweating, dark complexion or flushing, the tongue is red or pale with little coating, and the pulse is thready and taut or thready and uneven. Dietary Therapy should be administered to nourish and tonify the Liver and the Kidney, nourish the Blood and regulate menstruation.

The recommended diet is an infusion made with Chinese wolfberry 50 g, Chinese angelica root 15 g, and grapes 100 g, steeped in 1000 g of distilled alcohol for 7 days. Take the wine each night before going to bed, one small cup at a time. Chinese wolfberry and grapes tonify the Liver and the Kidney, Chinese angelica nourishes the Blood and regulates the periods, while distilled alcohol can activate the circulation of Blood.

Weak Qi and Blood

Symptoms include diminishing menstruation which results in total amenorrhea, a pale or sallow complexion, dizziness, palpitations, shortness of breath, reluctance to speak, lassitude or loss of appetite, loose stool, pale lips, pulse thready and weak or thready, slow and weak. Dietary Therapy should be administered to replenish Qi and Blood by using, for example, a thick mutton soup with Chinese angelica (see Dysmenorrhea).

Stagnation of Qi and Blood stasis

Symptoms are absent menstruation for months, mental depression, restlessness, stuffiness in the chest and the hypochondrium, distension and pain or tenderness in the lower abdomen, tongue dark at the edges or spotted, pulse deep and taut or deep and uneven. Dietary Therapy should be administered to regulate Qi and activate Blood circulation.

The recommended diet is Chinese rose decoction (BCGM) made with Chinese rose flowers 15 g and some brown sugar, decocted, to be taken in one session.

Chinese rose flower and brown sugar used together can activate Blood circulation and regulate the periods. The recipe can be modified by using equal amounts of Chinese rose flower with crystal sugar, steeped in wine to make an infusion for drinking. The wine used in the recipe can enhance the effects of activating Blood circulation, resolving stasis, regulating Qi and invigorating the periods.

ABNORMAL UTERINE BLEEDING (BENG-LOU)

Beng-Luo refers to bleeding other than a normal menstrual flow. Beng, or 'gushing', is usually sudden bleeding in large amounts, while Luo refers to dribbling of smaller quantities of blood.

The cause of this disease is usually Heat in the Blood, Blood stasis, weak Spleen or Kidney, leading to impairment of the Chong and Ren meridians and agitation of the Sea of Blood which fails to control menstruation. Cases caused by Heat and Blood stasis are Full, while those caused by weak Spleen or Kidney are Deficient.

Recommended foods

In general, it is desirable to have nutritious food. For Full cases, use foods that have a light and mild flavor and have the action of arresting bleeding, such as capsella, day lily, purslane, wood-ears and celery. For Deficient cases, take foods that can nourish and replenish Yin and Blood, such as chicken, cuttlefish, finless eel, hairtail, mussels and turtle meat. Foods that have the effect of arresting bleeding (as given above) can also be used in this group.

Foods to avoid

In both groups of cases, pungent and irritating foods, such as chillies, wine, pepper, ginger and garlic, are to be avoided. Deficient cases should also avoid raw and Cold foods, while Full cases should not eat foods that are Warm, tonifying, fatty or greasy.

Diet recipes

Blood Heat

Symptoms are sudden vaginal bleeding in large amounts, or protracted dribbling vaginal bleeding which is dark in color, together with a dry mouth and a desire to drink, dizziness, a red complexion, restlessness and insomnia, a red tongue with a yellow coating, and a slippery and rapid pulse. Dietary Therapy should be directed at clearing Heat, cooling Blood and arresting bleeding.

The recommended diet is a soup made with capsella and purslane 100 g each, decocted in water, seasoned with salt, vinegar and sesame, to be taken complete. Capsella and purslane used together can be effective in arresting bleeding, while vinegar is astringent and helpful in arresting bleeding.

Blood Stasis

Symptoms include dribbling vaginal bleeding or sudden vaginal bleeding in large amounts, with clots in the blood, together with tenderness and pain in the lower abdomen which lessens after the clots are excreted. Tongue is dark red or spotted at the edges, and the pulse is deep and uneven or taut and tense. Dietary Therapy should be directed at activating Blood circulation and resolving Blood stasis.

The recommended diet is Peach Kernel Gruel (see Epigastric Pain for the recipe).

Weak Spleen

Symptoms are sudden vaginal bleeding or dribbling vaginal bleeding which is pale red in color and thin in texture, a pale or puffy complexion, lassitude, cold limbs, shortness of breath and reluctance to speak, stuffiness in the chest, loss of appetite, loose stool, a tongue that is enlarged and tender or with tooth marks. Tongue coating is thin or greasy, and the pulse is thready and weak or hollow. Dietary Therapy should be directed at reinforcing the Spleen and replenishing Qi.

The recommended diet is dumplings made with Chinese yam and poria (peeled) 100 g each, powdered, and flour 300 g, mixed well and made into a dough. White sugar 200 g, lard, and dates (stoned) are used as fillings. Steam the dumplings before eating.

Chinese yam, poria and dates reinforce the Spleen and replenish Qi.

Another recommended diet is milkvetch root gruel, which is effective in replenishing Qi and assisting control of Blood.

Deficiency of Kidney Yin

Symptoms are small amounts of bleeding or dribbling vaginal bleeding, which is bright red, together with dizziness, tinnitus, a hot sensation in the chest, palms and soles, insomnia, night sweats, soreness and weakness in the back and knees, a red tongue with little or no coating, and a thready, rapid and weak pulse. Dietary Therapy should be directed at nourishing Yin to fortify the body's resistance.

The recommended diet is cuttlefish 250 g, tinned turtle soup and organic hen bones (such as good quality free-range chicken, or bantam) stewed till well cooked and eaten after seasoning with table salt.

Cuttlefish nourishes the Blood and nurtures the Yin; turtle meat nourishes Yin and cools Blood, while organic hen bones tonify the Essence.

Deficiency of Kidney Yang

Symptoms include large amounts of bleeding or dribbling vaginal bleeding, which is pale red, together with mental dullness, emptiness in the head and dizziness, intolerance to cold, cold limbs, a dark and dull complexion, frequent and profuse urination, loose stool, a pale tongue with thin white coating, and a deep and thready or weak pulse, especially at the Chi (proximal) region. Dietary Therapy should be directed at warming and tonifying the Kidney Yang.

The recommended diet is a soup (YSZY) made with Chinese wolfberry 30 g, mutton 250 g and two pairs of goat's kidneys boiled with condiments till the mutton is well done. The soup, mutton and kidneys are eaten with salt added for flavor.

The three used together can warm and tonify the Kidney Yang. For cases with large amounts of bleeding, add 10 g of preserved ginger and 6 g

of notoginseng to the recipe to help warm the channels and arrest bleeding. For cases with extreme deficiency of Kidney Yang, add 30 g of chopped typhonium tuber to help warm the Kidney.

LEUKORRHEA

In this section we only deal with leukorrhea in its narrow sense, i.e. vaginal discharge which is copious or abnormal in color, texture or odor or accompanied by systemic symptoms.

Leukorrhea is mainly due to a weak Spleen and stagnation of the Liver Qi leading to the downward flow of Damp-Heat, or to deficiency of Kidney Qi and exhaustion of the Lower Burner. Leukorrhea from Kidney deficiency may give off a fishy smell, while that involving Damp and Heat will smell leathery or rotten. Occasionally there are cases which are caused by exposure to toxic Damp, i.e. a recognized infection.

Recommended foods

For patients with leukorrhea of the Deficient type, it is desirable to have foods that can tonify the Spleen, consolidate the Kidney and arrest leukorrhea, such as euryale seeds, lotus seeds, Chinese yam, walnuts and ginkgo nuts. For cases with leukorrhea of the Full type, use foods that can clear up Heat and dissolve Damp. Examples are cluster mallow, water spinach, wax gourd, soya bean sprouts, purslane and coix seeds.

Foods to avoid

For Full cases, foods that are heating, fatty or tonifying should be avoided. Examples are fermented glutinous rice, and mussels. Deficient cases should not eat raw and Cold foods.

Diet recipes

Weak Spleen

Symptoms are continuous leukorrhea, which is white or light yellow, thick, sticky and odorless, together with a pale or sallow complexion, cold limbs, lassitude, loss of appetite, loose stool, edema in the insteps, a pale tongue with white or greasy coating, and a slow and weak pulse. Dietary Therapy should be directed at reinforcing the Spleen and resolving Damp.

The recommended diet is Jitou Zhou (YSZY) made with euryale seeds and non-glutinous rice 50 g each, boiled to make a gruel and seasoned with sugar.

Euryale seeds can reinforce the Spleen, resolve Damp and nourish the Stomach.

Kidney deficiency

Symptoms are profuse, dribbling leukorrhea, which is thin and white, together with soreness in the back, a cold sensation in the lower abdomen, frequent and profuse urination especially at night, loose stool, a pale tongue with white coating, and a deep and slow pulse. Dietary Therapy should be aimed at tonifying the Kidney and reinforcing the Spleen, consolidating and arresting the leukorrhea.

The recommended diet is Euryale Seed Gruel (BCGM) made with euryale seeds 30 g, walnuts (crushed) 15 g and five dates (stoned). Powder the euryale seeds, mix with cold water and beat well into a paste. Add boiling water and the walnuts and dates to make a gruel after adding sugar for flavor.

Euryale seeds tonify the Kidney and consolidate the Jing, reinforce the Spleen and arrest leukorrhea; walnuts help to tonify the Kidney, while dates reinforce the Spleen and fortify the Middle Burner.

Toxic Damp

Symptoms are profuse leukorrhea which looks like yellowish green pus or rice water, sometimes containing blood clots, with a foul odor, together with itching around the genitals, pain in the lower abdomen, scanty and dark urine, a bitter taste, a dry throat, a red tongue with yellow coating, and a rapid or slippery and rapid pulse. Dietary Therapy should be directed at clearing up Heat, removing toxins, resolving Damp and arresting leukorrhea.

The recommended diet is the Three-Green Salad made with purslane, houttuynia and celery in equal amounts, blanched in boiling water and drained, seasoned with salt, sugar, vinegar and sesame seed oil.

All three items have the effects of clearing away Heat, resolving Damp and removing toxins. When used together, these effects are enhanced.

PROLAPSE OF THE UTERUS

Prolapse of the uterus is marked by the sensation of heaviness in the vagina with tissues dropping or protruding out of the vaginal orifice. Because the problem mostly occurs after childbirth, it is also known as postpartum prolapse.

The disease is mainly due to deficiency of the Central Qi, or to impairment and exhaustion of the Kidney Qi, leading to disharmony of the Chong and Ren meridians and the failure of the Girdle Vessel (Dai Mai) to control Qi.

Recommended foods

Patients with prolapse of the uterus should have foods that are nourishing and tonifying, such as organic hen bones, eggs, crucian carp, finless eel, mussels, sea cucumber, black beans, soya beans, chestnuts, peanuts, dates and Chinese yam.

Foods to avoid

Foods that are Cool, Cold, raw and have the nature of sending down the Central Qi are to be avoided. Examples are turnips and onion.

Diet recipes

Qi deficiency

Symptoms are prolapse which is aggravated by physical exertion, heaviness in the lower abdomen, weakness in the limbs, shortness of breath, reluctance to speak, a dull complexion, frequent urination, profuse leukorrhea which is liquid and white, a pale tongue with thin coating, and a weak and thready pulse. Dietary Therapy should be directed at replenishing the Central Qi which will then perform its lifting function.

The recommended diet is chicken steamed with milkvetch (see Excessive Sweating for recipe).

Kidney deficiency

Symptoms include prolapse of tissues from the vagina together with soreness and weakness in the back and knees, heaviness in the lower abdomen, frequent urination (particularly at night), dizziness, tinnitus, a pale tongue, and a deep and weak pulse. Dietary Therapy should be directed at tonifying the Kidney and replenishing Qi.

The recommended diet is Steamed Beef (TPSHF) made with beef 250 g, washed to remove the blood, chopped into strips and boiled in water with ginger, spring onion and yellow rice or millet wine. Chicken meat and leg of pork 150 g each are boiled separately with ginger and spring onion before simmering on a low heat. Put the beef, chicken and pork into a large bowl, and add 10 g of Chinese wolfberry, 5 g of rehmannia root, 5 g of asparagus and 1 g of liquorice wrapped in a cloth. Then add the stock and some pepper. After steaming, discard the bag of herbs, add salt to season, drink the soup and eat the meat.

Beef can reinforce the Central Qi, warm the Kidney and tonify the Yang Qi. Chinese wolfberry, rehmannia and asparagus tonify the Kidney and replenish the Essence, while chicken and leg of pork replenish Qi and Blood and tonify the Kidney and the Essence.

MORNING SICKNESS

This is an ailment of pregnant women marked by nausea and vomiting, dizziness, anorexia or vomiting right after eating. It is one of the most common problems during the first stages of pregnancy.

The problem is mainly due to a weak Spleen and Stomach, disharmony of the Liver and the Stomach, leading to malfunction of the Stomach in sending down the Counterflow Qi from the Chong meridian.

Recommended foods

Women during pregnancy should have foods that are nutritious and easy to digest, that can replenish Qi and Blood, reinforce the Spleen and the Stomach, nurture the fetus and prevent threatened miscarriage. Such foods include cow's milk, eggs, bean products, lean pork, pig's liver, crucian carp, carrot, spinach, tomatoes, lemons, oranges and plums.

Foods to avoid

Fishy foods and foods that have unfamiliar flavors and are disagreeable to the patient are to be avoided.

Diet recipes

Weak Spleen and Stomach Deficiency

Symptoms are nausea, vomiting and anorexia after the onset of pregnancy, vomiting up clear saliva, dullness and sleepiness, a pale tongue with white coating, and a slow, slippery and weak pulse. Dietary Therapy should be directed at reinforcing the Spleen and the Stomach and sending down the Counterflow Qi to arrest vomiting.

The recommended diet is Crucian Carp cooked with Amomum Fruit (see Hiccups for the recipe).

Disharmony of the Liver and Stomach

Symptoms are vomiting up acid or bitter liquid during the first stages of pregnancy, together with stuffiness in the chest and pain in the hypochondrium, belching and sighing, heaviness in the head and dizziness, thirst, a bitter taste, a pale tongue with slightly yellow coating, and a taut and slippery pulse. Dietary Therapy should be directed at regulating the Liver and harmonizing the Stomach, sending down the Counterflow Qi and arresting vomiting.

The recommended diet is a tea made with red bay berries 30 g and plum blossoms 6 g, steeped in boiling water. Add some sugar and drink as tea.

Red bay berries can send down Counterflow Qi, harmonize the Stomach and arrest vomiting, while plum blossoms can regulate the Liver and harmonize the Stomach. Red bay berries are also used alone for the purpose.

VAGINAL BLEEDING DURING PREGNANCY AND THREATENED MISCARRIAGE

Vaginal bleeding during pregnancy is marked by dribbling vaginal bleeding without soreness in the back, abdominal pain or heaviness and distension in the abdomen. Threatened miscarriage is marked by the feeling of the fetus moving downwards, followed by soreness in the back, distension in the abdomen or slight vaginal bleeding.

These diseases are due to weakness of the Chong and Ren meridians which fail to control Blood and nurture the fetus. The causes of the weakness include weak Qi and Blood, Kidney deficiency, Blood Heat or traumatic injuries.

Recommended foods

For the deficient cases, it is desirable to have foods that replenish Qi and Blood and nurture the Liver and the Kidney. Examples are Chinese wolfberries, grapes, litchi, longan, sesame, peanuts, walnuts, liver, kidney, chicken eggs, chicken meat, cow's milk and fish. For cases with Blood Heat, use foods with a mild and light flavor which have the effect of cooling the Blood. Examples are capsella, turnips, egg plants, lotus rhizome and wood-ears.

Foods to avoid

It is not desirable to have pungent or irritating foods, such as dried ginger, spring onion, garlic and chillies in cases of Blood Heat. In either group, alcohol should be avoided. Foods that should be avoided by pregnant women are also be taken with care (see Chapter 4). For deficient cases, raw and Cold foods are to be avoided.

Diet recipes

Weak Qi and Blood

Symptoms are a sensation of the fetus coming downwards during the first stages of pregnancy, together with a small amount of vaginal bleeding which is pale red and liquid, dullness, lassitude, a pale complexion, palpitations, shortness of breath, or soreness in the back, distension in the abdomen, a pale tongue with thin white coating, and a pulse that is thready and slippery and weak on pressure. Dietary Therapy should be directed at replenishing Qi and Blood and calming the fetus.

The recommended diet is a thick soup made with one chicken egg, beaten well and mixed with boiling water to make a soup. Add 9 g E Jiao and salt for flavor.

E Jiao can arrest bleeding, nurture the Blood and calm the fetus, while chicken eggs can nourish the Yin and Blood. Milkvetch root 30 g can also be used to make a decoction, which is added to the soup. This herb is employed for enriching the body Qi.

Weak Spleen Qi

Symptoms are soreness in the back and heaviness in the abdomen during the first stages of pregnancy; vaginal bleeding, frequent urination or incontinence, a past history of repeated miscarriage, a pale tongue with white coating, and a deep and weak pulse. Dietary Therapy should be directed at tonifying the Kidney to secure the fetus.

The recommended diet is pig's kidney sauteed with eucommia bark (BCQD). Make a thick decoction using cold water and eucommia bark 12 g. Add starch, yellow rice or millet wine, soy sauce, table salt and white sugar, mixed well for use. Chop 250 g pig's kidney and saute on a high heat. Add spring onion, garlic, ginger and Sichuan pepper, pour in the eucommia bark decoction and some vinegar before turning off the heat. Stir well before serving.

Eucommia bark can tonify the Liver and the Kidney to calm the fetus. Pig's kidney can lead the herbs to the kidney, thus enhancing the effect of the recipe in tonifying the Kidney.

For cases with bleeding, this recipe is to be used alternately with the thick soup made with E Jiao and chicken egg (see Weak Qi and Blood above).

Blood Heat

Symptoms include bright red vaginal bleeding during pregnancy, a sensation of the fetus moving about and downwards, restlessness, a hot sensation in the palms, a dry mouth and throat, with hectic fever, scanty yellow urine, constipation, a red tongue with yellow dry coating, and a slippery and rapid or taut and slippery pulse. Dietary Therapy should be directed at clearing Heat, cooling down Blood, arresting bleeding and calming the fetus.

The recommended diet is the Fetus-Calming Carp Soup (adapted from the Fetus-Calming Carp Gruel, TPSHF). Boehmeria root 30 g (60–90 g if fresh) is decocted and strained. Boil 250 g carp (gutted) in the decoction till cooked. Add oil, salt and pepper to season. Eat the fish and drink the soup.

Boehmeria root can clear away Heat, cool down Blood, arrest bleeding and calm the fetus, Carp resolves edema and calms the fetus.

DIZZINESS AFTER CHILDBIRTH

This condition is marked by sudden dizziness after delivery, with an inability to sit up, nausea or even loss of consciousness.

This problem is caused by deficiency of Blood and exhaustion of Qi, due to constitutional weakness in Qi and Blood, plus loss of Blood during childbirth. It may also be due to stasis of Blood inside the body, obstructing Qi and Blood, hampering the clear Yang from rising and the turbid Yin from descending.

Recommended foods

For cases owing to exhaustion of Qi and Blood after childbirth, it is desirable to have foods that strongly tonify Qi and Blood, such as sea cucumber, mussels, finless eel, chicken, cow's milk, liver, grapes, dates and longan. For cases owing to Blood Stasis, take foods that are clear and light in flavor or that have the effects of activating Blood circulation and dissolving Blood stasis. Examples are Chinese hawthorn, rose flower and Chinese chives.

Foods to avoid

Tonifying foods can be used after the symptoms of Blood stasis are relieved, but be careful not to use foods that are *too* tonifying. In either case, raw and Cold foods are to be avoided.

Diet recipes

Exhaustion of Qi and Blood

Symptoms are heavy vaginal bleeding, sudden collapse and loss of consciousness, a pale complexion, palpitations, sweating, cold limbs, a soft abdomen, a pale tongue with scanty coating, and a weak or floating, large and weak pulse. Dietary Therapy should be aimed at replenishing Qi and restoring consciousness.

The recommended diet is a decoction of magnolia vine fruit (YSZY, perilla stem omitted). Magnolia vine fruit and ginseng 30 g each and granulated sugar 100 g are decocted for drinking during the day.

Ginseng replenishes Qi and restores consciousness, magnolia vine fruit replenishes Qi, promotes the production of Body Fluids and arrests sweating. For cases where bleeding continues, preserved ginger should be added to the recipe. Relevant tonifying foods are to be used after the symptoms are relieved or alleviated.

Blood stasis

Symptoms include sudden dizziness after delivery or even loss of consciousness; persistent or difficult lochia, pain and tenderness in the lower abdomen, dark lips, and a taut and slippery pulse. Dietary Therapy should be directed at activating Blood circulation and dissolving Blood stasis.

The recommended diet is a wine made with safflower 10 g and rose flower 15 g, steeped in 500 g wine for 7 days. Take the wine 10 ml at a time. Safflower and rose flower used together are effective in activating Blood circulation and dissolving Blood stasis. Wine enhances the effect of activating Blood circulation.

INSUFFICIENT MILK PRODUCTION (HYPOGALACTIA)

Hypogalactia is a disease marked by little or no milk in women after childbirth. The problem is caused by constitutional weakness and deficiency of the Stomach and Spleen or by suppressed Liver Qi, leading to obstruction in milk flow.

Recommended foods

For patients with hypogalactia, it is desirable to have foods that replenish Qi and Blood and activate the flow of milk such as chicken, eggs, pig's trotters, crucian carp, peanuts, mushroom and figs. For cases owing to suppressed and stagnant Liver Qi, use foods that regulate the Liver Qi, such as orange cakes, grapefruits, Cantonese orange, rose flower and jasmine.

Foods to avoid

Foods that are pungent, raw or Cold should not be taken.

Diet recipes

Weak Qi and Blood

Symptoms are little or no milk after delivery, milk thin when there is any, breasts soft without the sensation of distension, a pale complexion, lethargy and loss of appetite, a pale tongue, and a weak and thready pulse. Dietary Therapy should be directed at replenishing Qi, nurturing Blood and activating the flow of milk

The recommended diet is two pig's trotters, washed well, 200 g peanuts and 100 g milkvetch root (wrapped in a cloth), stewed in water till the trotters are well done. Discard the milkvetch root, add salt to season and eat the meat and drink the soup.

Pig's trotter and peanuts can replenish Blood and activate the flow of milk while milkvetch can replenish Qi. When Qi and Blood are abundant, adequate milk will be produced.

Depressed Liver Qi

Symptoms are little or no milk after delivery, dis-

tension in the chest and the hypochondrium, mental depression, slight fever and loss of appetite, a normal tongue with thin yellow coating, and a taut and thready or rapid pulse. Dietary Therapy should be directed at regulating the Liver and relieving the depression, unblocking the collaterals and activating the flow of milk.

The recommended diet is Pig's Trotter Soup (adapted from the Pig's Trotter Gruel contained in SQYLXS). Take two pig's trotters, 5 g Sichuan clematis stem, 15 g globe thistle (wrapped in cloth), 10 g finger citron and two stalks of spring onion and stew in water till the trotters are well done. Add salt to season.

Pig's trotter replenishes Blood and activates milk flow, while finger citron, Sichuan clematis stem and globe thistle regulate the Liver Qi, unblock the collaterals and activate the flow of milk.

HYSTERIA

Hysteria is a disease in women marked by mental depression, restlessness, unpredictable laughter and crying, and frequent yawning.

The term 'hysteria' is not as sexist as it might appear. The root of the word is the Greek *hustera*–the womb, used because the condition was considered to occur mainly in women. Although in TCM it covers a broader range of symptoms than in Western medicine, there are sound reasons for including it under women's conditions. Women lose Blood through menstruation and deplete it by breastfeeding and they lose both Blood and Jing through childbirth. Compared with men (who tend more to Qi deficiency), women are much more prone to problems associated with deficient Blood and/or Yin. Men have their equivalent problems, but they are less often associated with these symptoms.

Hysteria is due mainly to the patient's poor physical condition, overanxiety and sorrow which tend to impair the Heart, or fatigue impairing the Spleen. When the Heart and the Spleen are impaired, there will be a deficiency of the sources for the regeneration and transformation of Blood and Essence. It may also be due to impairment of the body's Yin by illnesses, or to loss of blood after childbirth. When Blood and Essence are exhausted and the five Zang Organs are malnourished, the mental Fire will move upwards to disturb the Mind and Spirit, leading to symptoms of hysteria.

Recommended foods

For patients with hysteria, it is desirable to have foods that can nourish and reinforce the Heart and the Spleen, such as wheat, dates, lily bulb, lotus seeds, mulberry, day lily and wood-ears. Fresh vegetables and fruits are also advisable.

Foods to avoid

Foods that are pungent, Warm and Dry, such as chillies, Sichuan pepper, pepper, garlic and wine, are to be avoided.

Diet recipes

Deficiency of Blood impairing the Spirit

Symptoms are dullness, confusion, restlessness, restless sleep, frequent yawning, uncontrollable laughter or crying and other mental symptoms, a dry mouth, constipation, a red tongue with little coating, and a thready pulse, weak and rapid or taut and thready. Dietary Therapy should be directed at nourishing the Heart and reinforcing the Spleen, moistening the Dryness and calming the Mind.

The recommended diet is dates cooked with liquorice and wheat (see Depression).

Deficiency of Liver and Kidney Yin

Symptoms include dizziness, tinnitus, soreness and weakness in the back and knees, hot sensation in the palms and soles, restlessness, palpitations, or confusion, a red tongue, and a taut, thready and rapid pulse. Dietary Therapy should be directed at nourishing the Liver and Kidney, nurturing the Heart and calming the Mind.

The recommended diet is a thick soup made with 30 g Chinese wolfberry and 60 g lily bulb, boiled in 1000 ml of water reduced down to 300 ml. Add two egg yolks beaten well and some crystal sugar for flavor. Take the soup twice a day.

Lily bulb clears the Heart and tranquilizes the Mind, Chinese wolfberry tonifies the Liver and Kidney and replenishes the Essence and Blood, while egg yolks nourish the Yin, nurture Blood and tranquilize the Mind.

Pediatric diseases 15

Children are full of vitality and growing vigorously, but their Vital Organs are still delicate and immature. They are physically fragile and any negligence will lead to illnesses. Pediatric diseases are mostly exogenous or due to impairment from improper diet. Therefore it is important for children to learn good eating habits. They need to be careful about cleanliness, avoid nibbling between meals and not be 'picky' or eat too much of one type of food (Wuwei Pianshi – partiality for one type of food), which may lead to the excess of that taste having a one-sided effect in the body. Their diet should be diversified, nutritious and easy to digest. Raw and Cold foods are to be taken with care.

For sick children, diet should be administered in accordance with the specific diseases. Children with exogenous epidemic diseases should have foods that help relieve the exterior syndrome, clear away Heat and remove the toxins. For children with impairment from improper diet, use foods that reinforce the Spleen, restore appetite, aid digestion and regulate the Middle Burner. Children with retarded growth and a fragile physical condition should have foods that reinforce the Spleen, replenish Qi, tonify the Kidney and nourish the body as a whole. It is important to tonify without causing stagnation, to aid digestion and purge without impairing the body's resistance.

Children, as 'Young Yang', are capable of changing rapidly. They are affected much more easily than adults and dietary changes alone will often produce striking improvements. In younger children it is particularly important to make mild tasting foods the central part of their normal diet and to avoid the more medicinal action of strongly flavored food unless it is needed.

MEASLES

Measles is caused by exposure to the measles toxin and is marked by fever, coughing, running nose, watery eyes and red eruptions over the body.

Measles occurs due to deficiency in the Spleen and the Stomach and fragility of the Lungs, which allow the epidemic toxins to invade via the mouth and the nose into the Lungs and the Spleen, i.e. at the Tai Yin level. When the Lungs fail to perform their normal functions and the toxins rage in the Spleen, measles develops.

Recommended foods

For children with measles, it is desirable to administer foods according to the patient's condition and different stages of the disease, choosing foods that can promote eruption, remove the toxins, nourish the body's Yin and replenish Qi, Examples are coriander, stalk of spring onion, mushroom, carrot, spinach, powder of lotus rhizome, water chestnuts, soya bean milk, cow's milk, and crucian carp.

Foods to avoid

Foods that are raw, Cold and spicy are to be avoided and greasy foods should be taken sparingly.

Diet recipes

Before eruption of spots

Symptoms are slight intolerance to wind and cold, nasal obstruction, running nose, sneezing, coughing, red eyelids, watery eyes, yawning, depression, redness in the mouth with white eruptions on the mucosa, or vomiting, diarrhea, a red tongue with thin white coating, and a floating and rapid pulse. This period lasts about 3 days. Dietary Therapy should be directed at relieving the exterior syndrome by using foods that are pungent and Cold.

The recommended diet is a tea made with mulberry leaves and peppermint (see Headache for the recipe).

During the eruption period

Normal cases

Symptoms are high fever, restlessness, thirst, aggravating coughs, red eyes with profuse discharge, measles spots erupting behind the ears and spreading to the whole body, which then get denser, turn from red to dark and can be easily felt by touch; a red tongue with yellow coating, and a rapid pulse. This period lasts about 3 days. Dietary Therapy should be directed at clearing Heat and removing toxins.

The recommended diet is Pueraria Root Gruel (SYXJb) made with pueraria root, chopped and ground with water to obtain the starch. Use 30 g of this starch at a time to make a gruel with 50 g of non-glutinous rice and drink after adding some crystal sugar.

This recipe has the effects of relieving the exterior syndrome and reducing fever, promoting the production of Body Fluids to ease thirst, facilitating the eruption of measles and arresting diarrhea.

Cold obstruction

Symptoms are measles failing to fully erupt or disappearing shortly after coming out after 3 days of fever, together with chills, lack of sweating, a pale complexion, a pale tongue with white coating, and a floating and tense pulse. Dietary Therapy should be directed at promoting the eruption of measles by using foods that are pungent in taste and Warm in nature.

The recommended diet is a soup made with one pig's lung, washed and chopped, ginger and spring onion 30 g each, boiled till the lung is cooked. Add 50 g of coriander (chopped), bring to the boil and season with salt.

Spring onion, ginger and coriander are pungent in taste, Warm in nature and effective in promoting the eruption of measles, while pig's lung has the effects of fortifying the body's resistance and helping to remove the toxins.

Heat obstruction

Symptoms are measles failing to fully erupt, dark purple eruptions, fever, thirst, possibly delirium, constipation, dark urine, a red tongue with yellow dry coating, and a vigorous and rapid pulse. Dietary Therapy should be directed at clearing away Heat and promoting the production of Body Fluids.

The recommended diet is a gruel made with gypsum and reed rhizome (see Epidemic Febrile Diseases for the recipe).

The recovery period

Symptoms are receding fever and cough, a slightly hoarse voice, improving appetite, rashes becoming red, flaking skin, pigmentation, a red tongue with little coating, and a thready and rapid pulse. This period lasts about 3 days. Dietary Therapy should be directed at nurturing the Yin, replenishing Qi and clearing away the remnants of toxins.

The recommended diet is glehnia root 100 g, sugarcane 1000 g and fresh cogongrass rhizome 500 g, squeezed to obtain the juice. Mix the juices together for drinking as desired.

Glehnia root and sugarcane replenish body Qi and nurture the Yin while cogongrass clears away the residual Heat.

To prevent measles, a drink made with arnebia root and the three beans (mung bean, black bean and red bean) can be used.

SMALLPOX

Smallpox is an epidemic skin disease marked by oval bean-shaped rashes with watery blisters.

This disease involves accumulation of Damp-Heat in the Spleen and the Lungs, plus exposure to epidemic toxins via the mouth and nose, which are transmitted to the Spleen and the Lungs to react with the accumulated Damp-Heat.

Recommended foods

For patients with smallpox, it is desirable to have foods that will help clear away Heat and remove Damp, remove the toxins and relieve the exterior syndrome. Examples are wax gourd, balsam pears, mung beans, red beans, soya bean sprouts, coix seeds and bamboo shoots.

Foods to avoid

Foods that are pungent, fragrant, Dry, fatty and greasy, such as ginger, garlic, chillies, fermented glutinous rice, fat pork and turtle meat, are to be avoided.

Diet recipes

Accumulation of Damp-Heat

Symptoms are a slight fever, nasal obstruction, running nose, scattered rashes which are pearly bright like dew, having no areola at the base of the eruption, rashes erupting succesively, with papules, blisters and scabs seen at the same time, mostly on the trunk; thin and white tongue coating, and a floating and rapid pulse. Dietary Therapy should be directed at clearing away Damp-Heat.

The recommended diet is Lophatherum Gruel (TPSHF) made with 30 g of lophatherum and 10 g of oriental wormwood, decocted and strained. Add 50 g of non-glutinous rice to make a gruel. Season with white sugar to taste.

This recipe is effective in clearing away Damp-Heat. For cases with only slight fever, oriental wormwood can be omitted.

Excessive Toxic Heat

Symptoms include persistent high fever, restlessness, red complexion and eyes, dense rashes with turbid fluids in the dark purple blisters, sores inside the mouth and on the tongue, a red tongue with yellow dry coating, and a vigorous and rapid pulse. Dietary Therapy should be directed at cooling the Ying level of the body and removing toxins.

The recommended diet is Bianque's drink with Three Beans (adapted from *The Compendium of Materia Medica*). Mung beans, red beans and black beans 50 g each, arnebia root, cimicifuga rhizome and liquorice 10 g each (wrapped in cloth) are boiled in water till well done. Discard the wrapped herbs, add some white sugar to flavor the decoction, eat the beans and drink the liquid.

This recipe is effective in clearing away Heat, cooling down the Ying level of the body and removing the toxins. The recipe will clear Qi, cool down the Ying and Blood and remove toxins more effectively when it is used in combination with the gruel made with gypsum and reed rhizome.

INFANTILE CONVULSIONS

This disease is caused by exposure to epidemic pathogens, improper breastfeeding or sudden alarm. This may lead to the generation of pathogenic Wind, Fire and Phlegm. These tend to agitate Liver Wind and obstruct the clear orifices and thus cause acute convulsions.

Congenital insufficiency plus feverish diseases, or protracted vomiting and diarrhea may cause deficiency of Yin and uncontrolled Yang Qi. This in turn can give rise to chronic convulsions as the Yang rises.

When the Earth (the Spleen and the Stomach) is deficient, Wood (the Liver) will not be properly controlled via the Controlling Cycle in the Five Element system. Liver Yang may develop into Liver Wind and once again manifest as chronic convulsions. 'Acute' convulsions are characterized by violent and Full symptoms, while 'chronic' are distinguished by their weak nature. Neither term is strictly accurate in terms of the duration of symptoms.

Recommended foods

For children with acute convulsions, it is desirable to have foods that can help clear away pathogenic Fire, dissolve Phlegm and calm pathogenic Wind. Examples are bamboo shoots, pears, sugarcane, watermelon, wax gourd, turnip and turtle. For children with chronic convulsions, use foods that are helpful in nurturing the Yin, warming the Yang or replenishing Qi, such as mutton, cow's milk, eggs, lotus seeds or dates.

Foods to avoid

Fried foods which tend to impair the body Fluids or raw and Cold fruits which tend to impair the Yang should be avoided by children with chronic convulsions. For acute cases, foods that are pungent, fatty and aid Damp and increase Heat, such as ginger, Chinese chives, mutton and beef, should not be eaten.

Diet recipes

Acute convulsions

Symptoms are a high fever, crying as if alarmed, restlessness, semiconsciousness, excessive saliva,

the eyes looking upwards, lockjaw, a stiff neck and back, jerking of the limbs, a red tongue with yellow coating, and a rapid pulse. Dietary Therapy should be directed at clearing away Heat, dissolving Phlegm and relieving convulsion.

The recommended diet is a gruel made with gypsum and hooked uncaria 15 g each, decocted and strained. Make a gruel with 50 g of non-glutinous rice in the decoction. Add 10 ml of bamboo juice and some honey when the gruel is nearly cooked and stir well till the gruel is done. Take the gruel as often as desired.

Gypsum and bamboo juice clear away Heat and dissolve Phlegm while hooked uncaria relieves convulsions and calms down pathogenic Wind.

Chronic convulsions

Agitation of Fire owing to Yin deficiency

Symptoms are restlessness, fatigue, flushing, a hot sensation in the palms and soles, spasm or stiffness in the limbs, constipation, a dry tongue which is livid with no coating, and a thready and rapid pulse. Dietary Therapy should be directed at nourishing Yin and relieving the Wind syndrome.

The recommended diet is a soup made with oyster (or mussels) 100 g, chopped and boiled. Add one egg yolk, beaten well, bring to the boil and season with salt. Drink the soup and eat the meat.

Oyster and egg yolk nourish the Yin and relieve the Wind syndrome.

Deficiency of Earth (Spleen) and hyperactivity of Wood (Liver)

Symptoms are lethargy and fatigue, a sallow complexion, crying from time to time, sweating, cold limbs, tremor in the extremities, sleepiness with eyes heavy, a pale tongue with a thin white coating, and a deep and weak pulse. Dietary Therapy should be aimed at reinforcing Earth and controlling Wood.

The recommended diet is blackboned chicken with wine and herbs (SJZL). One blackboned chicken, killed, gutted and clawed; cooking wine, stalk of spring onion, pepper, dried ginger, cinnamon bark and cloves are stewed on a low heat till the chicken is well cooked. Eat the meat and drink the soup.

This recipe is a combination of the Black Boned Chicken Wine (SJZL) and the Cold-expelling and Convulsion-Relieving Decoction (FYXB) and has the effects of tonifying the deficiency, relieving spasm, expelling Cold and relieving convulsions.

WHOOPING COUGH (PERTUSSIS)

Pertussis is a disease marked by a paroxysmal convulsive cough, followed by a sucking sound, ending in spitting up of foamy saliva.

This disease is caused by exposure to epidemic pathogenic Wind which invades the Lung system and becomes Heat, which reacts with Phlegm to obstruct the air tract. When the Lungs are no longer clear, other internal organs are impaired – the Stomach, the Liver, the Heart and the Kidney are affected in their turn.

Recommended foods

Patients with pertussis should take foods that help dissolve Phlegm, moisten the Lungs and nourish the Yin, such as turnip, bamboo shoots, oranges, loquats, pears, persimmon, lily bulb, sugarcane, crystal sugar, maltose, honey, tremella and duck meat.

Foods to avoid

Fried and sauteed foods and pungent foods should be avoided.

Diet recipes

The first coughing period

Symptoms are sneezing, a running nose, a cough with liquid sputum, or a cough with unclear sounds; symptoms being aggravated at night, fever and intolerance to wind, a white or thin and yellow tongue coating. This period lasts about 1 week. Dietary Therapy should be directed at expelling Wind pathogens and regulating the Lungs.

For cases with Wind-Heat syndrome, the recommended diet is a fresh reed rhizome gruel (see Cough for the recipe) and for cases with Wind-Cold syndrome, the recommended diet is candied ginger. Take glutinous rice flour 500 g, ginger juice 200 ml and brown sugar 200 g and make into a dough. Steam till cooked, cut into strips and take as often as desired.

The recipe can dispel the Wind-Cold syndrome and arrest coughing.

Convulsive cough

Symptoms are frequent coughs which are aggravated at night, vomiting with each spell of coughing, a red complexion, arching the back, watery eyes, cough often accompanied by sucking sounds and possibly spasm of the extremities. Dietary Therapy should be directed at purging the Lungs and arresting coughing.

The recommended diet is a drink made with the two 'whites'. White turnip 500 g and fresh stemona root 50 g, squeezed (or decocted) to obtain the juice. Add some maltose and mix it well with boiling water for drinking.

Turnip used with stemona root can clear away Heat, dissolve Phlegm and arrest coughing.

The recovery period

Symptoms include a diminished cough but one that is still dry and choking, sweating easily, a red tongue with a thin clear coating; or coughing that is not vigorous with a low sound, lethargy, a pale tongue with white coating. Dietary Therapy should be directed at moistening the Lungs and arresting cough.

The recommended diet (BCGM) is lily bulb 30 g and non-glutinous rice 50 g, cooked to make a gruel. Add some crystal sugar when the gruel is done.

Lily bulb is effective in moistening the Lungs and arresting cough.

INFANTILE MALNUTRITION

Infantile malnutrition is a chronic disease in children with symptoms of deficiency of Qi and

Blood and exhaustion of Body Fluids, such as emaciation, dry hair or enlargement of the abdomen with venous engorgement.

Infantile malnutrition may develop from improper feeding, early weaning, an imbalanced diet or overfeeding which leads to retention of food and impairs the Spleen and Stomach. The Spleen and Stomach may also suffer from lack of proper care after illness or from protracted vomiting or diarrhea. Once the Earth is affected, it is unable to nourish the internal organs and the body as a whole.

Recommended foods

It is desirable to have foods that are easy to digest and nutritious, replenishing Qi and Blood, such as Chinese hawthorn, sugarcane, water chestnuts, spinach, turnip, carrot, lily bulb, lotus seeds, flat beans, cow's milk, quail, chicken, chicken's liver and pig's liver.

Foods to avoid

Foods that are raw, Cold or greasy are to be avoided.

Diet recipes

Qi deficiency type

Symptoms are sallowness, lethargy, reluctance to speak, thin hair, slight emaciation, anorexia, loose stool, restlessness, thin and white tongue coating and a weak pulse. Dietary Therapy should be aimed at reinforcing the Spleen and replenishing Qi.

The recommended diet is a gruel (YXCZL) made with rice crust, lotus seeds (plumule removed) and white sugar 50 g each, cooked to make a gruel. Take the gruel three times a day between meals, 3–5 tablespoonfuls a time.

Lotus seeds reinforce the Spleen and replenish Qi, while rice crust reinforces the Spleen and restores appetite.

Food retention type

Symptoms are lethargy, emaciation, sallowness, thin dry hair, restlessness and crying, an enlarged abdomen with venous engorgement, itching all over, nail-biting, teeth-grinding, a red tongue with little coating, and a thready and rapid pulse. Dietary Therapy should be directed at dissolving the retention and regulating the Spleen.

The recommended diet is stewed pig liver (TPSHF). One pig's liver, cut open and stuffed with 3 g Ulmus macrocarpa*, is roasted with wet paper wrapped around it.

The recipe can kill parasites, dissolve the retention and regulate the Spleen.

Dry type

Symptoms are an aged-looking figure, dry skin, emaciation, drumlike abdomen, dry hair, lethargy, crying feebly, loss of appetite, loose stool or constipation, an occasional low fever, a dry mouth and lips, a tenderly red or pale tongue with sparse and dry coating, a deep, thready and weak pulse, and visible venules in the index finger. Dietary Therapy should be directed at reinforcing the Spleen, replenishing Qi, killing parasites and dissolving the retention.

The recommended diet is the Essence Nourishing Powder (JYQS) made with glutinous rice 2500 g, drained after soaking in water overnight. Toast it over a low heat till cooked and then powder it with Chinese yam, euryale seeds and lotus seeds 100 g each (toasted), Sichuan pepper 10 g (toasted till wet with oil), quisqualis fruit (shelled) and Chinese hawthorn (kernel and peel removed) 100 g each. Take the powder when hungry, 50–100 g at a time with some white sugar, mixed with boiling water.

Chinese yam, euryale seeds and lotus seeds can reinforce the Spleen and replenish Qi, while Sichuan pepper, quisqualis fruit and Chinese hawthorn kill parasites and dissolve food retention. The recipe is purging as well as reinforcing.

Another recommended diet is mutton gruel as recorded in Notes on the Use of Foods and Drinks (YZFSJ), which is composed of mutton, powdered ginseng, poria, dates, milkvetch root, non-glutinous rice and salt.

---

* Ulmus macrocarpa (= U. parvifolia) is a semi-evergreen tree. It is more commonly used as an external dressing on wounds and ulcers.

THE FIVE TYPES OF RETARDATION

The five types of retardation refer to five types of delayed development in infants, including retardation in standing, walking, hair growth, teeth development and the faculty of speech.

This group of problems arises from congenital deficiency and lack of proper care after birth. When the Liver and the Kidney (Kidney Jing) are insufficient and Qi and Blood are weak, the marrow is not able to sustain growth, and the muscles, the hair and the mind are not sufficiently nourished and retardation results.

Recommended foods

Children with retardation should have foods that help reinforce Qi and Blood, nourish the Liver and the Kidney and strengthen the bones and muscles, such as longan, peanuts, sesame, black beans, Chinese wolfberry shoots, spinach, chestnuts, walnuts, cow's and sheep's milk, chicken, chicken eggs, crucian carp, yellow croaker, eel, pig's kidney, and ox's spinal cord.

Foods to avoid

Raw and Cold melons or fruits are to be taken with care and it is advisable not to use much spicy condiment in preparing foods for these children.

Diet recipes

Deficiency in the Liver and the Kidney

Symptoms include slow growth with retarded sitting, standing, walking and growth of teeth, a dull complexion, physical weakness, fatigue, dullness, lassitude, a pale or red tongue with little coating, and a thready and rapid pulse. Dietary Therapy should be directed at replenishing and tonifying the Liver and the Kidney.

The recommended diet is Xuanwu Bean (JYQS) made with goat's kidney 250 g (chopped), Chinese wolfberry 100 g, psoralea fruit 30 g, star anise fruit and common fennel fruit 10 g each, desert cistanche 15 g, blue salt (Qingyan), all decocted together thoroughly. Remove the residue, boil 1000 g of black beans in the decoction and cook till the liquid is dry. Take out the beans and air-dry for chewing from time to time.

The recipe is neither dry nor greasy and is good for reinforcing the Liver and the Kidney.

Deficiency of Heart Blood

Symptoms are low intelligence, dullness, quiet demeanor, slow or blurred speech, a pale complexion, thin, dry yellow hair, a poor appetite, loose stool, and a smooth tongue with little coating. Dietary Therapy should be directed at reinforcing the Heart and replenishing Blood.

The recommended diet is a soup (BCSGY) made with grassleaved sweetflag rhizome 3 g and one pig's heart, washed clean and chopped, stewed in water and seasoned with salt. Drink the soup and eat the heart.

Grassleaved sweetflag rhizome refreshes the clear orifices while pig's heart reinforces the Heart and replenishes the Blood.

Another recommended diet for the purpose is a thick soup made with grassleaved sweetflag rhizome (see Wind-Stroke for the recipe).

External diseases and traumas 16

External diseases, sores and carbuncles are mostly caused by exposure to external pathogens and toxins which will in due course turn into Heat and obstruct Ying and Wei, or by overeating spicy, fatty, rich food, resulting in Heat accumulated in the Stomach and Intestines. Dietary Therapy should help to relieve the exterior syndrome, disperse pathogenic factors, clear away Heat, remove toxins, dissolve Damp and cool the Blood. For cases due to Qi stagnation and Phlegm accumulation, it is advisable to have foods that can help to regulate Qi, dissolve Phlegm and soften hard masses. Generally, patients with external diseases should have foods with a mild or light flavor, while foods that are spicy, fatty, greasy or tonifying should be avoided. For cases with sores or carbuncles failing to come through or be healed owing to weak Qi and Blood, use foods that can reinforce Qi and nourish Blood to fortify the body's resistance and expel the pathogens. In cases of trauma, there is probably stagnation of Qi and Blood and impairment of the bones and muscles. Dietary Therapy should be administered to help activate the flow of Qi and Blood circulation or reinforce the Liver and the Kidney, aid the regeneration of bones and related tissues. Raw and Cold foods that tend to impair the Stomach and Spleen or Warm and Dry foods that tend to impair the Yin should be avoided.

SORES, CARBUNCLES AND FURUNCLES

Sores, carbuncles and furuncles are acute external carbuncles in the skin. Generally, those with relatively small bases are called sores, those with larger bases are called carbuncles, while those that look like millet and have a tough deep root are called furuncles.

The disease involves the overintake of rich, fatty foods, pungent-spicy foods and wine, leading to accumulation of Damp-Heat inside the body. Otherwise it may be due to exposure to external pathogens or summer-Damp which invade the skin to cause stagnation of Qi and Blood followed by ulceration and suppuration.

Recommended foods

For patients with external diseases, it is desirable to have foods that can help clear away Heat, remove toxins, cool the Blood and activate Blood circulation. Examples are towel gourd, balsam pears, mung beans, red beans, bamboo shoots, spinach, water spinach, celery, purslane, acanthaceous indigo, houttuynia, and chrysanthemum.

Foods to avoid

Pungent-spicy, fragrant, Dry and Warm foods, such as coriander, ginger, chillies and mutton, should not be eaten. Fish and shrimps tend to cause an allergic reaction, so they should also be avoided.

Diet recipes

Full cases

Symptoms involve the formation of nodules at the onset, with redness, swelling, heat and pain. Then the nodules become soft and suppurate, with thick yellow pus and rotten tissue which comes off easily. In these cases, the sores are easily healed. Accompanying symptoms are fever, thirst, constipation, dark urine, a red tongue and rapid pulse. Sores have a shallow root and local-ized focus and are usually found in the head, face and the neck; carbuncles are deep-rooted, affect larger areas and are usually found in the neck and the back; and furuncles look like millet and have deeply seated roots which are extremely tough. These are usually found in the head, face and the extremities. Dietary Therapy should be directed at clearing away Heat and removing toxins.

The recommended diet is a salad made with purslane 500 g, washed, chopped and blanched in boiling water, seasoned with crushed garlic, salt, white sugar, vinegar, and sesame seed oil, to be eaten with meals.

Purslane is effective in clearing away Heat, removing toxins and reducing inflammation.

Deficient cases

Symptoms are flat sores which have widely spread bases, dull purple coloring, retarded sup-puration with liquid pus, the suppuration fails to discharge and the sores are not easily healed. There is a pale complexion, lethargy, a pale tongue with little coating, and a thready, rapid and weak pulse. Carbuncles are seen in these cases, but rarely sores and furuncles. Dietary Therapy should be directed at reinforcing the body's resistance and expelling the toxins.

The recommended diet is a thick soup made with duck meat (SLBC). One white duck, gutted and cleaned, with a suitable amount of fermented soya beans is stewed on a low heat. Add 15 g stalk of spring onion, bring to the boil and season with salt. This makes several servings.

Duck meat has the effects of tonifying the deficiency, replenishing Qi and expelling toxins. The stalk of spring onion also has the effect of removing toxins.

YIN CARBUNCLES

Yin carbuncles are sores in the skin characterized by flatness, light coloring and little fever or pain. They tend to develop in the deeper tissues.

This problem is mostly due to constitutional deficiency of Qi and Blood, plus exposure to toxic Heat and toxins which tend to obstruct the flow of Qi and cause pathogens to accumulate in the Ying Blood; or to Cold-Damp remaining in the channels and collaterals and entering the Blood circulation.

Recommended foods

For patients with Yin carbuncles, it is desirable to have foods that help to replenish Qi and Blood, reinforce the body's resistance and expel the toxins. Such foods include dates, peanuts, walnuts, rabbit meat, eel, crucian carp and duck meat.

Foods to avoid

Patients should avoid raw and Cold melon and other Cold fruits and foods that are spicy, pungent and irritating, such as peach, water-melon, coriander and chillies.

Diet recipes

The first symptoms are milletlike nodules, hard, red, swollen, hot or painful. A few days later, the sore develops a large flat base, with no protruding tip, dull in color. Then it will ulcerate, with dark purple coloring, rotten tissue, liquid pus and a wound that is not easily healed. Other symptoms are often yellowish-dark complexion, lethargy, chills, desire for warmth, a pale tongue with white coating, and a thready and weak pulse. Dietary Therapy should be directed at replenishing Qi and Blood, reinforcing the body's resistance and expelling toxins.

The recommended diet is Milkvetch Gruel (see Deficiency syndrome for the recipe).

Another useful recipe is a thick soup made with four pig's trotters, Chinese angelica root 15 g and stalk of spring onion 30 g, stewed on a low heat till the trotters are well cooked. Add some salt and eat as often as desired. This recipe can replenish Qi and Blood and reduce sores and inflammation.

ACUTE MASTITIS

Acute mastitis is an acute suppurative disease in the breasts.

The disease is due to overintake of fatty, rich foods resulting in the development of Damp-Heat and accumulation of Stomach Heat; or due to excessive anger or mental depression causing stagnation of Liver Qi and Blood stasis. There are also other cases which are caused by injury to breasts, by obstruction of milk or by exposure to toxins which result in excess of Heat and degenerating tissues.

Recommended foods

Patients with acute mastitis should have foods that will help regulate the Liver, clear the Stomach Heat and remove the toxins. Examples are tangerines, kumquats, red beans, mung beans, sprouts, eggplant, towel gourd, houttuynia, capsella and purslane.

Foods to avoid

Foods that are greasy, Warm and Dry are to be avoided. Examples are pork, mutton, mustard greens, coriander and chillies.

Diet recipes

In the first stages

Symptoms are swelling, distension and tenderness in the breasts, local skin uncolored or slightly red masses, episodic obstruction or hesitancy of milk flow, chills and fever, soreness in the joints, with stuffiness in the chest, thirst, a thin and yellow tongue coating, floating and rapid or thready and rapid pulse. Dietary Therapy should be directed at clearing Heat, removing toxins and dissolving hard masses.

The recommended diet is a soup made with red beans 250 g, stalk of spring onion and dried mandarin peel 30 g each, boiled till the beans are done and seasoned with salt for eating at meals.

Red beans can clear Heat and remove toxins, dried mandarin peel and stalk of spring onion regulate Qi and dissolve hard masses.

In the developing stage

Symptoms are a persistent high fever, enlarged inflammed masses and obvious hard nodules, heat and redness in the skin; or masses gradually becoming soft, creating a wave motion when touched, a red tongue with yellow greasy coating, and a taut and rapid pulse. Dietary Therapy should be directed at clearing Heat, removing toxins, unblocking milk flow and promoting suppuration.

The recommended diet is Dandelion Gruel (ZP) made with fresh dandelion 30 g, washed, decocted and strained. Make a gruel with 50–100 g non-glutinous rice cooked in the decoction. Add some crystal sugar before drinking.

The recipe is effective in clearing Heat, removing toxins, reducing swelling and dissolving hard masses.

After ulceration

When the swelling and pain are all aleviated, the fever is receding and the mastitis nearly cured,

Dietary Therapy should be directed at clearing away the residual Heat and reinforcing the body's resistance.

The recommended diet is a gruel made with 10 g bamboo leaves and 30 g glehnia root, decocted and strained. Make a gruel with 100 g non-glutinous rice cooked in the decoction.

The recipe is effective in clearing away Heat and replenishing Qi.

For cases in which the mastitis has suppurated but the swelling and pain fail to be alleviated, with persistent fever, continue with the dandelion gruel. For cases with unhealing ulceration, shortness of breath and reluctance to speak, a recommended diet is the Thick Soup of Pig's Trotters (see Yin carbuncles for the recipe).

INTESTINAL ABSCESS

An intestinal abscess is the development of a suppurative abscess inside the intestines caused by the accumulation of toxic Heat.

An intestinal abscess may be caused by dietetic intemperance, overeating of rich fatty foods or raw and Cold foods, overfatigue and traumatic injuries, emotional disturbance and maladaptation to changes in temperature, leading to impairment of the Stomach and the Intestines which then fail to perform their functions. When this happens the Qi will be interrupted, leading to Qi stagnation and Blood stasis, which will turn to Heat and burn the Qi and Blood.

Recommended foods

Patients suffering from this disease should exercise temperance in diet. Foods that can help purge the Fu Organs, clear away Heat and remove toxins are recommended. Examples are turnip, shepherd's purse, spinach, lotus rhizome, potatoes, egg plant, wax gourd, towel gourd, purslane, mung beans and red beans.

Foods to avoid

Foods that are heating, pungent or irritating, such as ginger, mustard greens, chillies and mutton, are to be avoided.

Diet recipes

Before suppuration

Symptoms include paroxysmal abdominal pain, the abdomen is slightly tense and very tender, distension and pain in the upper abdomen, nausea, fever and chills, constipation, a red tongue with thin white coating or thin yellow coating, and a taut and tense pulse. Dietary Therapy should be directed at purging the Heat and moving the stasis.

The recommended diet is made with coix seeds, mung beans and red beans 100 g each and liquorice 20 g, decocted in water till the beans are well done. Season with salt before eating the beans and drinking the decoction.

Mung beans and red beans can clear away Heat and remove toxins, while coix seed can remove Damp and promote suppuration.

Suppuration

Symptoms are severe abdominal pain, a rigid abdomen, a palpable mass in the right lower abdomen which is very tender, high fever, sweating, constipation, scanty dark urine, a red tongue with yellow dry coating, and a rapid pulse. Dietary Therapy should be aimed at clearing away Heat, removing toxins, dissolving stasis and unblocking the Fu Organs.

The recommended diet is a gruel (SJZL) made with moutan bark, peach kernels and wax gourd seeds 15 g each, decocted and strained. Make a gruel by cooking coix seeds 50 g and non-glutinous rice 50–100 g in the decoction and season with white sugar before eating.

This recipe is adapted from the Coix Seed Decoction, plus non-glutinous rice and white sugar, and is effective in clearing away Heat, removing toxins, removing Damp and stagnation and promoting suppuration. Moutan bark can be omitted from the recipe.

After suppuration

Symptoms are severe pain extending to the whole abdomen, which is rigid and very tender, stuffiness and fullness in the chest, chills and high fever, a red tongue with yellow coating, and a rapid pulse. Generally, fasting should be implemented but when necessary, Dietary Therapy can be administered so as to dredge and purge the Intestines, clear away Heat and remove toxins.

The recommended diet is a gruel made with coix seeds and peach kernel (see above). A salad made with purslane can also be administered (see Sores, carbuncles and furuncles for the recipe).

SCROFULA

Scrofula is tuberculosis, carbuncles and fistulae which are like strings of beads and develop around the neck and under the arms.

The disease is due to emotional disturbances and chronic Liver depression, or to exhaustion of Lung or Kidney Yin, leading to deficiency of Water and excessive Fire which burns the Body Fluids into Phlegm, plus exposure to toxic Wind and Heat and the invasion of the muscles and Blood Vessels by tuberculosis worms.* When Phlegm and pathogenic Fire entangle with Qi and Blood and result in disharmony of Ying and Wei, scrofula will develop where the body's resistance is weak.

Recommended foods

For patients with scrofula, it is desirable to have foods that help dissolve Phlegm and hard masses. Examples are celery, crown daisy chrysanthemum, three-colored amaranth, mustard greens, laver, seaweeds and taro. Patients in a fragile condition should have foods that can nourish the Liver and Kidney, reinforce the body's resistance and expel the toxins. Examples are river snails, oysters, turtle, eel, crucian carp, and pigeons.

Foods to avoid

Foods that are fragrant and Dry and tend to impair body Yin are to be taken with care.

---

* The character 'Chong', literally meaning worms, is an old term used medically in several diseases which Western medicine would view as involving microbes.

Diet recipes

In the first stages

Symptoms are subcutaneous nodules around the neck, chest, armpits and groin, which are as big as peas or finger tips, scattered, fairly hard, movable, not red or painful. Other symptoms are alternating chills and fevers, stiffness and pain in the head and neck, a red tongue with little coating, and a rapid pulse or with a normal tongue picture and pulse. Dietary Therapy should be directed at relieving the Liver depression and dissolving the hard masses.

The recommended diet is taro gruel (LNCYL) made with fresh taro 50 g, peeled, washed and chopped, non-glutinous rice 50–100 g and some brown sugar, boiled in water to make a gruel.

The recipe has the effects of reinforcing the Spleen and the Stomach and extinguishing scrofula.

Intermediate phase

Symptoms are enlarged nodules which are like strings of beads, fixed and with increasing pain. When the local skin turns dark red, slightly hot and pitted, then the nodules have suppurated. The tongue is red, the pulse thready and rapid. Dietary Therapy should be administered to help expel the toxins and promote draining of the pus.

The recommended diet is Chinese rose flower, genkwa and eagle wood 3 g each, one large crucian carp, gutted and scaled, cooked in water and wine in equal amounts till the fish is well done. Eat the fish and drink the soup.

Crucian carp reinforces the body's resistance and helps expel the toxins, while Chinese rose flower, genkwa and eagle wood used together can activate Blood and regulate Qi to facilitate the draining of pus and reduction of swelling.

In the late stages

Symptoms are persistent ulceration of the scrofula which looks grayish on the surface, with persistent liquid pus and degenerating tissue, and the local skin being dark purple. Other symptoms are usually a pale complexion, fatigue, emaciation, hectic fever, night sweat, loss of appetite, a red tongue with little coating or a pale tongue with thin coating, and a thready and rapid pulse. Dietary Therapy should be directed at reinforcing the Qi and Blood, promoting the drainage of pus and regeneration of new tissues.

The recommended diet is pigeon steamed with millet wine (BCQZ). One pigeon, gutted, cleaned and roughly chopped, seasoned with some soy sauce, white sugar and 1–2 tablespoons of millet or rice wine, is steamed till the meat is well cooked. Eat the meat and drink the soup.

This recipe can replenish Qi and Blood to help drainage and aid the regeneration of tissues.

ERYSIPELAS

Erysipelas is an acute dermatosis marked by clear-edged swellings that are hot and scarlet red. Those occurring in the head area are called erysipelas of the head (Bao tou huo dan), those which occur under the hypochondrium, the waist area and around the hips are called internal erysipelas (Nei fa dan du), those in the legs are called erysipelas of the shank (Liu huo) and those wandering around the whole body are called wandering erysipelas (Chi you dan).

The main causes are invasion of toxic Fire causing Heat at the Blood level which in turn causes stagnation in the surface tissues; or injury to mucous membranes, where toxins can most easily penetrate.

Symptoms in the head area usually involve Wind-Heat; around waist and hips Liver Fire may be involved; in the legs there will probably be Damp-Heat, and if the whole body is affected in infants, it will often be combined with excessive internal Heat.

Recommended foods

For patients with erysipelas, administer foods which help clear away Heat and remove toxins or those that are good for cooling the Blood and dissolving stasis, depending on the actual symptoms. Examples are cluster mallow, water spinach, shepherd's purse, day lily, eggplant, towel gourd, houttuynia, purslane, red beans and mung beans. For deficient cases, it is desirable to have foods that can nourish the body Yin, such as turtle meat, oyster and duck meat.

Foods to avoid

Foods that are pungent, Warm and Dry, such as mustard greens, coriander, spring onion, garlic and mutton, are to be avoided.

Diet recipes

Acute cases

Symptoms are sudden onset, chills and fever, heat, redness and swelling on the local skin, which turns pale on touch. The dermatosis spreads rapidly.

The tongue is red with a yellow coating, and the pulse is rapid. Dietary Therapy should be directed at cooling the Blood and removing toxins.

The recommended diet is a soup (SJZL) made with boehmeria root 15 g, decocted and strained. Cook 100 g of red beans in the decoction till the beans are well done. Add some salt before serving.

Boehmeria root can clear away Heat, remove toxins and cool the Blood. The effects are enhanced when used with the red beans.

Chronic cases

Symptoms include recurrent dermatosis, usually in the lower limbs, with redness, heat and swelling at the onset, possibly firm swelling of the legs, a thick and greasy tongue coating, and a soft pulse. Dietary Therapy should be directed at nourishing the Yin, replenishing Blood, reinforcing the body's resistance and expelling the toxins.

The recommended diet (BCSY) is fresh oysters (shelled) 250 g, boiled in water, flavored with ginger, salt and vinegar.

Oyster is employed for its effects of nourishing the Yin, replenishing Blood, reinforcing the body's resistance and removing toxins. When there is Heat and Damp to be cleared away, mustard greens can be added to the recipe.

SCABIES AND RINGWORM

Small spots of very itchy dermatosis occurring in skin wrinkles and folds are called scabies. Those that are invisible in the first stages and then infiltrate and spread, forming clear-edged rings of urticaria which are very itchy and painful, are called ringworm (tinea).

Both diseases are due to Heat in the Blood, pathogenic Wind and Dryness, plus exposure to Wind-Damp, Heat and parasites, leading to accumulation of toxins in the channels and collaterals, manifested as skin lesions.

Recommended foods

Care should be taken to prevent infection. Dietetically, it is best for the patients to have foods that help clear Heat in the Blood, remove Damp and moisten Dryness, such as mustard greens, houttuynia, water spinach, towel gourd, mung beans, honey, pig's tripe, turtle meat, eel, and jellyfish.

Foods to avoid

Foods that tend to dry the Blood and agitate pathogenic Wind, increase Damp and cause infection are to be avoided. Examples are chillies, pepper, fish and shrimps.

Diet recipes

Scabies

Symptoms are itching starting from between the fingers, spreading to skin folds in the wrist, elbow, knee and pubic area. The skin lesions are light red, as big as mustard seeds, in wet eruptions with dry bases. There may be grayish or dark rings. The lesions are very itchy, especially during sleep or when encountering heat. Dietary Therapy should be directed at eliminating parasites and expelling pathogenic Wind.

The recommended diet is pig's tripe cooked with gleditsia pod (BCGM). Wash one pig's tripe and stuff with one gleditsia pod which is roasted till crisp. Boil the two together till the tripe is cooked. Remove the pod, cut the tripe into strips, season with salt and soy sauce.

Pig's tripe can rectify deficiency, while gleditsia can expel pathogenic Wind, eliminate parasites and ease itching.

ABNORMAL HAIR LOSS (ALOPECIA AREATA)

Alopecia areata is the sudden fall of hair in round or irregular shaped areas on the head.

This problem is due to mental depression impairing the Heart and the Spleen which fail to nourish the hair; or to impairment and exhaustion of the Liver and the Kidney, and deficiency of Yin and Blood, leading to malnutrition of the skin and hair plus invasion of pathogenic Wind, causing Dryness of Blood.

Recommended foods

Patients with alopecia areata should eat foods that help to tonify the Liver and the Kidney and nourish the Blood, such as grapes, litchi, longan, dates, mulberry, Chinese wolfberry, walnut, sesame, black beans, wheat, soya beans, day lily, oyster and finless eel.

Foods to avoid

Foods that are pungent, Warm and Dry and tend to impair body Yin are to be avoided.

Diet recipes

Symptoms are sudden onset and loss of hair in round or irregular shapes with clear margins. There are no blisters, eruptions or papules. The patches enlarge or the number of patches increases in a very short time. In most cases, there are no subjective symptoms. With a few cases, there may be itching or tingling pain in the affected area before onset. The problem often occurs after mental distress. Dietary Therapy should be directed at tonifying the Liver and the Kidney, nourishing the Blood and expelling Wind pathogens.

The recommended diet is black sesame gruel

(BCGM). Black sesame seeds 30 g, pounded after baking, and non-glutinous rice 50–100 g are boiled to make a gruel, seasoned with white sugar. Black sesame seeds and mulberry electuary can also be employed for this condition.

ECZEMA

Eczema is a dermatosis with infiltrating, wet pimples which occur symmetrically or in irregular patches and are very itchy. The term eczema in Western medicine covers a much wider range of symptoms than this.

The disease is due to pathogenic Wind, Damp and Heat lodged in the muscles and skin, obstructing the striae. There is more Damp-Heat with acute cases, while chronic cases often include Blood deficiency and are caused by exhaustion of Blood after protracted illness.

Recommended foods

For patients with eczema, it is desirable to have foods that help reinforce the Spleen, remove Damp and clear away Heat, such as mung beans, red beans, coix seeds, soya bean sprouts, bamboo shoots, purslane, houttuynia, towel gourd and wax gourd.

Foods to avoid

Foods that are fatty, rich, Warm and Dry are to be avoided.

Diet recipes

Eczema owing to Damp-Heat

Symptoms include sudden onset and short duration, with red and swollen skin rashes, infiltration, ulceration, scabs, itching, thirst, scanty urine, constipation, a red tongue with white greasy coating, and a slippery and rapid or taut, slippery and rapid pulse. Dietary Therapy should be directed at clearing away Heat and removing Damp.

The recommended diet is Prostrate Knotweed

Gruel (SYXJb) made with prostrate knotweed 30 g, decocted and strained. 100 g of non-glutinous rice and 15 g of fermented soya beans are boiled in the decoction to make a gruel. Season it with salt.

Prostrate knotweed can clear away Heat, remove Damp and relieve itching and is good for curing scabies and eczema.

Other recommended diets are purslane gruel and dandelion gruel.

Eczema owing to weak Spleen deficiency

This is characterized by its long duration, patchy infiltrating skin lesions, thickened skin, pigmentation, eruptions covered with scabs or scales, sometimes with erosion, exudation, paroxysmal severe itching, fatigue and lassitude, loss of appetite, a pale tongue with white coating or white greasy coating, and a soft and thready pulse. Dietary Therapy should be directed at reinforcing the Spleen and removing Damp.

The recommended diet is Coix Seed Gruel (see recipe under Bi syndrome).

PRICKLY HEAT

Prickly heat is a type of skin rash with dense, milletlike eruptions which are very itchy and have red bases.

The problem occurs in a hot summer and autumn, when the heat and sweat obstruct the sweat glands and produce skin rashes.

Recommended foods

In the treatment of the problem, use foods that are effective in clearing away Heat, removing summer-Heat and Damp, such as mung beans, red beans, flat beans, coix seeds, soya bean sprouts, watermelon, cucumber, balsam pears and wax gourd.

Foods to avoid

Foods that are Dry and Warm or tend to increase Damp-Heat, such as fried foods, beef, mutton and coriander, are to be avoided.

Diet recipes

The symptoms occur after exposure to the sun, with redness on the skin, heat and itching, eruption of red milletlike rashes or blisters, mostly around the upper body and the limbs, which will settle when the weather turns cooler. Accompanying symptoms may be stuffiness in the upper abdomen, loss of appetite, dark urine, a red tongue with yellow coating, and a soft and rapid pulse. Dietary Therapy should be directed at clearing away Heat and expelling summer-Heat.

The recommended diet is mung bean decoction (JYQS) made with mung beans 100–200 g, boiled in water till the beans are well cooked. Add some white sugar for eating and drinking when cool.

The recipe clears away Heat, expels summer-Heat and relieves the sensation of heat. Honeysuckle flower (30 g, wrapped in cloth) can be added to the recipe to enhance its effects.

IMPETIGO

Impetigo is an infectious skin disease characterized by pimples filled with pus, which will turn into a yellow liquid to infiltrate the surrounding skin. When the problem occurs in deeper tissues, it is called pitted impetigo (Nong wo chuang).

The problem is usually due to accumulation of Damp-Heat in the Spleen and the Stomach, plus exposure to summer-Heat and toxins, which invade the Lung channel.

Recommended foods

Patients with impetigo should have foods that can help clear away Heat, relieve Damp and toxins, such as flat beans, mung beans, red beans, soya bean sprouts, towel gourd, wax gourd, balsam pears, watermelon, young dandelion, purslane, houttuynia and duck meat.

Foods to avoid

Rich, fatty, fried or pungent foods, such as shrimps, coriander and spring onion, should be avoided.

Diet recipes

Impetigo is most likely to occur in the summer or autumn. First, there may be the sudden appearance of red spots or blisters on the head, face and the limbs which are very itchy. These rapidly form pimples with pus, as big as the size of a finger tip, surrounded by red skin. These later form waxy yellow or grayish yellow scabs. The problem goes when the scabs come off. The pus is infectious. Dietary Therapy should be directed at clearing away Heat, removing Damp and aiding the drainage of pus.

The recommended diet (YYJC) is trichosanthis root 15 g and red beans 100 g boiled in water till the beans are well cooked. Add some salt before eating the beans and drinking the liquid.

Trichosanthis root clears away Heat and helps drainage of pus, while red beans reinforce the Spleen and remove Damp.

BURNS AND SCALDS

Burns and scalds are traumatic injuries from high temperature including boiling water or fire.

Burns and scalds, if severe, may cause injury to the skin and deeper tissues or even impairment of the internal organs by toxic Heat, bringing about systemic symptoms.

Recommended foods

For patients with burns or scalds, it is desirable to have foods that help clear away Heat, remove toxins, nourish the Yin and promote the production of Body Fluids. Such foods include mung beans, red beans, watermelon, pears, grapes, sugarcane, red bay berry, persimmon, turnip, tremella, wood-ear, honey and egg yolk.

Foods to avoid

Foods that are pungent, fragrant and Dry are to be avoided.

Minor cases

Symptoms are smaller and shallow injury, with

redness and pain in the affected skin, or development of a blister after injury. When the superficial skin comes off, the flesh underneath is red. The injury is healed when the blister dries. Generally there are no systemic symptoms. The tongue is red and the pulse rapid. Dietary Therapy should be directed at clearing away Heat and removing toxins.

The recommended diet is 250 g of mung beans, boiled in water. When the beans are nearly cooked, add 30 g of honeysuckle flower and 20 g of liquorice (wrapped in cloth). Boil further till the beans are well cooked. Discard the wrapped herbs and add some honey.

The recipe is effective in clearing away Heat and removing toxins.

Serious cases

Characterized by larger and deeper injury of the muscles, tendons and bones which produces blisters. When the superficial skin comes off, there is grayish white or dark red flesh underneath or even rotten or scorched skin or flesh with running liquid or pus. There may be high fever, restlessness or even loss of consciousness and delirium, or fatigue and shallow breathing. Loss of fluids is a major factor. Dietary Therapy should be directed at clearing away Heat, removing toxins, nourishing the Yin and nurturing the Blood.

The recommended diet is Rehmannia Root Decoction made with rehmannia root and honeysuckle flower 30 g of each, decocted and strained. Add 150 g honey for drinking when cool.

Honeysuckle clears away Heat and removes toxins, while rehmannia root nourishes the Yin and Ying.

HEMORRHOIDS

Hemorrhoids are varicose veins around the lower end of the colon. They are often inflamed and if there is a perforation which discharges fluid, it is known as a fistula.

The problem is caused by accumulation of Damp-Heat, overeating of Dry and Warm foods, straining to produce a bowel motion leading to downward flow of Damp-Heat and the stagnation of turbid Qi and stasis of Blood around the anus. Protracted hemorrhoids will lead to exhaustion; healed carbuncles may leave behind uncleared toxins which will infiltrate and perforate to form a fistula.

Recommended foods

For cases of the Full type, it is desirable to have foods that help clear away Heat, remove Damp, cool the Blood and remove toxins, such as spinach, purslane, egg plant, three-colored amaranth, water spinach, houttuynia, torreya nuts, persimmon, banana and figs. For cases of the Deficient type, use foods that help nourish the Yin, moisten Dryness and replenish Qi, such as kelp, wheat, wood-ear, catfish, finless eel, crucian carp and snakehead mullet.

Foods to avoid

In either case, foods that are spicy; pungent and irritating should be avoided. Examples are pepper, ginger, chillies and fermented glutinous rice. Excessive tea or coffee consumption should be curbed.

Diet recipes

Full cases

Symptoms are a sensation of obstruction at the anus, blood in the stool or dribbling or gushing bleeding after stool, itching, distension and pain in and/or around the anus, fistula running with foul pus, a red tongue with yellow coating, and a rapid pulse or with normal tongue and pulse picture. Dietary Therapy should be directed at clearing away Heat, cooling the Blood and removing Damp.

The recommended diet is steamed dried persimmon (SJBC). 100 g of large dried persimmons are steamed in a cooking pot till well done for eating warm before meals.

The recipe is effective in cooling the Blood and moistening Dryness.

Another recipe for the purpose is purslane gruel (BCGM) which is effective in cooling the

Blood, arresting bleeding, clearing away Heat and removing Damp (see Diarrhea for recipe).

Deficient cases

Symptoms are a protracted hard sore, which is grayish white and tends to prolapse at stool and cannot be restored by itself, a fistula failing to heal, with liquid pus, a sallow complexion, palpitations, shortness of breath, a pale tongue with white coating, and a thready and rapid pulse. Dietary Therapy should be directed at replenishing Qi and Blood.

The recommended diet is 100 g of figs, 50 g of milkvetch root (wrapped in cloth) and 250 g of lean pork, stewed on a low heat in water till the meat is dried and browned. Discard the milkvetch root and add some salt.

The combination of the three items can replenish Qi and Blood. Figs can also moisten the intestines and help relax the bowels.

INJURIES

Injuries refers to trauma resulting in the stagnation of Qi and Blood leading to swelling, pain, hemorrhage and restricted movement.

Recommended foods

Patients with acute injuries should have foods that are mild in flavor and help activate Qi and Blood, relieve pain and dissolve Blood stasis, such as the stalk of spring onion, oranges, rose flower and crabs. For cases of chronic injuries, it is desirable to have foods that help reinforce the Liver and the Kidney, such as grapes, black soya beans, chicken, beef, mutton and turtle meat.

Foods to avoid

For patients with acute injuries, raw and Cold foods are to be avoided.

Diet recipes

Acute injuries

Symptoms are sudden pain in the injured muscles, restricted movement such as bending, stretching and turning, or pain on movement. There may be swelling, bruising, cuts or bleeding in the local area. The tongue is either red with yellow coating or normal, and the pulse is rapid. Dietary Therapy should be directed at activating Blood circulation and dissolving Blood stasis.

The recommended diet is Peach Kernel Gruel (see Epigastric pain for the recipe).

Chronic injuries

This refers to injuries which have not healed within a reasonable time, with dull pain and restricted movement which is aggravated with changes of weather or fatigue, palpable knotted tissues or swelling, discoloration on the tongue with a thin white coating, and an uneven or deep pulse. Dark spots on the tongue reflect stagnant Blood and are more likely to be present after severe trauma, remaining for years if the stagnation has not cleared. The position on the tongue will often relate to the area of the body affected. If the stagnation is minor, it may not clearly reflect in pulse or tongue. Dietary Therapy should be directed at reinforcing the Liver and Kidney, warming and unblocking the Channels and Blood Vessels.

The recommended diet is one chicken, gutted and cleaned, 60 g of eucommia bark, 30 g of Chinese angelica root, 15 g of cinnamon twig (wrapped in cloth), ginger, pepper, dried mandarin peel, yellow rice or millet wine and water, stewed on a low heat till the chicken is well cooked. Discard the wrapped herbs, season with salt, eat the meat and drink the soup.

Eucommia bark, Chinese angelica and chicken can reinforce the Liver and Kidney, while Chinese angelica and cinnamon twig can warm and unblock the Channels and Collaterals.

FRACTURE

Fracture is mostly caused by traumatic injury but there are also cases of fractures which are caused by only slight external force because of the existence of a bone tumor or bone and joint tuberculosis.

Recommended foods

Cases of fracture in the first stages are Full. It is desirable for the patients to have foods that help activate Blood circulation and dissolve Blood stasis, relieve swelling and pain. Examples are onion, shepherd's purse, spring onion, Chinese chives and crabs. Cases in the late stages are Deficient and patients should have foods that help reinforce Qi and Blood, reinforce the Liver and Kidney, strengthen the bones and tendons. Examples are Chinese wolfberry, longan, chestnut, black bean, quails, pork, beef, mutton and ox's bone.

Diet recipes

In the first stages

Symptoms are local swelling, dislocation, severe pain, restricted or abnormal movement, bony crepitus on touch, together with fever, a dry mouth, dark urine, a red tongue and rapid pulse. There may also be tiredness, a pale complexion, cold limbs, a pale tongue, and a thready, rapid and weak pulse. Dietary Therapy should be aimed at activating Blood circulation, dissolving Blood stasis, relieving swelling and pain.

The recommended diet (BCGM) is drynaria rhizome 10 g, decocted and strained, with 100 g of millet cooked in the decoction and made into a gruel. Add some brown sugar to season.

Drynaria rhizome activates Blood circulation, arrests bleeding, dissolves Blood stasis and relieves pain.

Albizia bark can be added to the recipe to enhance the effects of easing the tendons and activating Blood circulation, relieving depression and tranquilizing the Mind.

In the late stages

There may be no distortion or swelling in the local area, but there is a soreness which is aggravated with changes of weather, restricted movement, weakness, emaciation, a pale tongue and a weak pulse. Dietary Therapy should be directed at replenishing Qi and Blood and strengthening the bones and tendons.

The recommended diet is a thick soup of ox's bones (SJZL) made with the ox's bones, crushed, and millet 500 g, boiled in water till the bone is well done. Add two lamb's kidneys and boil further till the kidneys are cooked. Strain the decoction. Stew the kidneys (chopped) with stalk of spring onion, salt, thick soy sauce, Sichuan pepper and sugar to make a thick soup.

The recipe can tonify the Kidney and strengthen the bones and tendons. To replenish Qi and Blood, add 30 g of milkvetch root and 12 g of Chinese angelica root to the recipe.

Complaints of the eye, ear, nose and throat

17

Traditional Chinese medicine holds that 'When there is illness in the internal parts of body, there are bound to be external manifestations', because the diseases in the external parts of the body are the reflection of the mechanism of the internal Vital Organs. Therefore, Dietary Therapy in the treatment of complaints of the eye, ear, nose and throat should follow the idea of perceiving the condition of the Vital Organs through changes in the external sensory organs and administer diet recipes accordingly. For Deficient cases, tonifying diets should be given while Cold and Cool diets should be avoided. For Full cases, Cold and Cool diets should be administered, while Warm and tonifying diets should be avoided.

NIGHT BLINDNESS

Night blindness, also known as bird's blindness (Que mang), is marked by normal vision in the day but loss of vision after dusk or in the dark.

Congenital night blindness is also known as pigmentary degeneration of the retina, with the pupil golden in color (Gao feng que mu). It is due to deficiency of the Liver and Kidney, malfunction of the Spleen and exhaustion of the Yang Qi. Acquired night blindness is due to Liver deficiency, which is often caused by protracted illness leading to physical fragility and deficiency of Qi and Blood; or to improper diet impairing the Spleen and the Stomach, resulting in Liver deficiency and scanty Blood supply which in turn lead to malnutrition of the eye.

Recommended foods

For patients with night blindness, it is desirable to have foods that tonify the Liver and Kidney, replenish Qi and Blood. Examples are liver, cow's milk, eggs, carrot, spinach, black beans, mulberry and Chinese wolfberry.

Foods to avoid

Foods that are pungent, Warm and Dry, such as Chinese chives, chillies, garlic and wine, are to be avoided.

Diet recipes

Differentiation is unnecessary as both types of night blindness have the same dietary requirements.

Symptoms may include a sallow complexion at the onset of the visual symptoms, dim vision or dry eyes with photophobia. There may be frequent blinking, loss of vision in dim light and in grave cases, the pupil color will be golden. Dietary Therapy should be directed at replenishing the Blood, nourishing the Liver and promoting the acuity of vision.

The recommended diet is a thick soup (TPSHF) made with 150 g of pig's liver, washed well and sliced, boiled in water on a low heat till the liver is cooked. Add three stalks of spring onion and two chicken eggs and bring to the boil. Season with salt, drink the soup and eat the liver and the eggs. This diet should be repeated from time to time.

Pig's liver replenishes the Blood, reinforces the Liver and promotes acuity of vision. Chicken eggs replenish the Blood and nourish the Yin.

Another recommended diet is pig's liver sauteed with the young shoots of Chinese wolfberry.

CONJUNCTIVITIS

Conjunctivitis is known in TCM as Wind-Heat eye trouble. It is mainly caused by exposure to external Wind-Heat or epidemic toxins, which tend to remain in the Lung channel and disturb the normal activities of the Lungs. The Heat thus produced, plus constitutional accumulation of Lung Heat or Stomach Heat or excessive Lung Fire, lead to aggravation of the disease.

Recommended foods

Useful foods are those with a plain flavor, such as Chinese cabbage, celery, fresh lotus rhizome, mung bean sprouts, balsam pears, shepherd's purse, tomato, water chestnuts, pears and river snails.

Foods to avoid

Foods that are pungent and irritating are to be avoided. Examples are wine, spring onion, garlic, pepper and chillies.

Diet recipes

Invasion of pathogenic Wind and Heat

Symptoms are redness and swelling of the eyelids, redness in the white of the eye, heat with tears, photophobia, dryness, profuse discharge in the eye. Other symptoms are headache, nasal obstruction, chills and fever, thirst, dark urine, a thin and yellow tongue coating, and a floating and rapid pulse. Dietary Therapy should be directed at clearing away Heat, expelling pathogenic Wind and promoting acuity of vision.

The recommended diet is an infusion made with chrysanthemum and roasted cassia seed 10 g each, baked and steeped in boiling water. Add white sugar to flavor for drinking as a tea.

Chrysanthemum is good for clearing away Heat, expelling pathogenic Wind and promoting acuity of vision, while cassia seeds can clear Liver Heat and aid vision.

Excess Heat in the Lung and Stomach

These cases show similar symptoms, with a more profuse discharge, a red tongue and a headache reflecting the more advanced condition. Dietary Therapy should be directed at purging Heat in the Lungs and Stomach, plus cooling the Blood.

The recommended diet is an infusion of chrysanthemum and gypsum. Gypsum 50 g and cogongrass rhizome 30 g are decocted and strained. Steep 10 g of chrysanthemum in the decoction. Add some white sugar to flavor for drinking as a tea.

Gypsum is very effective in purging Heat from the Lungs and the Stomach, cogongrass clears away Heat and cools the Blood; while chrysanthemum clears away Heat and promotes acuity of vision.

SORE THROAT

This term covers a wide range of conditions in TCM, from mild soreness due to Wind-Heat through to severe symptoms accompanying toxic Heat invading the Vital Organs. To simplify treatment through Dietary Therapy, we may divide sore throats into acute, excess cases and chronic, deficient cases.

Acute sore throat is usually due to invasion of the Lungs by pathogenic Wind-Heat and toxins resulting in malfunction of the Lungs. When this happens, the toxic Heat will burn upwards along the Lung channel and accumulate at the throat, obstructing the Vessels and Collaterals, burning up the Body Fluids and causing redness, swelling and soreness. Otherwise it could be caused by excessive Heat in the Lungs tending to burn upwards and attack the throat, or to overeating of pungent and fried foods leading to accumulation of Heat in the Spleen and the Stomach. When Fire and Heat in the Spleen and the Stomach rise upwards along the channel and attack the throat, the excessive Heat will cause Qi stagnation and Blood stasis; when there is swelling from the Fire-Heat, Blood and flesh will be affected and form carbuncles.

When there is excess of toxic Phlegm-Heat and epidemic toxins accumulated in the throat, there will also be stagnation of Qi and Blood, with obstruction of the Channels and Collaterals and the air tract.

Chronic sore throat is mostly caused by toxic Heat impairing the Yin or by deficiency in the Lungs and the Kidney, leading to the rising of deficient Fire.

Recommended foods

For patients with an acute sore throat, it is desirable to have foods that are light and mild in flavor and have the effects of clearing away Heat, expelling toxins and easing the throat. Examples are arhat fruit, carambola fruit, dried persimmon, olives, figs, turnip, towel gourd, peppermint and honeysuckle flower. For cases of chronic sore throat, take foods that are effective in nourishing Yin, clearing the Heat and promoting the production of Body Fluids. Examples are pears, water chestnut, tremella, lily bulb and pig's skin.

Foods to avoid

Foods that are pungent, Warm and Dry are to be avoided in both cases.

Diet recipes

Acute sore throat

In cases caused by invasion of pathogenic Wind-Heat, with Heat in the Lung channel, symptoms are a dry throat, a sensation of heat, pain, difficulty in swallowing, redness and swelling in the throat and the uvula, possibly with granules at the base of the throat. Systemic symptoms are fever, intolerance to cold and a headache.

When the toxic Heat has entered into the interior and there is excess Heat in the Lungs and the Stomach, symptoms will be severe pain, redness and swelling in the core of the throat, with red and white suppurating spots on the surface, which gradually turn to pseudomembrane (that is, something like membrane, formed as spots coalesce), or even redness and swelling in the isthmus of the fauces, a hard mass below the jaw which is markedly tender, swelling in the uvula, enlargement of follicles at the base of the throat, together with high fever, thirst, coughing up thick yellow sputum, a red tongue with thick yellow coating, and a full, large and rapid pulse.

When it is caused by retropharyngeal abscess, symptoms will be redness and swelling in the throat, severe pain, difficulty in swallowing and with speech, with the fauces turning red, swelling and protruding.

In acute laryngeal infection, symptoms will be a sore throat, difficult breathing, profuse sputum, difficulty with speech and swallowing.

For any of the above cases, Dietary Therapy should be directed at clearing away the Heat, expelling the toxins and easing the throat.

The recommended diet is the Blue-Dragon White-Tiger decoction (WSYA) made with seven Chinese olives and 250 g of turnip, decocted. Add some crystal sugar, drink the decoction and eat the olives and the turnip.

Chinese olives are effective in clearing away Heat, expelling toxins and easing the throat, turnip can expel toxins and dissolve hot Phlegm, and crystal sugar is effective in reducing Heat and promoting the production of Body Fluids. For cases due to invasion of pathogenic Wind-Heat, peppermint can be added to the recipe to expel the Wind-Heat and relieve the exterior syndrome.

When there is toxic Heat entering the interior parts and excess of Lung Heat, gypsum can be added to help reduce the Heat in the Lungs and the Stomach.

With retropharyngeal abscess, add honeysuckle flower and houttuynia to clear away Heat, remove toxins and reduce the abscess.

In acute laryngeal infection, use this recipe only after prompt medical treatment.

Chronic sore throat

Mainly caused by the rising of deficient Fire, symptoms are a dry soreness in the throat, discomfort, redness on and around the core of the throat, with yellow and white suppurated spots. Alternatively Hard masses may be felt below the jaws, there may be discomfort in the throat, slight pain, dryness and itching, a sense of heat or a foreign body stuck in the throat, a chronic low dry cough, congestion at the base of the throat with eruptions which are scattered or in dense strings. The tongue is red, the pulse is thready and rapid. Dietary Therapy should be aimed at nourishing the Yin, moistening the Dryness and easing the throat.

The recommended diet (SHL) is pig's skin 250 g, boiled till well done. Add 50 g of honey, eat the pig's skin and drink the soup. (Rice powder was added for regulating the Middle Burner and arresting diarrhea in the original recipe, but it may be omitted here.)

Pig's skin is sweet and slightly Cold and can nourish the Yin and moisten Dryness, while honey clears away Heat, moistens Dryness and eases the throat.

MOUTH ULCERS

Mouth ulcers are shallow ulcerated spots occurring in the oral cavity.

Clinically there are Full and Deficient cases. Full cases are mostly due to overconsumption of pungent and rich foods and wine, leading to accumulation of Heat in the Heart and the Spleen, plus exposure to pathogenic Wind, Fire and Dryness. When these are excessive, they will turn into Fire to attack upwards along the channels and develop sores in the mouth.

These cases may also be caused by uncleanness of the mouth or injury, which will facilitate the invasion of toxins, resulting in ulceration of the mucosa.

The Deficient cases are usually due to constitutional deficiency of the Yin, plus exhaustion of the genuine Yin by illnesses or fatigue. The Heart and the Kidney will in their turn be impaired and the Yin fluids will be insufficient, leading excessive deficient Fire to burn upwards.

Recommended foods

Patients with mouth ulcers should have eggs, soya bean products, balsam pears, turnip, Chinese cabbage, spinach, three-colored amaranth, persimmon, watermelon and honeysuckle flower.

Foods to avoid

Foods that are pungent, Warm and Dry should not be eaten.

Diet recipes

Accumulation of pathogenic Heat

Symptoms are the development on the lips, cheeks, gums and the tongue surface of yellowish white ulcerative spots, which are round or oval, as big as peas, with a depression in the centre and redness and slight swelling in the mucosa around. The ulcerative spots are numerous or even joined together to form patches, with sensations of heat and pain. Other symptoms may be fever, thirst, foul breath, a red tongue with yellow coating, and a rapid pulse. Dietary Therapy should be directed at purging the accumulated Heat.

The recommended diet is a tea made with 6 g of unfolded young bamboo leaves, 15 g of reed rhizome and 10 g of lilyturf root steeped in boiling water. Add some white sugar to the infusion, to be drunk as a tea.

Unfolded young bamboo leaves clear Heart Fire, induce urination and are good for treating mouth ulcers. Reed rhizome helps clear away Heat and promote the production of Body Fluids, while lilyturf root nourishes the Yin, reinforces the Stomach and clears Heart Fire.

The combination of the three items can purge the accumulated Heat.

Hyperactivity of Fire due to deficiency of the Yin

Symptoms are scattered, relatively pale ulcerative spots in the mouth, which do not fuse but tend to be recurrent. There may be slight pain, which is more obvious at meals. The tongue is red with little moisture or coating, and the pulse is thready and rapid. Dietary Therapy should be directed at nourishing Yin and sending down pathogenic Fire.

The recommended diet is an infusion of dendrobium 15 g and unfolded young bamboo leaves 6 g, decocted and strained. Add white sugar to the decoction, to be drunk as a tea.

Dendrobium can nourish Yin and clear away Heat, while young bamboo leaves clear away Heart Fire, induce urination and purge pathogenic Fire.

BLEEDING GUMS

The Yangming channel travels along the teeth and gums. Gum bleeding is usually due to excessive Stomach Fire burning upwards along the Yangming channel, causing the Blood to rise with the Fire; or to deficiency of the Liver and Kidney Yin, leading to the rise of deficient Fire, impairing the Collaterals in the gum.

Recommended foods

Patients with bleeding gums should eat foods that can clear away Heat, cool down Blood and nourish the Yin. Examples are shepherd's purse, bitter gourd, turnip, cluster mallow, water spinach, towel gourd, celery, tomato, watermelon, lotus rhizome, day lily and wood-ears.

Foods to avoid

Foods that are pungent and tend to irritate pathogenic Fire, such as chillies, pepper, fried food and wine, are to be avoided.

Diet recipes

Excessive Stomach Fire

Symptoms include bleeding from the gum, the blood being bright red, swelling and redness of the gums, headache, foul breath, a red tongue with yellow coating, and a full and rapid pulse. Dietary Therapy should be directed at purging the Stomach Fire, cooling down Blood and arresting bleeding.

The recommended diet is an infusion of gypsum and cogongrass rhizome 50 g each, decocted and strained. Add white sugar and drink as a tea.

Gypsum purges Stomach Fire while cogongrass rhizome cools Blood and arrests bleeding.

Hyperactivity of Fire owing to deficiency of the Yin

Symptoms are bleeding from the gum with pale red blood, loose teeth, a red tongue with little coating, and a thready and rapid pulse. The problem is often triggered off when the patient encounters heat or is fatigued. Dietary Therapy should be directed at nourishing the Yin and cooling the Blood.

The recommended diet is 150–200 g of Chinese wolfberry shoots and two pig's kidneys, cut open, washed well and chopped, sauteed together with some wood-ears.

Pig's kidney used together with Chinese wolfberry shoots can nourish the Liver and the Kidney and clear away deficient Fire, while wood-ears cool the Blood and arrest bleeding.

SINUSITIS

Sinusitis or rhinorrhea with profuse turbid discharge is a commonly seen disease marked by nasal obstruction, running nose, dull headache, and impaired sense of smell.

Full cases of the disease are usually due to

pathogenic Wind, Heat and toxins invading the Lungs or exposure to Wind and Cold which become stagnant and turn into Heat. The pathogenic Heat, attacking upwards along the channel, impairs the nasal sinuses. Otherwise Damp-Heat may develop inside, which tends to stagnate and affect the Spleen and the Stomach. The Damp-Heat and the toxins rise upwards along the Channel, carrying the Heat to the brain and impairing the nasal sinuses.

Deficient cases are usually due to deficient and Cold Lung Qi. When the Lung Qi is weak, the toxins will persist, allowing the problem to occur repeatedly.

Recommended foods

Patients with sinusitis should eat foods that can clear away Heat, such as houttuynia, balsam pears, mung bean sprouts, towel gourd, egg plant, persimmon, loquat, pears, banana and Chinese olives. For cases with deficiency of Spleen and Lung Qi, use foods that can reinforce the Spleen and the Lungs. Examples are dates, coix seeds, Chinese yam, duck's eggs, duck's meat and pig's lungs.

Foods to avoid

Rich, fatty, pungent or irritating foods are to be avoided and wine is strictly prohibited.

Diet recipes

Wind-Heat in the Lung channel

Symptoms are profuse yellow or white and sticky nasal discharge which runs downwards from above the nasal cavity, intermittent or continuous nasal obstruction, impaired sense of smell, redness and swelling inside the nose, tenderness between the eyebrows or in the cheek area. Systemic symptoms can include fever, intolerance to cold, headache, stuffiness in the chest, a cough, a red tongue with slightly yellow coating, and a floating and rapid pulse. Dietary Therapy should be directed at expelling the pathogenic Wind and Heat and awakening the clear orifices by using fragrant drugs.

The recommended diet is a tea made with chrysanthemum and gardenia 10 g each, peppermint 3 g and stalk of spring onion 3 g, steeped in boiling water. Add honey to season and drink as a tea.

Chrysanthemum is employed to expel pathogenic Wind and clear away Heat, gardenia purges Heat in the Lungs, peppermint disperses pathogenic Wind-Heat while stalk of spring onion awakens the clear orifices.

Deficiency of Spleen Qi and Lung Qi

Symptoms are nasal discharge that is white and sticky or yellow and thick, nasal obstruction, impaired sense of smell, light red nostril lining, general weakness, confusion, heaviness in the head, loss of appetite, loose stool, nasal obstruction and nasal discharge being aggravated when encountering Wind and Cold, a pale tongue with thin white coating, and a slow and weak pulse. Dietary Therapy should be aimed at reinforcing the Spleen and the Lungs.

The recommended diet is milkvetch root and lotus seeds 50 g each, with one pig's lung, washed, stewed with condiments till the pig's lung is well cooked. Add salt for flavor, drink the soup and eat the lung and the lotus seeds.

Milkvetch root is an important drug for reinforcing the Lung Qi, lotus seeds reinforce the Spleen, while pig's lung reinforces its human counterpart.

For cases with nasal obstruction, add the stalk of spring onion.

Glossary of herbs

COMMON NAME	PHARMACEUTICAL/LATIN	PINYIN
Acanthopanax bark	*Cortex Acanthopanacis Radicis*	Wu Jia Pi
Achyranthes root	*A. Bidentata*	Huai Niu Xi
Aconite	*Radix Aconiti Lateralis Praeparata*	Fu Zi (restricted use)
Agastache	*Herba Agastachis*	Huo Xiang
Albizia bark	*Cortex Albizziae*	He Huan Pi
Albizia flower	*Flos Albizziae*	He Huan Hua
Amomum fruit	*Fructus Amomi*	Sha Ren
Anemarrhena asphodeloides	*Rhizoma Anemarrhenae*	Zhi Mu
Areca nut (Betel nut)	*Semen Areca*	Bing Lang
Arisaema root	*Rhizoma Arisaematis*	Tian Nan Xing
Arnebia root	*Radix Arnebiae*	Zi Cao
Asparagus cochinchinensis	*Radix Asparagi*	Tian Men Dong
Aucklandia root	*Radix Aucklandia*	Mu Xiang
Badian (eggplant)	*Solanum Melongena*	Que Zi
Barley	*Fructus Hordei Germinatus*	Mai Ya
Bitter cardomom	*Alpinia Oxyphylla*	Yi Zhi Ren
Bletilla tuber	*Rhizoma Bletillae*	Bai Ji
Boat-fruited sterculia seed	*Semen Sterculiae Scaphigerae*	Pang Da Hai
Boehmeria root	*Radix Boehmeriae*	Zhu Ma Gen
Bupleurum root	*Radix Bupleuri*	Chai Hu
Bur-reed tuber	*Rhizoma Sparganii*	San Leng
Canger leaves	*Coptis*	Huang Lian Ye
Cassia seeds	*Semen Cassiae*	Jue Ming Zi
Chaenomeles fruits	*Fructus Chaenomelis*	Mu Gua
Cherokee rosehip	*Rosa Laevigata*	Jing Ying Zi
Chicken's gizzard membrane	*Endothelium Corneum*	Ji Nei Jia
Chinese hawthorn apple	*Crataegus Cuneata*	Shan Zha
Chinese olive	*Canarium Album*	Qing Guo
Chinese rose	*Rosa Chinensis*	Yue Chi Hua
Chinese wolfberry	*Fructus Lycii Chinensis*	Gou Qi Zi
Chinese wolfberry shoots	*Folium Lycii*	Gou Qi Ye

COMMON NAME	PHARMACEUTICAL/LATIN	PINYIN
Chinese yam	*Dioscorea Opposita*	Shan Yao
Chrysanthemum	*Flos Chrysanthemi*	Ju Hua
Chuanxiong rhizome (see Ligusticum)		
Cimicifuga rhizome	*Rhizoma Cimicifugae*	Sheng Ma
Cinnamon bark	*Cortex Cinnamomi*	Gui Pi or Rou Gui
Cinnamon twigs	*Ramulus Cinnamomi*	Gui Zhi
Clematis root	*Radix Clematidis*	Wei Ling Xian
Cluster mallow	*Malva Verticillata*	Dong Kui Zi
Cogongrass	*Imperata Cylindrica*	Bai Mao Gen
Coix	*Semen Coicis*	Yi Yi Ren
Cordyceps	*Cordyceps*	Dong Chong Xia Cao
Costus root	*Radix Aucklandia*	Mu Xiang
Crown daisy chrysanthemum	*Chrysanthemum Coronarium*	Tong Hao
Croton	*Semen Croton Tiglium*	Ba Tou
Curcuma root	*Radix Curcumae*	Yu Jin
Cynanchum	*Radix Cynanchi Atrati*	Bai Wei
Dahurian angelica	*Radix Angelicae Dahuricae*	Bai Zhi
Dandelion	*Herba Taraxaci*	Pu Gong Ying
Day lily	*Hemerocallis Fulva*	Huang Hua Cai
Dendrobium	*Herba Dendrobii*	Shi Hu
Desert cistanche	*Herba Cistanchis*	Rou Cong Rong
Dodder seed	*Semen Cuscutae*	Tu Si Zi
Dog thorn	*Ilex Cornuta*	Zhou Gu
Dogwood	*Fructus Corni*	Shan Zhu Yu
Donkey-hide gelatin	*Colla Corii Asini*	E Jiao
Dried ginger	*Rhizoma Zingiberis*	Gan Jiang
Drynaria	*Rhizoma Drynariae*	Gu Sui Bu
Dwarf lilyturf	*Radix Opophiogonis*	Mai Men Dong
Eagle wood	*Lignum Aquilariae Resinatum*	Chen Xiang
Eclipta	*Herba Ecliptae*	Han Lian Cao
Epimedium	*Herba Epimedii*	Yin Yang Huo
Eucommia bark	*Cortex Eucommiae*	Du Zhong
Euryale seed	*Semen Euryalis*	Qian Shi
Fennel fruits (seedpods)	*Fructus Foeniculii*	Xiao Hui Xiang
Finger citron	*Fructus Citri Sarcodactylis*	Fo Shou Gan
Five juice mix	*Water chestnut, fresh pears, Lu Gen, Mai Men Dong, lotus root*	
Fragrant mushroom (Shiitake)	*Lentinus Edodes*	Xiang Gu
Fragrant solomonseal	*Polygonatum odoratum*	Yu Zhu
Fresh ginger	*Rhizoma Zingiberis Recens*	Sheng Jiang
Fritillary bulb	*Bulbus Fritillariae Cirrhosa*	Chuan Bei Mu
Galangal	*Rhizoma Alpiniae Officinarum*	Gao Liang Jiang
Gastrodia	*Rhizoma Gastrodiae*	Tian Ma
Genkwa flower	*Flos Genkwa*	Yuan Hua
Ginseng	*Radix Ginseng*	Ren Shen
Gleditsia pod	*Fructus Gleditsiae*	Zao Jiao
Glehnia root	*Radix Glehniae*	Bei Sha Shen

COMMON NAME	PHARMACEUTICAL/LATIN	PINYIN
Globe thistle root	*Radix Rhapontiei*	Lou Lu Gen
Glossy privet fruit	*Fructus Ligustri Lucidi*	Nu Zhen Zi
Gorgon fruits	*Euryale Ferox*	Qiam Shi
(Gracilaria)	*Gracilaria Verrucosa*	Jiang Li
Grassleaved sweetflag rhizome	*Rhizoma Acori Graminei*	Shi Chang Pu
Gypsum	*Gypsum Fibrosum*	Shi Gao
Hemp seed	*Fructus Cannabis*	Huo Ma Ren
Honeysuckle	*Lonicera*	Jin Yin Hua
Hooked uncaria	*Ramulus Uncariae*	Gou Teng
Houttuynia	*Herba Houttuyniae*	Yu Xing Cao
Hyacinth bean	*Dolichos Lablab*	Bian Dou
Immature bitter orange	*Fructus Aurantii Immaturus*	Zhi Shi
Japanese bindweed	*Calystegia Japonica Choisy*	Da Wan Hua
Japanese raisin tree	*Fructus Hovenia Dulcis*	Qi Qu
Jujuba seeds (wild)	*Semen Ziziphi Spinosae*	Suan Zao Ren
Katsumadai seed	*Semen Alpiniae Katsumadai*	Cao Doukou
Kelp	*Thallus Eckloniae*	Kun Bu
Kiwi fruit	*Actinidia Chinensis*	Xian Hou Tao
Knotweed	*Polygonum Multiflorum*	He Shou Wu
Kudzu vine fruits	*Pueraria Lobata*	Ye Ge
Largeheaded atractylodes	*Atractylodes Macrocephela*	Bai Zhu
Ligusticum quanxiong rhizome	*Rhizoma Chuanxiong*	Chuanxiong
Lilyturf	*Radix Opophiogonis*	Mai Men Dong
Liquorice	*Radix Glycyrrhizae*	Gan Cao
Longspur epimedium	*Herba Epimedii*	Yin Yang Huo
Lophatherum	*Herba Lophatheri*	Dan Zhu Ye
Loranthus mulberry mistletoe	*Ramulus Loranthi*	Sang Ji Sheng
Lotus rhizome	*Nelumbo Nucifera*	He Ye
Lygodium spores	*Spora Lygodii*	Hai Jin Sha
Magnolia bark	*Cortex Magnoliae Officinalis*	Hou Po
Magnolia vine fruit	*Fructus Schisandra*	Wu Wei Zi
Maize tassel	*Zea Mays*	Yu Mi Xu
Mandarin peel	*Pericarpium Citri Reticulatae*	Chen Pi
Milkvetch	*Radix Astragalus*	Huang Qi
Monkshood	*Aconitum Carmichaeli*	Chuan Wu (**poisonous**)
Mountain rorippa	*Roripa Dubia*	Wu Ban Han Cai
Moutan bark	*Cortex Moutan Radicis*	Mu Dan Pi
Mugwort	*Folium Artemisiae Argyri*	Ai Ye
Mulberry bark	*Morus Alba*	Sang Bai Pi
Mume flower	*Flos Mume Albus*	Mei Hua
Notoginseng	*Radix Notoginseng*	San Qi
Notopterygium root	*Radix Notopterygii*	Qiang Huo
Old mandarin peel	*Pericarpium Citri Reticulatae*	Chen Pi
Oriental wormwood	*Herba Artemisia Capillaris*	Yin Chen Hao
Oyster mushroom	*Pleurotus Ostreatus*	Cap Pi Ce Er
Pagoda tree flower	*Flos Sophorae*	Huai Hua
Peony (white or herbaceous)	*Paeonia Albiflora*	Bai Shao Yao

COMMON NAME	PHARMACEUTICAL/LATIN	PINYIN
Persimmon calyx	*Calyx Kaki*	Shi Di
Perilla leaves	*Folium Perillae*	Zi Su Ye
Phellodendron bark	*Cortex Phelodendri*	Huang Bai / Bo
Pilose antler	*Cornu Antelopis*	Lu Rong
Pilose asiabell root	*Radix Codonopsis*	Dang Shen
Pinellia tuber	*Rhizoma Pinellia (processed)*	Fa Ban Xia
Pink	*Herba Dianthi*	Qu Mai
Plantain seed	*Semen Plantaginis*	Che Qian Zi
Platycodon	*Radix Platycodi*	Jie Geng
Plum blossoms	*Flos Mume*	Mei Hua
Poria	*Poria*	Fu Ling or Fu Shen
Prostrate knotweed	*Herba Polygoni Avicularis*	Bian Xu
Pseudoginseng	*Radix Notoginseng*	San Qi
Psoralea fruit	*Fructus Psoralea*	Bu Gu Zhi
Pueraria	*Radix Puerariae*	Ge Gen
Puffball	1. *Lasiophaera Seu* 2. *Calvatia*	1. Mao Giu Ma Bo
		2. Tu Ma Bo
Purple-flowered peucedanum	*Radix Peucedani*	Qian Hu
Purslane	*Portulaca Oleracea*	Ma Chi Xian
Radish seed	*Semen Rephani*	Lai Fu Zi
Rangoon creeper fruit	*Fructus Quisqualis*	Shi Jun Zi
Red sage root	*Radix Salvia Miltiorrhizae*	Dan Shen
Red tangerine peel	*Exocarpium Citri Reticulatae*	Hong Jie Pi
Reed rhizome	*Rhizoma Phragmitis*	Lu Gen
Rehmannia root (dried)	*Radix Rehmannia*	Sheng Di Huang
Rehmannia root (cooked)	*Radix Rehmannia Preparatae*	Shu Di Huang
Ricepaper pith	*Tetrapanax papyferus*	Tong Cao
Rosehip	*Fructus Rosa Roxburghii*	Luo Si Hua
Round cardamom	*Amomum Compactum*	Bai Dou Kou
Rush pith	*Medulla Junci*	Deng Xin Cao
Safflower	*Flos Carthami*	Hong Hua
Saline cistanche	*Herba Cistanchis*	Rou Cong Rong
Sargassum	*Sargassum spp.*	Ma Wei Zao
Schizonepeta	*Herba Schizonepetae*	Jing Jie
Scrophularia root	*Radix Scrophulariae*	Xuan Shen
Selfheal	*Spica Prunellae*	Xia Ku Cao
Shepherd's purse	*Capsella Bursa-Pastoris*	Qi Cai
Sichuan aconite	*Radix Aconitum Lycotonum*	Chuan Wu (**poisonous**)
Sichuan clematis stem	*Caulis Clematidis Armandii*	Chuan Mu Tong
Sichaun pepper	*Xanthoxylum*	Hua Jiao
Snakegourd fruit	*Fructus Trichosanthes*	Gua Luo
Snakegourd root	*Radix Trichosanthes*	Tian Hua Fen
Soft shelled turtle		Bie Jia
Spinach	*Basella Rubra*	Luo Kun
Spreading hedyotis	*Hedyotis (Oldenlandia) Diffusa*	Bai Hua She She Cao
Star anise	*Fructus Anisi Stellati*	Ba Jiao
Stemona root	*Radix Stemonae*	Bai Bu

COMMON NAME	PHARMACEUTICAL/LATIN	PINYIN
Straight ladybell roots	*Radix Adenopohorae Stricta*	Nan Sha Shen
Sweet sedge	*Herba Acorus Calamus*	Shui Chang Pu
Sword bean	*Canavalia Gladiata*	Tao Tou
Talc	*Talcum*	Hua Shi
Thorny eleagnus	*Eleagnus sp.*	Hu Tu Zi
Three-colored amaranth	*Amaranthus Tricolor*	Xian Cai
Tortoise plastron		Gui Ban
Torreya	*Semen Torreya*	Fei Zi
Towel gourd	*Retinervus Luffae Fructus*	Si Gua Luo
Tribulus fruit	*Fructus Tribuli*	Bai Ji Li
Trichosanthis root	*Radix Trichosanthes*	Tian Hua Fen
Tsaoko	*Fructus Tsaoko*	Cao Guo
Tuckahoe (outer skin)	*Poria*	Fu Ling
Tuckahoe (whole fungus)	*Poria*	Fu Shen
Typhonium tuber	*Rhizoma Typhonii*	Bai Fu Zi
Water chestnut	*Heleocharis Dulcis/plantaginea*	Qi Shao / Po Qi
White plum blossoms	*Flos Mume*	Mei Hua
(Wildford's cynanchum)	*Cyanchum Wildfordii*	Ge Shan Xiao
Wild jujube seeds	*Semen Ziziphi Spinosae*	Suan Zao Ren
Wild rice	*Zizania Aquatica*	Jiao Sun
Wolfberry bark	*Cortex Lycii Radicis*	Di Gu Pi
Yellow-root yam	*Dioscorea Bulbifera*	Huang Yao Zi
Zedoary	*Curcuma Zedoaria*	Wo Shu
Zhuru (bamboo shavings)	*Caulis Bambusae in Taenis*	Zhu Ru

Note

Every effort has been made to ensure that the information supplied in this glossary is as accurate and complete as possible. The publisher would welcome correspondence on any missing herb names.

Bibliography abbreviations

BCBS (Ben cao bie shuo, *A Different Herbal*)

BCCX (Ben cao cong xin, *New Compilation of Materia Medica*) Wu Yiluo, 1757

BCGM (Ben cao gang mu, *The Great Compendium of Materia Medica*) Li Shizhen, 1578

BCGMSY (Ben cao gang mu shi yi, *Supplement to the Compendium of Materia Medica*) Zhao Xuemin, 1765

BCHY (Ben cao hui yan, *On Materia Medica*) Ni Zhumo, 1624

BCJa (Bai cao jing, *Herbal Mirror*)

BCJb (Ben cao jing, *Shennong's Herbal Classic*) See SNBCJ

BCJJZ (Ben cao jing ji zhu, *Collective Notes to the Canon of Materia Medica*) Tao Hongjing, cal. 536

BCJS (Ben cao jing shu, *Annotation to the Herbal*) Miu Xijong, 1625

BCQD (Ben cao quan du, *The Herbal Weighed and Measured*) Huang Jizhi, 1535

BCQY (Ben cao qiu yuan, *Tracing the Origin of the Herbal*)

BCQZ (Ben cao qiu zen, *Herbal Truths*) Huang Gongxiu, 1769

BCSGY (Ben cao shu gou yuan, *An Expoundation on the Origin of the Herbal*) Yang Shitai, 1842

BCSY (Ben cao shi yi, *A Supplement to the Herbal*) Chen Cangqi, the Tang Dynasty

BCYY (Ben cao yan yi, *Amplified Materia Medica*) Kou Zongshi, 1116

BCZX (Ben cao zai xin, *A Newly Revised Materia Medica*)

BHJJF (Bin hu ji jian fang, *Binhu's Collection of Simple Prescriptions*)

BJFY (Ben jing feng yuan, *The Origin of the Canon of Materia Medica*) Zhang Lu, 1695

BQZHF (Bu que zhou hou fang, *A Supplement to the Handbook of Prescriptions for Emergencies*)

CDGWRL (Chong ding guang wen re lun, *Revised General Treatise on Febrile Diseases*) He Lianchen, the Qing Dynasty

CFQY (Cheng fang qie yong, *Set Recipes of Practical Value*) Wu Yiluo, 1761

DNBC (Dian nan ben cao, *Medical Herbs in Southern Yunnan*) Lan Mao, mid-15th century

DPBC (De pei ben cao, *Well Combined Herbs*) Yan Je, Shi Wen, Hong Wei, 1761

DXF (Du xing fang, *Single-drug Remedies*)

DXXF (Dan xi xin fa, *Danxi's Experiential Therapy*) Zhu Zhenheng, 1347

FMZZ (Fang mai zheng zong, *Orthodox School of Recipes and Pulse Study*)

FQYLS (Feng qin yang lao shu, *A Book on the Care of Aged Relatives*) See YLFQS

FQYLXS (Feng qin yang lao xin shu, *A New Book on the Care of Aged Relatives*) Zhou Hong, 1307

FRLF (Fu ren liang fang, *Useful Prescriptions for Women*) Chen Ziming, 1237

FSJF (Fu shou jing fang, *Selected Prescriptions for Longevity*) Wu Min, 1530

FYXB (Fu you xin bian, *A New Book on the Care of Children*)

GJYTDQ (Gu jin yi tong da quan, *A Complete Work of Medical Traditions*) Xu Chunfu, 1556

HDNJ (Huang di nei jing, *Huangdi's Internal Classic*) according to legend, by Huangdi, or the Yellow Emperor, between the Waring States Period and the Qin or Han Dynasties

HJJF (He ji ju fang, *Heji Official Prescriptions* or *Prescriptions of Peaceful Benevolent Dispensary*) The Imperial Medical Institute, 1078

HYBC (Hai yao ben cao, *Chinese Materia Medica*) Li Xun, the Tang Dynasty

HYRZ (Huan you ri zha, *Journals of an Official*)

JBDF (Jian bian dan fang, *Simple and Single-drug Prescriptions*)

JHBC (Jiu huang ben cao, *Herbal for Relief of Famines*) Zhu Su, the Ming Dynasty

JJF (Ji jian fang, *A Collection of Simple Recipes*)

JKY (Jin kui yi, *A Supplement to the Synopsis of Prescriptions of the Golden Chamber*) You Zaijing, 1768

JKYL (Jin kui yao lue, *Synopsis of Prescriptions of the Golden Chamber*) Zhang Ji, cal before 206

JSML (Ji sheng mi lan, *A Secret Book of Succouring the Sick*)

JYBC (Jia you ben cao, *Jiayou Herbal*) Zhang Yuxi, the Song Dynasty

JYF (Jing yan fang, *Proven Recipes*)

JYQS (Jing yue quan shu, *Complete Works of Zhang Jingyue*) Zhang Jiebin, 1624

KBBC (Kai bao ben cao, *Kai-Bao Herbal*) Liu Han et al, 973

LCBC (Lu chuan ben cao, *Land and Water Herbs*)

LCCJYF (Liu chang chun jing yan fang, *Liu Changchun's Proven Prescriptions*)

LKZS (Liu ke zhun sheng, *Standards for the Six Branches of Medicine*)

LLHY (Lao lao heng yan, *Common Sayings for Senile Health*)

LLYH (Leng lu yi hua, *Medical Talks from the Deserted House*) Lu Yitian, 1897

LNCYL (Ling nan cai yao lu, *Records of Collecting Lingnan Herbs*)

LNCYZ (Ling nan cao yao zhi, *Records of Lingnan Herbs*)

LS (Ling shu, *The Miraculous Pivot*) Part of Huang di nei jing. See HDNJ

MSJYF (Mei shi ji yan fang, *Master Mei's Collection of Proven Prescriptions*) Mei Wenmei, the Sui Dynasty

MYBL (Ming yi bie lu, *Records of Famous Physicians*) Tao Hongjing (456–536), cal. late Han Dynasty

NJ (Nei jing, *The Internal Classic*) See HDNJ

PJF (Pu ji fang, *Prescriptions for Universal Relief*) Zhu Su et al, 1381

PWL (Pi wei lun, *Treatise on the Spleen and Stomach*) Li Gao, 1249

QJF (Qian jin fang, *Prescriptions Worth a Thousand Gold*) Sun Simiao, cal. 650

QKSY (Qian kun sheng yi, *A Book for Improving Life*) Zhu Quan, late 14th century

RHZBC (Ri hua zi ben cao, *Rihuazi's Herbal*) Rihuazi, the Tang Dynasty

RMSQ (Ru men shi qin, *Confucians' Duties to Their Parents*) Zhang Congzheng, 1228

RYBC (Ri yong ben cao, *Daily Herbal*)

RZTJYF (Rui zhu tang jing yan fang, *Proven Prescriptions from the Ruizhu House*) Sha Tu Mu Su, cal. 1326

RZZZF (Ren zhai zhi zhi fang, *Renzhai's Effective Prescriptions*) Yang Shiying, 1264

SCSS (Shi cai san shu, *Shicai's Three Books*) Li Zhongzi, 1667

SHF (Sheng hui fang, *Peaceful Holy Benevolent Prescriptions*) See TPSHF

SHL (Shang han lun, *Treatise on Febrile Diseases*) Part of Shang han za bing lun. See SHZBL

SHTJF (Si he ting ji fang, *Collected Recipes from the Siheting*)

SHZBL (Shang han za bing lun, *Treatise on Exogenous Febrile Diseases and Internal Diseases*) Zhang Ji, cal. before 206

SJBC (Shi jian ben cao, *Verified Dietetic Herbs*) Chai Yi, 1741

SJZL (Sheng ji zong lu, *Complete Collection for Holy Relief*) Governmental institution of the Song Dynasty 1111

SLBC (Shi liao ben cao, *Dietetic Materia Medica*) Meng Shen, the Tang Dynasty

SNBCJ (Shen nong ben cao jing, *Shennong's Herbal Classic*) author unknown, cal. between the Qin and the Han Dynasties

SPJ (Shi pin ji, *A Collection of Diets*) Wu Lu, the Ming Dynasty

SQYLXS (Shou qin yang lao xin shu, *A New Book on Caring for the Aged Relatives*) Chen Zhiyuan, 1307

SSBY (Shou shi bao yuan, *Longevity and Health Preservation*) Gong Tingxian, 1615

SW (Su wen, *Plain Questions*) Part of Huang di nei jing. See HDNJ

SWBC (Shi wu ben cao, *Dietetic Herbal*) 1. Lu He, 17th century 2. Wang Ying, 1620 3. Li Dongyuan, cal. after 1641

SWBCHZ (Shi wu ben cao hui zuan, *Collection of Dietetic Herbs*) Shen Lilong, 1691

SXBC (Shi xing ben cao, *Properties of Diet*)

SXJYSP (Sui xi ju yin shi pu, *Recipes of Suixiju*) Wang Shixiong, 1861

SYSD (Sui yuan shi dan, *Diet Recipes from the Suiyuan Garden*) Yuan Mei, the Qing Dynasty

SYSS (Shi yao shen shu, *Ten Effective Remedies*) Ge Kejiu, 1348

SYXJa (Shi yi xin jian, *Dietician's Understandings*) Zan Yin, cal. 853

SYXJb (Shi yi xin jing, *Dietician's Mirror*)

TJYSB (Tiao ji yin shi bian, *A Study on Diets for Correcting Ailments*) Zhang Mu, 1813

TPSHF (Tai ping sheng hui fang, *Peaceful Holy Benevolent Prescriptions*) Wang Huaiyin et al, 992

TSL (Tong shou lu, *Records on Life Preservation*)

TWFZ (Tai wan fu zhi, *Annals of Taiwan Prefecture*)

TXJXF (Tan xian jie xiao fang, *Tanxian's Effective Prescriptions*)

TYJYF (Tang yao jing yan fang, *Tangyao's Proven Prescriptions*)

TYWSYF (Tan ye weng shi yan fang, *Tanyeweng's Proven Prescriptions*)

WBTB (Wen bing tiao bian, *Treatise on Differentiation and Treatment of Epidemic Febrile Diseases*) Wu Jutong, 1798

WTMY (Wai tai mi yao, *The Medical Records of an Official*) Wang Tao, 752

WKZZ (Wai ke zheng zong, *Orthodox Manual of External Diseases*) Chen Shigong, 1617

WRJW (Wen re jing wei, *Essentials of Febrile Diseases*) Wang Mengying, 1852

WSYA (Wang shi yi an, *Wang's Medical Records*) Wang Shixiong, cal. 1843

WSYJF (Wei sheng yi jian fang, *Simple Recipes for Health Preservation*) Hu Ying, 1410

WYDF (Wu yao dan fang, *Simple Recipes Without Drugs*)

XXBC (Xin xiu ben cao, *The Newly Revised Materia Medica*) Su Jing et al, 659

XYL (Xing yuan lu, *Records from the Awakening Garden*)

YCSY (Yi chun sheng yi, *Medical Truths Newly Discovered*)

YJ (Yi ji *Medical Steps*) Dong Xiyuan, 1777

YKLML (Yan ke long mu lun, *Miraculous Ophthalmology*) author unknown, cal. between the Sui and the Tang Dynasties

YLFQS (Yang lao feng qin shu, *Caring for Aged Relatives*) Chen Zhi, the Song Dynasty

YLJY (Yi lin ji yao, *A Collection of Important Medical Books*)

YPXC (Yin pian xin can, *Herbal Pieces Prepared for Decoctions*)

YSBL (Yin shi bian lu, *The Verified Records of Diets*) See TJYSB

YSJCF (Yang shi jia cang fang, *Yang's Family Prescriptions*) Yang Tan, 1178

YSXZ (Yin shi xu zhi, *A Dietetic Handbook*) Zhu Benzhong, 1676

YSZY (Yin shan zheng yao, *The Essence of Diet*) Hu Sihui, 1330

YXCZL (Yin xue cong zhong lu, *Popular Medicine*) Chen Nianzu, 1820

YXL (Yao xing lun, *Properties of Drugs*)

YXSJL (Yi xue sui jin lu, *Scattered Medical Golds*)

YXZZCXL (Yi xue zhong zhong can xi lu, *Records of Traditional Chinese and Western Medicines in Combination*) Zhang Xichun, 1909

YYJC (You you ji cheng, *A Complete Work on Pediatrics*) Chen Fuzheng, 1750

YZFSJ (Yin zhuan fu shi jian, *Notes on the Use of Foods and Drinks*) Gao Lian, the Ming Dynasty

YZHB (Yi zong hui bian, *A Compilation of Important Medical Books*)

YZJJ (Yi zong jin jian, *The Golden Mirror of Medicine*) Wu Qian et al, 1742

ZGYYZJ (Zhong guo yao yong zhen jun, *Chinese Medicinal Fungi*)

ZHBJF (Zhou hou bei ji fang, *Prescriptions for Emergencies*) Ge Hong, cal. before 363

ZP (Zhou pu, *A Manual of Gruels*)

ZSJYF (Zhu shi ji yan fang, *Zhu's Collection of Proven Prescriptions*)

ZYCSC (Zhong yao cai shou ce, *Manual of Materia Medica*) Renmin Weishing Press, 1959

ZYF (Zhai yuan fang, *Selected Medical Prescriptions*)

ZYNKX (Zhong yi nei ke xue, *Traditional Chinese Internal Medicine*) 1964

ZYYKLJFY (Zhong yi yan ke liu jing fa yao, *Ophthalmology in Traditional Chinese Medicine According to the Six Classics*)

ZZYJ (Zheng zhi yao jue, *Gists of Diagnosis and Treatment*) Dai Sigong, 1443

Indexes

There are three indexes, broadly corresponding to the three sections of the book.

The General index covers primarily the introduction and Part 1, dealing with the concepts and principles of TCM Dietary Therapy.

The Foods index covers primarily Part 2, which deals with foods, their properties and applications.

The Symptoms index covers the diagnoses and symptoms as found in Part 3. This section deals with diets under the headings of the symptoms and diagnoses for which they are recommended. The user may need to cross-refer between the Foods and Symptoms indexes to obtain maximum information e.g.: for a patient presenting with palpitation, the user may seek 'palpitation' in the Symptoms index, but may then wish to go to the Foods index to find fuller information on the specific foods recommended.

General Index

Age
  variations of Blood and Qi with,
    33–34
Alcohol, 16
  liquor, 129–130
  wines, medicinal, 28
Allergies and appetite, 6
Animal
  feed, 10
  products, 26, 103
    see also Foods Index for individual
    references
Antagonism, food combinations, 24
Antibiotics
  in cow's milk, 10
  natural, in seaweeds, 68
Antifungal sprays, 7
Appetite, 5–6
Artificial flavouring, 6–7
Autumn, recommended diet for, 33

Baby food, 10
Baking, 3
Balanced diet, 16, 25
Ben, 6
Biao, 6
Blood
  containing, 38
  cow's milk for deficiency, 9
  meat for deficiency, 9
  methods of enriching, 38–39
  tonics, 2
  variations with age, 33–34
Body fluids, promoting, 40
Boiling, 3
Bottling, 7
Bovine spongiform encephalopathy,
  10
Brazil nuts, quantities consumed, 6
Breastfeeding, diet prohibitions, 30
  see also Symptoms Index:
    Hypogalactia

Candied fruits, 28

Canning, 7
Cereals, generally, 91–95
Channel propensities, 4, 20–21
Chelation of heavy metals, 68
Childbirth
  diet prohibitions following, 29–30
China, regional variations, 33
Clam, 113, 123
Cleanliness and hygiene, 41–42
Climate, adapting diet to, 32–33
Cold and iced drinks, 3
Combination of foods, 2–3, 23–24
Condiments, 27, 125–131
Control Cycle, 5
Cooked dishes, 27
Cooking methods, 26
  effect on nature of foods, 3
Cooling and Heating properties *see*
  Nature of foods
Coordination of Internal Organs, 32
Cow's milk, 9–10, 110
Crab, 113, 122–123

Dairy products, 10–11 *see also* Milk
Damp
  effect of milk, 9
  removal of, 38
Decoctions, 27
Diet
  adaptation to individual needs,
    33–34
  balanced, 16, 25
  fads in, 8
  methods of therapy, 37–40
  principles of therapy, 31–35
  prohibitions, 29–30
  therapy, concept and origins, 15–17
  unbalanced, 7, 25–26
  Yin and Yang, adjustment of, 31–32
Dietetic hygiene, 41–42
Diets for illness, 34–35
  see also Symptoms Index for illnesses
Drinks, 27–28
  iced, effects of, 3

Dryness, moistening, 40

Electuaries, 28
Elements, Five, 4–5
Essence, tonifying, 40

Fads and diets, 8
Fasting, 5–6
Fats, addition of, 7
Fish, 113–124
Five Elements, 4–5
Five Tastes, 4–5, 20
Flavour
  cereals, nuts and pulses, generally,
    91
  Five Tastes, 4–5, 20
  of food and medicine, 1–3
  fruits, generally, 73
  as indication of Qi, 6
  overconsumption of one type, 25
  regional variations in, 33
Flavouring, artificial, 6–7
Food
  fads, 8
  hygiene, 41–42
  for nourishment, 1
  preparation of, 3, 26–29
  preservation of, 7–8
  production, in West, 6–7
  properties *see* Properties of food
  Qi, 5, 6, 7
  seasonal, 8, 32–33
  taste *see* Taste
Foods
  choice of, 26
  combination of, 2–3, 23–24
  cooking methods, 26
  and medicines, during illness, 29
  nature of, 2–3, 19–20, 45, 73, 91, 103,
    113
  with toxic effects, 42, 46, 58, 59
  Yin and Yang classification, 4
  'the Four Natures', 19–20
Fowls, 103–107

Foods Index

Symptoms Index